Brain at Work

Neuroexperiential Perspectives

C.R. Mukundan

ATLANTIC

PUBLISHERS & DISTRIBUTORS (P) LTD

Published by

ATLANTIC

PUBLISHERS & DISTRIBUTORS (P) LTD

7/22, Ansari Road, Darya Ganj, New Delhi-110002
Phones: +91-11-40775252, 23273880, 23275880, 23280451
Fax : +91-11-23285873
Web : www.atlanticbooks.com
E-mail : orders@atlanticbooks.com

Branch Office
5, Nallathambi Street, Wallajah Road, Chennai-600002
Phones: +91-44-64611085, 32413319
E-mail : chennai@atlanticbooks.com

Printed in India at Nice Printing Press, A-33/3A, Site-IV, Industrial Area, Sahibabad, Ghaziabad, U.P.

Foreword

Philosophically and historically, India occupies the premier position in the creation of knowledge of concepts of the mind. In terms of modern scientific thinking, institutions in the country are only in the early stages of progress in such efforts. The scientific knowledge of the functioning of the brain has contributed extensively and deeply to the standards, values and controls applied by individuals in their living styles, habits, and pursuits in life. There is constant need to engage the brain for creating and understanding new relationships, which helps to construct new realities, as well as understand the mysteries of the brain, the human mind, and the physical realities. Prof. C.R. Mukundan is one of those who laid the foundation for clinical and cognitive neuropsychology in India; he standardized clinical examination procedures, and set up electrophysiological experiments. His work emphasizes the need to address the issues of the brain and the mind with multidisciplinary approach, which is the hallmark of this book.

Emergence of the human mind from the processes in the brain and the associated behavior form the foundation of human civilization. The strengths and weaknesses of the human mind therefore, have deep origin in the functioning of the brain. The book brings out issues related to the interdependence of the brain-mind and behavior, which facilitates the process of socialization and its controlling effects in the brain, the absence of which manifests as criminal behavior. Study of criminal behavior requires applications of knowledge of clinical and cognitive neuropsychology. Prof. C.R. Mukundan has experimented upon such interface at the Directorate of Forensic Sciences and the Gujarat Forensic Sciences University,

Gandhinagar for extracting remembrance of experiential knowledge in individuals.

Knowledge of the multiple functional modules at work in the brain is, therefore, an important requirement for understanding normal and abnormal behavior whether clinical or criminal. There is a need to strengthen the assets, and to overcome and reduce the weaknesses. Knowledge of these processes and control over them are needed for achieving these effects, which form the goals of many institutions developed and nourished by humankind. The multidisciplinary understanding required to study the brain-mind interface is well reflected in this book. It contains extensive discussions on various complex brain functions, which we consider constitute the mind. I trust these will inspire others, especially the younger scientists, to take these works and ideas forward.

Dr. J.M. Vyas
Director General,
Gujarat Forensic Sciences University,
Gandhinagar, Gujarat, India

Preface

Knowing the functions of the brain and its processing methods forms the foundations of neuroscience. This knowledge is essential for mastering its processing abilities, and for enhancing skills for achieving optimum performance. Traditionally, maximum information of brain functions was acquired during examination of patients with diseases and lesions of the brain. Animal brain experiments too have immensely contributed to the understanding of brain structure and functions, though the human brain has comparatively extraordinary acumens compared to animal brains. Neuroimaging studies have not only supported the findings from earlier lesion studies, but also opened an umbrella of knowledge of intra-structural connectivity and functional participation of different brain regions. Understanding the brain performance and achieving mastery over it have become an inevitable need, especially during early years of growth and education, in diseases and injuries of the brain, and for facilitating neurogenesis during ageing. Neuroscientists working on brain structures and their connectivity and those who have been developing parallel computing systems have contributed richly to the understanding of the functional capabilities of the brain. These streams of knowledge have helped us to understand the enigma of human mind and its inseparable nature from the brain.

I came to know of neuropsychology, when Dr. G.N. Narayana Reddy, the neurosurgeon at the erstwhile All India Institute of Mental Health (AIIMH), Bangalore enquired about my knowledge of the specialty, just after he had returned from a visit to Minnesota University in 1975, where he had met Dr. Brenda Milner and a few others. Listening to "neuropsychology" as the name of the specialty, which was hitherto unknown to me, started the long journey to explore and know more about it. Luria's *Higher Cortical Functions* was the only practical remedy and the greatest source of knowledge for the adventure, though I had never examined a patient in the lines explained by Luria in his book. The recourse was to examine normal individuals and later gradually learn to observe and quantify the deficits in patients. Dr. K.S. Mani and Dr. H.N. Murthy were the two other stalwarts and pillars of knowledge, who helped me to understand and work on the new specialty—from its elementary basics—to the higher levels of understanding the mystery of functioning of the brain. The next 5 years marked the era of explorations, constructions and reconstructions of clinical examination procedures for eliciting neuropsychological deficits, changes in emotional responses and the controls of behavior in patients, with and without brain lesions. I am deeply indebted to the faculties of the Departments of Neurology, Neurosurgery, Neuroradiology, Psychiatry, and Clinical Psychology at the National Institute of Mental Health and Neuro Sciences (formerly AIIMH) for their patients, interest, and willingness to accept and utilize the neuropsychological examination profiles. Soon neuropsychology became a subject of immense academic and clinical interest at NIMHANS, Bangalore The data collected in several studies from mid-1970s formed the database of the several results cited in this book.

Clinical neuropsychological examination is a procedure, which a trainee has to acquire through practice under supervision. There is no alternative to the examination skills that one has to master and use in everyday clinical practice for determining the neuropsychological dysfunction in patients. One must learn to identify absence to subtle changes in psychological functioning and behavior in a patient, compared to premorbid level, which would yield the clinical neuropsychological profile of the patient. This was indeed a long journey, and I am especially thankful to Prof. Oliver Louis Zangwill, in Cambridge University, for personally assuring me and giving me confidence in the clinical approach of patient examination for detecting the cognitive and behavioral deficits in patients. This contributes to the clinical acumen of a clinician and further helps to identify the subtle constituents of a functional system, using which we can rebuild a functional capability.

I am deeply indebted to my colleagues, who helped me in the completion of this book. Dr. P. Ajayan gave me valuable critical comments on various chapters of the book, especially discussions on patterns of stimulus inputs into the brain, drive and its effects on the initiation of actions, early socialization, and development of ability to learn response inhibition through control of drive inhibition. I am also thankful to Dr. C. Kamarajan, for his valuable comments. I could do my best because of the positive and critical comments and continuous support provided to me by Dr. Priyanka Kacker, in the review and discussion of several chapters, especially related to consciousness, awareness, and attention. She helped me with the complex and time-consuming job of proofreading from the point of view of a subject expert. I could not have accomplished the task of writing this book without the emotional, intellectual and material support from Chetan, Ashwin, Deepa, and Sumit, the neurocognitive software stalwarts at the Axxonet System Technologies, Bengaluru. Several of the issues discussed in the book have been closely connected with the cognitive neuroscience research projects carried out at this research center.

I am indeed grateful to Dr. J.M. Vyas, Director General of Gujarat Forensic Sciences University, where I completed the book. He provided me with all facilities, which enabled me to go for its quick completion.

C.R. Mukundan

Contents

1 The Human Brain

The book describes and discusses clinical and experimental research findings related to the origin of behavior and cognitive processing within the human brain, the unique capabilities that develop during the developmental process and processing states, and issues related to the development of such processing capabilities. Historically, properties of the brain have been described using different terms such as mind and consciousness, perception and other cognitive abilities related to learning and memory, simple and complex motor programming, emotions, and awareness. Behavior is explicit expression, in which a motor response is expressed involuntarily or voluntarily, in response to a stimulus with and without its perception, or triggered by an idea and action plan to achieve a goal and the navigation is controlled from within the brain. Cognitive processing related to complex visuospatial processing and semantic interpretations creating ideas take place within the brain, online with and without sensory inputs. Thinking and problem-solving often take place without behavioral accompaniments, which may follow them in a strategic manner. Brain receives external signals and they are processed within, online as well as offline, when they are retrieved and processed. The brain assigns meaning to the sensory signals creating information. Interpreted or assigned meanings are utilized for recognition of the world. One tends to learn to create new meanings, if available knowledge bank does not help to recognize a new entity. The interpretations of sensory-motor effects help control and regulate motor expressions, and help in the navigation of the individual to future. The chapters are organized to provide basic information on the various functional aspects of the brain related to attention, recognition, learning, memory, working memory, encoding, and transcoding, initiation and execution of motor acts, simple and complex motor programming, and cognitive control of emotions.

Structural Organization of the Brain starts with configurations of different types of neurons and the glial cells developing multiple processing capabilities, which become the foundation of sensory and motor events in the body, leading to cognitive functions and behavioral manifestations. Both cognition and behavior represent complex and dynamically interactive neural domains, requiring multiple and mediations for regulating the functional processes. The brain structures develop the functional capabilities to carry out mode and processing specific functions in the domains of skills and abilities, including regulation of functions related to sensory inputs and motor outputs, learn to encode signals for creating information and store, retrieve, and communicate the information created, and carry out problem-solving solutions. Equally important is the role of emotions—the fuel of life, without which the dynamic processing ceases to happen, and which can affect the quality of all cognitive processing and behavior. The multiple functional systems and their interactions may be happening almost as millions of people interact on the internet carrying out multiple jobs, who may share and/or differ in the meanings assigned in each processing.

Neurons and Glial Cells

The Brain is composed of two different types of cells called the neurons and the glial cells or neuroglia. The neurons are the signal processing units of the brain, while glial cells provide supportive help to the neurons by providing nutrition and maintenance of homeostasis in terms of fluid around the neurons for producing their electrical insulation. The fluid contains "myelin" which surrounds the neurons providing electrical insulation, as neuronal activation produces electrical activity, which is transmitted to surrounding and distant group of neurons, which may be involved in the deployment of same function. The glial cells carry nutrition and oxygen for the neurons, and electrically insulate one neuron from another. Emotions, sensory-motor functions, and cognitive abilities emerge from the activation of the neurons. Neurons contribute to the physical resource for the emergence of mind. During developmental stages of the brain and acquisition of new skills and abilities, groups of adjacent neurons are assembled together to form neural networks subserving a function or part of functional system. The brain of a newborn infant weighs between 300-400 grams and its weight increases to 1300-1400 grams through neurogenesis of neurons by adulthood. Estimates of the number of neurons in the brain range from 86 to 100 billion in the brain (Azevedo et al. 2009; Williams, Herrup 1988). The ratio of neurons to glial cells varies from part to part in the brain. The ratio is estimated to be 3.72 in the entire cerebral cortex whereas it is reported as 1.48 in cerebral cortex grey matter, and 11.35 in the basal ganglia, diencephalon and brainstem (combined) is reported as 11.35 (Azevedo et al. 2009). The cerebral cortex grey matter indeed has greater number of neurons. Neurons are identified based on the type of neurotransmitter they transmit and they are identified as Cholinergic, Gabbaenergic, Glutamatergic, Dopaminergic, and Serotonergic neurons. The neurons are classified into afferent and efferent neurons, based on their major functional roles. Afferent neurons form afferent fiber systems and carry signals from body tissues and organs to the central nervous system (CNS), while efferent neurons or the motor neurons form different efferent fiber systems and carry signals from the CNS to the effector cells. The interneurons interconnect neurons within specific regions especially the brain.

Cortex, Midbrain, and Hindbrain

The brain is anatomically divided into the cortex, the midbrain, and the hindbrain. The human cerebral cortex is about 2-4 mm (Kandel et al. 2000) in thickness and it contains the cell bodies of neurons, which makes the upper most layer of the brain grey in color, and hence it is named the grey matter.

The cerebral cortex forms average 77% of the volume of brain. The cortical thickness varies from region to region with the sensory areas being thinner than motor areas (Kruggel et al. 2003). It has been suggested that cortical thickness may be related to level intelligence (Narr et al. 2007). The cortex is divided into left and right halves and each hemisphere has four major areas called the cerebral lobes viz., the frontal lobe, the temporal lobe, the parietal lobe, and the occipital lobe. The cerebral cortex is further divided into isocortex or neocortex and allocortex, based on the number of structural layers seen during the developmental stages of the brain. The neocortex develops through 6 layers (e.g. Striate area), whereas the allocortex has less than 6 layers (e.g. hippocampus) during formative development. The two hemispheres are interconnected with connecting fibers called the corpus callosum, which allow inter transfer of signals from one hemisphere to the other.

Cortex and Subcortex

Yet another way of classifying the brain is to divide it into cortical and subcortical areas. Important subcortical structures are basal ganglia, thalamus, hypothalamus, amygdala, and hippocampus. The basal ganglia are associated with voluntary motor controls and learning motor skills. The hypothalamus, amygdala, hippocampus, and thalamus form the limbic system responsible for the control of emotional arousal. The thalamus and the hypothalamus form the diencephalon. The thalamus receives the sensory signals from the sensory receptors and relay them to the respective ipsilateral and contralateral primary sensory cortical areas. It is known as the major sensory relay center of the brain. The hypothalamus, which lies below the thalamus, regulates body temperature, hunger and thirst, sexual activity and body growth. It serves as the major center for the control of endocrine functions and integrates the parasympathetic (anterior part) and sympathetic (posterior part) activities of autonomic nervous system (ANS). Fight-flight behavior is connected with the hypothalamus and is one of the areas connected with experience of pleasure. The amygdala and the hippocampus play major roles in emotional experiences and expressions. The role of hippocampus in memory is well established and discussed in detail elsewhere. The hindbrain contains the cerebellum and the brainstem areas. The brainstem includes the medulla oblongata merging into the spinal cord and pons and the area has important role in the control of vital functions of the body. Occasionally the midbrain structures are also referred as included in the brainstem. The cerebellum meaning the "little brain" integrates sensory feedback with motor commands, thereby controlling and coordinating the smooth (voluntary) execution of movements. The brain stem is the seat of ascending reticular activating system (ARAS) and this vital brain center regulates breathing, swallowing, heart rate, and the wake-sleep cycles.

The cortex sends signals to the subcortex through efferent pathways and the subcortex sends up signals through afferent connections to cortex. Most of the sensory information is passed to primary sensory cortical areas through the thalamus. Intra connectivity across cortical areas is considered most extensive amounting to almost 99% whereas only the remaining may be with the subcortical structures (Braitenberg, Schüz 1991). Such cortical connectivity paves the routes for extensive cortical networks enabling participation of different cortical areas for supporting multiple processing modes in a given function or cognitive ability. This explains the involvement of extensive areas of the brain in problem-solving considering multiple relationships and for creating complex mental concepts. There are five major functional systems originating from the frontal cortex, of which three have primarily behavioral and cognitive regulations. These are discussed in detail elsewhere in the text.

If the body is divided into left and right halves, one side of the body is mainly controlled by the contralateral (opposite) cerebral hemisphere (for example the left side of the body is controlled by the right cerebral hemisphere). In the same manner, sensory inputs from one side of the body including eyes and ears are received and processed mainly in the contralateral hemisphere, though the ipsilateral (same side) hemisphere does get receive minimal inputs. Each cerebral hemisphere receives signals from the opposite hemisphere through the corpus callosum and thereby controls the processing in the other hemisphere. Therefore, with regard to any given cerebral function, even if it is mainly carried out by one hemisphere, there may be inputs from the other hemisphere controlling or mediating the same function. For example, even though major aspects of speech viz., listening and expressing are controlled mainly by the left hemisphere, there is simultaneous powerful right hemisphere mediation of some of the language functions. Dissection or disconnection of the corpus callosum can therefore cut off such interaction of the two hemispheres and the two will be forced to function independently without accessing and knowing the capabilities of the other hemisphere. This was demonstrated in split brain studies conducted by Roger Sperry and reported by Gazzaniga (1970).

Each mode specific sensory processing such as sensory registration takes place in the respective primarily cortex. The interpretation of the signals leading to their recognition is carried out by the respective secondary association areas and may additionally be processed by distant areas such as the frontal lobes. What we call information is created only when neural signals are interpreted and a meaning is created by the brain. A meaning is recreated when we hear a word or see an object using the meanings already stored as memory traces, or it is created afresh when the available knowledge bank does not help to identify a suitable meaning. Storing information and their retrieval are essential routine processing requirements of the brain for dealing with the external world. A stimulus is recognized when its meaning could be recreated by retrieving it from the memory by the brain. Understanding the meaning of a word or knowing a stimulus visually seen is recognition. The entire process of receiving the signals and their interpretive analysis for recognition is called perception. Therefore, the word perception has a larger contextual meaning as it refers to the meaning of a stimulus or condition understood by the perceiver. The visual (area 17) and auditory (area 41) primary

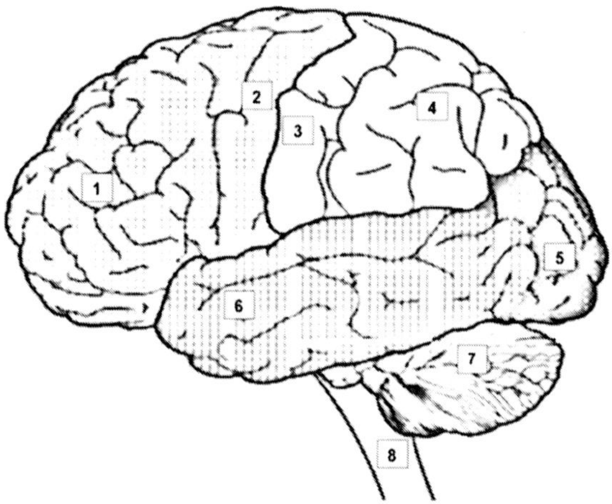

Fig. 1: Showing the Frontal Lobe (1), Primary Motor Cortex (2), Primary Sensory Cortex (3), Parietal Lobe (4), Occipital Lobe (5), Temporal Lobe (6), Cerebellum (7), and Spinal cord (8)

sensory cortices occupy relatively very small areas in the brain. Assigning meaning to the signals received in each primary sensory cortex is carried out by extensive secondary association areas, including frontal cortices. Therefore, interpretation or assigning meaning to signals is a colossal job in the brain, which explains the presence of much larger cerebral cortex in human brain. It is often considered that 80% of the information created by the brain is from the visual signals received in the brain and hence human being is often called a visual animal. With regard to the motor system, the primary motor cortex represents the one to one representation of body parts in the brain used for voluntary execution of motor acts. Additionally the supplementary motor cortex placed anteriorly in the frontal cortex represents the center for voluntary selection and regulation of sequences components of motor behavior. Voluntary movements are often made according to plans of action, created though thinking, symbolic processing, and emotional needs, and they are monitored and regulated as per anticipated and actual effects of action. The visual and kinesthetic feedbacks are important components for the regulation and therefore the motor areas interact with the respective sensory areas and acts are executed. Parietal cortex and dorsolateral prefrontal lobes play direct roles in such executions, whereas many more areas in the cerebral cortex may be indirectly involved in the generation and regulation of motor acts. Deep below the cerebral cortex lies grey matter nuclei called basal nuclei or basal ganglia consisting of corpus striatum (consisting of caudate nucleus and putamen), and globus pallidus, which interact with the motor cortex and substantia nigra of the midbrain for achieving motor regulation.

Frontal Functional Systems

2

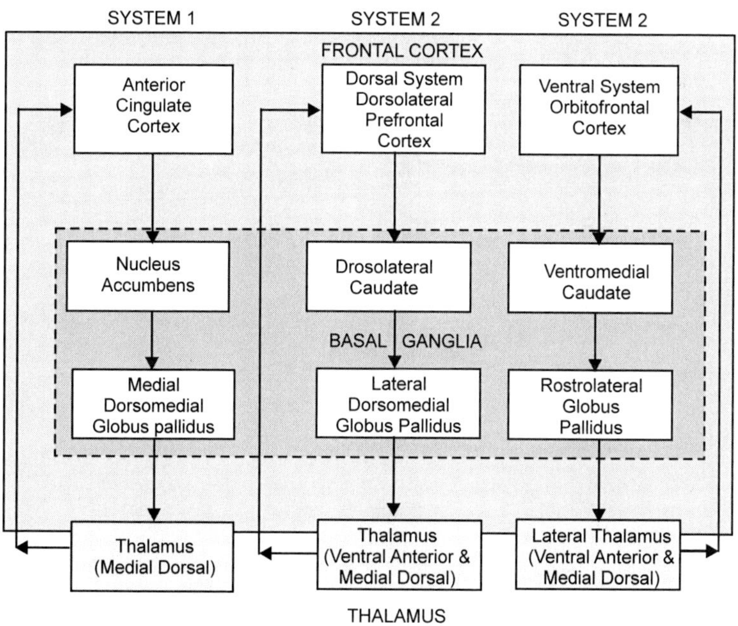

Fig. 2: Frontal Cognitive – Behavioral Functional Systems showing connectivity from Frontal Cortex to Thalamus through Basal Ganglia and directly from Thalamus to Frontal Cortex (Cummings, J.L. et al. 1995)

The frontal lobes have extensive interconnections with several other areas in the brain and some of them are those, which control emotions, mood, and cognitive processing. The frontal lobes are the highest control centers of these functional systems in the brain (Alexander, G.E. et al. 1986, 1990; Cummings, J.L. 1995; Groenewegen, H.I. et al. 1990; Nolte, J. 2002). There are three general anatomical divisions of the frontal cortex starting from the limbic, the precentral, and the prefrontal cortices, which have immense behavioral and psychological significance. The prefrontal cortex is subdivided into orbitolateral prefrontal cortex, dorsolateral prefrontal cortex, and anterior cingulate. The prefrontal cortex has extensive connections with various other areas of the cerebrum and subcortical areas. The interconnections of the prefrontal cortex with temporal, parietal, occipital areas of the cerebrum, and subcortically with basal ganglia, thalamus, and cerebellum, explain their extensive control on various segments of behavior. Of the five such circuits known, three have important behavioral and cognitive basis. Of the other two, one is a motor circuit and the other is occulomotor circuit originating from the frontal eye fields.

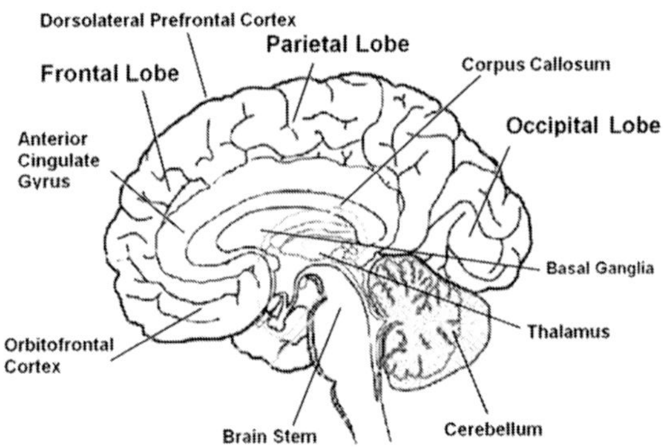

Fig. 3: Anterior Cingulate Cortex, Orbitofrontal Cortex and Dorsolateral Prefrontal Cortex

System 1: Anterior Cingulate Cortical (ACC) System

ACC is the anterior part of the Cingulate Cortex (Fig. 3) formed by the medial aspect of the cerebral cortex that lies immediately above the corpus callosum interconnecting the brain hemispheres. The cingulate cortex directly interacts with the thalamus, the neocortex, and the entorhinal cortex located in the medial temporal lobe. It plays crucial role in autobiographic memory related actions and providing the emotional arousal—drive required for all actions and responses (Hayden, Platt 2010). The origin of Anterior Cingulate Gyrus (Brodmann's area 24) projecting into the ventral or limbic striatum, which includes Nucleus Accumbens, and Ventromedial aspects of the

Caudate and Putamen as shown in the diagram above. Other limbic structures such as Hippocampus, Amygdala, and Enthorinal Cortex, also project into ventral striatum. Through the rostrolateral Globus Pallidus, the Striatum is connected to the mediodorsal Thalamus and there exists a direct link between the Thalamus and the Anterior Cingulate as in the case of the other two circuits discussed above (Cummings, J.L. 1995).

The most effective way of understanding the functional importance of a part of the brain has been to remove that part from the brain and observe the changes in the behavior and cognitive functions. A comparable picture is available in clinical conditions when specific areas of the brain are damaged and changes are detected in the behavior of the affected person. When ACC is damaged (lesion) and the patient has become dysfunctional, plethora of significant deficits are detected in the affected patient. Lesion or damage in the ACC produces severe arousal-activation related dysfunctions in a person. The patients may show one or more below mentioned deficits in varying degrees.

1. Akinetic mutism (patient is unable to speak though does not have expressive aphasia) in bilateral lesions
2. Transient akinetic mutism in unilateral lesions
3. Absence of spontaneous speech
4. Speaks in monosyllables if made to speak
5. Apathy—absence of emotion
6. Absence of emotion even when hurt and in pain
7. Absence of interest in self and surroundings
8. Absence of initiative in the patient and the patient becomes indifferent
9. Does not ask for food, eat and drink only if fed
10. Failure of response initiation
11. Patient becomes incontinent.

Akinetic mutism is a state in which the person is awake with eyes open, but lies mute, immobile, and unresponsive. The deficits described above indicate the absence of an arousal mechanism, which is essential prerequisite for the initiation of internally controlled movement and behavior in general. Absence of the various activities described above is not because of a dysfunction of the organs required for their execution, or because of absence of wakefulness in the patient. The concerned activity is not initiated in the patient, as the drive necessary for their initiation is not present. It shows merely being awake or knowing that one should initiate an action is not enough for one to either respond to a stimulus to start an action. The individual must experience the need state, when it can motivate or trigger to respond to the stimulus or start an action as part of a navigational strategy. In navigational movements, the goals are attained only at the end, when the goal is achieved. The individual must move forward hoping and wanting to reach the goal. It is as if a moving vehicle is stuck, if fuel is not injected into the engine. Having the fuel in the tank is not enough but it must be transferred into the engine. In the same manner, drive must be drawn and made available for the individual to respond and act. Dispensation of intense levels of fuel may be called emotional states, though an idle running condition is just considered being alive. Cognitive labeling of the increased or decreased presence of drive is carried out during its self-awareness and has been labeled by numerous names as fear, anxiety, sadness, etc. The anterior cingulate controls the availability and utilization of the drive for disposal. During brain development, one gradually learns toutilize the drive voluntarily, which can trigger responses and actions. During brain development, drive may not appear by itself, as it needs to be aroused through experiences, for which opportunities normally occur in the company of the parents, siblings, and peers. Excessive arousal on the other hand, may lead to clinically significant conditions of hyper-attention and hyperactivity as seen in ADHD children. Normally the child learns response inhibition, which is the most significant principle by which one learns to control activities induced by arousal.

Absence of emotional response to pain stimuli indicates that even normal biological survival response is absent when bilateral damage to the Anterior Cingulate takes place. Arousal or drive is therefore a basic requirement for the initiation of any motor activity or response. Emotional arousal is found to be a necessity for a human being (or for that matter even for animals) to respond to any stimulation from the external world as well as internal need states. Control and maintenance of this functional system is found to be the most important function of this part of frontal lobes, which is designated as the Anterior Cingulate. The Anterior Cingulate is connected to the remaining parts of the limbic system. The inputs from those structures of the limbic system make the Anterior Cingulate, the major area associated with emotional arousal, which is primarily required for the initiation of all forms of behavioral responses and actions. The functional system associated with arousal or injecting fuel into the piston and igniting has complex psychobiological mechanisms, which the brain has to cultivate during developmental stages. It is not enough to have high levels of arousal, but one has to learn to inject and fire it for initiating the actions, which one has carefully thought and strategy for action has been planned.

Emotion has the most debated phenomenology in history, as it involves experience and expression of variety of emotions. Experience of emotions related to achievements in life is considered the ultimate goal of life, by all. Emotions drive the individual, drive him through unexplainable stresses in life, and finally take him to the goal. Extreme emotional expressions are in the form of aggression, fight, flight, behavioral withdrawal, whereas experiences range from intense happiness to sadness, fear and anxiety. What fear is if one cannot explain it verbally? Even animals have the same fear, when they take to flight. What they cannot explain may be the experience or anticipation of an impending threat to life from which they may run away. On the other hand, a human being may not resort to flight, stay back, and experience the fear as a threat to life. If allowed or needed we will verbalize it using several words and try to convey the state of mind of having fear. One may experience intense happiness and become excited when one is in the close company of another person and learn to verbalize and differentiate differences in such experiences in terms of the closeness one could establish with the other person and anticipations. During such verbalization or transcoding, one may use words and ideas to make the experience a unique and extraordinary one or yet another threat to life. In this sense, emotions may be considered positive or negative in terms of their acceptance and their cognition and outcomes mark them unique to the individual. One learns to experience an emotion slowly according to the narration one has created and differentiate one emotional state from another. All emotional experiences and expressions have a direction and meaning interpreted by the brain. It is the cognitive interpretation, which makes one emotion different from the other. It is well established that fear can be aroused without perception and awareness of a stimulus as in preattentive emotions (LeDoux 1996, 1998; Morris et al. 1998; Whalen et al. 1998; Soares, Ohman 1998; Windmann, Kruger 1998). Reward, punishment, conflict, confrontation are cognitive interpretations of emotional experiences based on their specific effects on the individual, in which the associated emotional experience is either attractive and addictive or repulsive and threatening. States in which one can avoid negative emotions, fear, threat, and anxiety become psychologically and physiologically addictive. What the subject experiences is fear as described by the participants in the preattentive emotional experiments. Fear can be evoked without perception and awareness of a fear-provoking stimulus and it shows that a certain emotions, which help survival can be conditioned and automatically elicited by a stimulus in the external world without its perception, when the stimulus is detected by the brain. However, fear, even as a conditioned and unconscious emotional response is appraised as threatening to the system because of its threat to survival to the system. Without pain and some elementary cognitive component established sometime in the early part of life, the physiological arousal (activation of the brain and the body) will not be experienced as fear and threatening to the system. Fear is produced by self-awareness of threat, though it may be later aroused without the registration of the cause in the primary sensory cortex. Flight and fight on the other hand, can be elicited without perception and awareness of the threat, when emotional experience may be that of pain alone or threat (unconditioned response) of pain. Cognitive interpretations of pain and threat of pain and knowledge of impending danger can almost instantly follow a flight initiated after the detection of a threatening stimulus by other centers in the brain. The cognitive appraisal of fear would depend on how fast the nervous system has processed the cognitive component after the initiation of the flight. The same may attain colorful and vivid explanations when the original experience is transcoded, as one can transcode only the experience of flight after it is executed and perceived by the brain.

Emotional experiences and expressions may be considered primarily as markers of the physiological state of being alive and responsive to the world. We always consider being alive as a psychophysiological state, and accompanied by psychological or behavioral expressions. The psychological components of emotion have become more significant and their varied expressions have greater effects at inter and intra individual interactions. Emotions are classified in terms of the presence of psychological components in its experience and expression and the physiological accompaniment is often considered a common factor. The physiological activation varies in different emotional states, and the emphasis has been always on significant changes rather than on states when there is no appreciable increase or decrease in the emotional state. There is indeed an emotional arousal accompanying states of being merely awake, though non-receptive, though we do not label this state as emotional. Mental states with absence of interest, thrill, excitement, anxiety, fear, sadness, anger, etc. are considered non-emotional states. We consider only those states, which are subjectively pleasant or causing anxiety, sadness, or fear, etc., as emotional states. Emotions are either positive or negative. Qualitatively different psychological components have been identified and associated with different cognitive processing and behavioral expressions as emotions. Distinct psychological states and behavioral components of emotions are said to accompany states of excitement and hopelessness. This is considered an important function of the ACC as it gates the physiological activation produced by the autonomic nervous system with the cognitive labels used for the emotions. However, one cannot execute even the most simple response or action without drive. Without drive, one may not even turn around and press a button to switch on a light or fan. Without drive, one may wait for another person to come and do that job. This is the typical clinical profile described above, which we get to see in a patient with anterior cingulate lesion. A patient with large anterior cingulate lesion does not talk, eat food or drink water on his own, does not respond to pain, and does not have any initiative or interest in himself or the surroundings. It is the same drive in significantly varying levels of intensity and accompanied by varying cognitive labels, that are labeled as emotions. Emotions influence recognition of entities and events, and thinking, which could contribute to attitude to self and to others. State of intense anxiety may be accompanied by inability to terminate or give up a particular line of thinking; negative interpretations and inadequate encoding may characterize depression whereas incongruent thinking may characterize a psychotic state. Emotional arousal is a necessary component for the expression of conditioned behavior as well as self-initiated actions. Physiological activation and psychological alertness contribute to the emotional arousal required for initiation and execution of actions. Additional cognitive appraisals of the emotional arousal may occur rendering the emotional state distinct and complex. The psychological labeling is a subjective exercise making the physiological arousal become a unique experience to the person.

System 2: The Orbitofrontal System

The Orbitofrontal circuit has its origin in the inferolateral Prefrontal Cortex (Brodmann's area 10, 11, and 47; Kringelbach 2005) and projects to ventromedial Caudate Nucleus. The Caudate Nucleus projects directly to dorsomedial Pallidum and rostromedial Substantia Nigra, and indirectly to Globus Pallidus

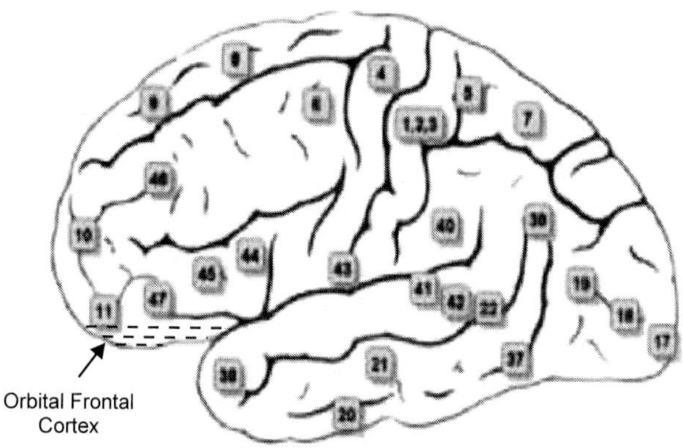

<table>
<tr><td>8</td><td>9</td><td>46</td><td>44</td><td>45</td><td>Lateral 47</td><td>Orbital 47</td><td>11</td><td>10</td></tr>
<tr><td>Posterior Dorsolateral</td><td colspan="2">Mid-Dorsolateral</td><td colspan="3" rowspan="2">Ventrolateral</td><td colspan="2" rowspan="3">Orbitofrontal, Ventromedial, Basal</td><td rowspan="3">Frontopolar Anterior, Rostral</td></tr>
<tr><td colspan="3">Dorsolateral</td></tr>
<tr><td colspan="6">Dorsal - Lateral</td></tr>
</table>

Fig. 4: Showing Brodmann's Areas—Lateral view

externa and subthalamic nucleus (Cummings 1995). The Pallidum and Substantia Nigra connect to the ventral anterior and medial thalamic nuclei and project back to the Orbitofrontal cortex. The system also has interconnection with amygdala and hypothalamus, and hippocampus. The Orbitofrontal functional system is associated with emotional regulation, personality, purposeful and goal directed behavior of individual. The thalamo-frontal circuits control the flow of sensory signals into the different frontal areas by which the functions of the respective cortical areas are mediated. The frontal control of the thalamus therefore can regulate the sensory inputs into the brain at the thalamic level. The controls that take place in the thalamo-cortico-thalamic circuits may be part of the regulation of sleep-wakefulness states and the state of consciousness and alertness of the individual on the one hand and dispensation of drive in varying emotional states.

Clinical lesion studies have shown that lesions in the Orbitofrontal and the interconnected areas in patients result in syndrome characterized by several deficits, which are discussed below.

Different personality changes are reported in patients with lesions in the Orbitofrontal system. Emotional changes are the most significant of these; they bring about drastic changes in the style of functioning and self-controls used by the individual. The changes may consist of being less worried about self, irritability, elevated mood, variable and inappropriate emotions, sexual disinhibition, excessively talkative and outspoken, less concerned about self and family, loss of tact, superficiality, difficulty to delay responses leading to consequent impulsivity, and need for immediate gratification leading to excessive and disinhibited activities, imitation and utilization behavior, and presence of primitive reflexes. Orbitofrontal cortex is involved in response inhibition and there are several circuits emerging from this region which connect to other centers. Several of the above deficits may therefore be present in varying degrees depending on the extensiveness of the lesion and the impairment produced in frontal circuits that connect to other cortical and subcortical regions. Loss of internal controls (response inhibition) make the patient become more environment dependent and imitation and utilization behavior (Lhermitte 1983, Lhermitte et al. 1986, Shallice et al. 1989) may be consequences of such dependency (Besnard, J. et al. 2011). Frontal lobe lesion patients may also presence of primitive reflexes (Vreeling et al. 1993; Zafeiriou 2004; Schott, Rossor 2003) and their presence in adult patients is a clear indicator of frontal pathology. Braver et al. (2001) proposed the ACC as the generic detector of processing conflicts. Impairment in spontaneous arousal of attention and ability to remain focused are other indicators of orbitofrontal pathology. These patients show impairment in being purposive and in state of motivation needed for goal directed activities. The debilities also lead to disruption of maintenance of mental set needed for appropriate response selection. The personality changes appear as a recent change in a person, which the relatives and friends would fail to understand. The changes in the personality make-up of an inflicted person are always taken note of by others. Some of the typical changes are reported below:

- Person who was known for his patience and tolerance becomes impatient and intolerant.
- Person who was shy and inhibited becomes outspoken and less inhibited in comments and behavior with others.
- Person who was actively involved in his professional life/occupation has become less or not concerned about the same.
- Person with an earlier serious disposition has become frivolous.
- Is not interested in the welfare of self, the family, and the cause for which he has been striving.

The functional role of the Orbitofrontal Cortex system that emerges from the findings of lesion studies can be summarized as that of control and maintenance of emotional drive, monitoring anticipated and actual effects of actions initiated and being executed for achieving personal goals in terms of social approval, maintenance of mental set for facilitating the actions being executed, and monitoring sensory inputs, which may include evaluation of the satisfactory effects in terms of reward appraisal and its effect on the emotional experiences (Lezak et al. 2004; Alvarez et al. 2006; Rolls et al. 2008).

The above indicate the importance of the orbitofrontal cortical areas in defining the emotional state of the individual, which affects his interpersonal relationships and navigational abilities in life. Emotional disposition must also match with the cognitive processing state of the individual. The system is considered to provide the platform required for the cognitive control of emotions. Patients with lesion in the ventromedial areas have difficulty in continuously maintaining their mental set required for persistent and continued pursuit of goals in life. The loss of focus in life will have devastating effect on the life affecting ability to take responsibilities and achieve goals. One of the most significant functional roles of the frontal lobes is in regulation of complex motor acts, in which the orbital frontal area plays important role. The distinct features of the motor control systems are discussed in detail elsewhere. The orbitofrontal lobes function in conjunction with the anterior cingulate lobes for cognitive control of emotions and direct the drive in a purposeful and directed manner for achieving goals in life.

The orbitofrontal areas required to conceptualize purposes and goals for the self. It has also the capacity to conceptualize the same in other individuals, thereby understanding and empathizing with them, which we refer to as the Theory of Mind capacity of the brain. Loss of motivation, purposiveness, planning, and initiative because of orbitofrontal lesion and pathogenesis of the area appear as a major personality impairment. It will derail social behavior, interpersonal relationship, as well as occupational interests of the individual. The orbitofrontal areas may be hypothesized to control the mind, with capacity to release the drive required to initiate actions and keep the actions executed control for achieving the goals. These negative symptoms could be further worsened by the presence of positive symptoms arising out of disinhibition and the consequential loss of frontal control on the other functional systems of the brain. Personality changes are usually coupled with emotional changes either in the form of excessiveness of emotions, emotional withdrawal, or inappropriateness and vacillations of emotions. It is the result of absence, impairment or loss of the mechanism of regulation, which leads to either excessive or under expression of emotional arousal. These changes may appear in an acute or insidious manner, depending on the actual onset and progress of pathology in the brain. What needs to be emphatically understood in this context is the fact that these functions need to be cultivated first in the brain during the brain developmental stages. The opportunities available for the cultivation of such functions and abilities may vary from child to child and the variations account for the differences seen in adult individuals in these domains. Developing these functions may be possible even in an adult brain, but may pose greater difficulties and problems unless the whole process is strategically managed. It must be apparent that these skills cannot be acquired in the classroom alone by a child, but needs to be acquired in the larger sphere of life.

Emotions are experienced in varied forms including as empathy, when one is capable of producing the same emotions seen in another person. Orbitofrontal Cortex and Anterior Cingulate Cortex is found to have a special role in emotional empathy (Decety, Jackson 2004; Jackson et al. 2006). Empathy is an important aspect of Theory of Mind (ToM), by which we explain social interactions at the affective and cognitive levels. Empathy is experienced at emotional and cognitive levels and the orbitofrontal cortex, especially right ventromedial areas are related to emotional empathy (Shamay-Tsoory et al. 2010, 2005; Baird et al. 2006).

System 3: Dorsolateral Prefrontal System

Dorsolateral Prefrontal Circuit originates in the dorsolateral aspect (Brodmann's areas 9 and 10) and projects to the dorsolateral head of the caudate nucleus. The dorsolateral caudate, in turn connects directly to dorsomedial Globus Pallidus Interna and rostral Substantia Nigra and indirectly to Globus Pallidus Interna and Substantia Nigra through Globus Pallidus Externa via Subthalamic nucleus. The Pallidum and nigra project to ventral anterior and medial dorsal thalamic nuclei. The thalamic structure in turn, connects back to the dorsolateral prefrontal cortex forming a total feedback loop. Lesion in the dorsolateral prefrontal cortex and the connecting circuits results in impairment of various controls needed for executive function and cognitive processing. Several of the original studies in which the dysfunctions of Dorsolateral prefrontal cortex were identified, based on which normal cognitive processing models were developed by Luria (1966a, b, 1969, 1973), Lezak (1995, 1982), Teuber (1964, 1963). Lesions in the circuit were found to affect impairment in the following functions:

Executive Functions and Working Memory
Motor Programming
Hypothesis Testing and Changing Mental Set
Verbal and Design Fluency
Organizational Capacity in Learning
Constructional Strategy for copying Complex Designs

The functional deficits seen in patients with dorsolateral prefrontal lesions clearly indicate that the system plays important role in the executive control of several cognitive and motor functions. Several of these cognitive regulatory functions are discussed in detail in the next chapters.

The three functional systems originating in the prefrontal cortex therefore decide major programming strategies in the life of an individual and activation of regulatory controls needed for various executive requirements. The regulatory controls start with the activation and utilization of the drive available within the system. The functional development of system represented by the Orbitofrontal cortex is considered responsible for one to learn defining purposes in life, ability to defining specific goals and also chalking out execution plans to achieve the goals. However, it may be wrong to assume that these abilities develop automatically in the developing brain of a child. The developing brain must be taken through those lines of actions where the growing child finds the need to indulge in and can cultivate the abilities in the brain. A growing child will find it easier to acquire the abilities if he is guided in these respects rather than left without such guidance. As the brain grows functionally, it learns to redefine the emotional arousal and excitement experienced in the early years and learns to label and use the same drive as specific motivations for achievements in life. Once the ability to be aroused and excited is present, it can be remolded and redefined as positive motivation and drive for achieving goals in life. However, one must learn to redefine and use the drive for achievement, without which the drive will go astray without allowing the person to achieve specific goals. This would mean that it is not enough to have the drive at disposal; one must learn to release it. Drive can be released and meaningfully employed only when one has learnt to define purposes in life and identify goals to achieve, and then learnt to chalk out action plans for achieving those goals. One must even learn to use the drive for initiation of actions and learn to perform goal directed activities, in addition to change the action plans in response to anticipated and actual effects of navigation until the goals are achieved. As can be seen from real life experiences, these faculties may not indeed develop just over a few years; they may take their own time depending on how fulfilling and rewarding the pursuits are for the concerned person.

Dysfunctions in Lesions of Fronto-Subcortical Circuits

The Frontal cortex is connected to the thalamus through subcortical structures viz., dorsal and ventral; caudate, nucleus accumbens, medial, lateral and rostrolateral globuspallidus. Lesions in the subcortical structures and thalamus can also breakdown the above functional systems and bring about certain characteristic neuropsychological deficits. These deficits are shown in the table below:

Neuropsychological Deficits Specific to Thalamus and Striatum

Lesion in Thalamus
Memory Deficits 1. Lesions of the anterior and medial parts of the thalamus can lead to memory dysfunction. Bilateral lesions may produce severe form of memory deficits. Unilateral lesions may produce material specific, verbal or visual type of memory disturbances (Speedie, Heilman 1982a, b; Bogousslavsky et al. 1988; Daum, Ackerman 1994a, b). 2. Verbal memory may often be spared after right thalamic lesions (Speedie, Heilman 1982b), and visuospatial memory may be preserved after left thalamic lesions (Daum, Ackerman 1994a). 3. Anteromedial thalamic lesions (both left and right) associated with long-term anterograde memory deficits and often accompanied by deficits in retrograde memory. Short-term memory is found to be unaffected, although may be impaired in large thalamic lesion. 4. In thalamic lesions, procedural memory remains intact and autobiographical memory either preserved or impaired for recent events (Speedie, Heilman 1982b).

(Contd...)

5. Behavioral changes concomitant to memory problems in thalamic lesions are increased irritability and disinhibition (Daum, I., Ackerman, H. 1994b; Bogousslavsky et al. 1988).
6. Lesions affecting the tuberthalamic structure result in the most severe form of cognitive deficits. The deficits include dysphasia, verbal paraphasia, comprehension deficits, impaired visuospatial processing, and verbal memory (Sala et al. 1997).
7. Daum and Ackerman (1994) reported a case of 63 years old woman with lesion (infarct) in the premedian thalamic area exhibiting impaired immediate recall in verbal and visual modalities in the presence of intact IQ and attentional function.
8. Sala et al. (1997) observed persistent global amnesia in right thalamic stroke.

Focal lesion in	Deficits
Striatum-dorsal	Confused, disinterested (Mendez et al. 1989).
Striatum-ventral	Disinhibited, euphoric, inappropriate (Mendez et al. 1989).
Caudate-medial	Mood disorder, irritability, explosive behavior, apathy, obsessive-compulsive features (Mendez et al. 1989). Deficits in Wisconsin Card Sorting test, decreased verbal fluency, poor recent memory (Cummings, Cunningham 1992; Butters et al. 1994; Fuster 1980). Correspond to the deficits in the three prefrontal circuits.
Nucleus accumbens	Apathy (Cummings 1995).
Globus pallidus	Apathy, psychic akinesia, reduced spontaneous activity, impaired initiative (Cummings 1995). Normal language, reasoning, intact mental control.

Frontal Inhibitory Controls

3

The Orbitofrontal cortex and the Basotemporal cortex have under their direct inhibitory control various other areas of the brain. The Orbitofrontal and the Basotemporal cortex are called the controlling centers and the remaining cortical and subcortical areas are the controlled areas of the brain. Release of inhibition is the necessary requirement for the controlled areas to get activated and function or process the tasks centered in their areas. Such inhibition facilitates optimum functioning of a functional system. The functional efficiency could be increased or decreased depending on the needs of situation by the controlling centers. Damage to the controlling centers and the connecting tracts would release the controlled centers from inhibitive control leading to hyperactivation of the controlled areas and the consequent deviations and abnormalities of functions associated with these areas. Disruption of frontal-subcortical circuits has been considered major cause of behavior disinhibition (Cummings 1993, 1995: Tekin, Cummings 2002), which prevents frontal control on behavioral manifestations. The two controlling areas are the Orbitolateral prefrontal cortex and the Basotemporal cortex (Starkstein, Robinson 1997). The release of inhibition leads to disinhibition of the controlled areas and the following are the major inhibitive circuits and disinhibition symptoms, when hyperactivation takes place because of lack of inhibitive controls. The afferent inputs into the Orbitofrontal areas help in the monitoring and regulation of the sensory and motor events and in the absence of such regulation these events become hyperactive. A breakdown of dorsal-ventral balance in the frontal cortex was hypothesized as the cause for disinhibition by Goldar et al. (1993).

Motor Inhibition—Disinhibition

Orbitofrontal-basotemporal areas have connectivity with Medial and Dorsal Frontal structures, and subcortically with Striatum. The Orbitofrontal cortex and the Basotemporal cortex share anatomical connections, which control the association between frontal-initiated volitional regulations and psychomotor behaviors, and Limbic-related emotional drive for initiation and execution of actions. Impulsiveness, loss of tact, uncontrolled speech, impersistence, inappropriate perseveration, restlessness, and hyperactivity, pressure of speech, decreased need for sleep and difficulty to focus attention intentionally (distractibility) are some of the frequently observed disinhibition symptoms seen in Orbitofrontal lesion patients. The schema theory proposed by Schmidt (1975) explains the need general rules of motor programming that can be applied in different environmental and situations contexts. The motor programming model put forth by Schmidt and Lee (2005) later explains the frontal control required for movement in their generalized motor program (GMP), which takes into account the nature and type of movements, their sequences, timing and the forces to be used. On the other hand, the model suggested by Goldberg (1985) explains the neural strategy for navigation across space and time, and the role of supplementary motor area and other brain centers in carrying out propositional and navigational movements across space and time. As against this, the conditioned responses, which are controlled from the Arcuate Premotor Areas (APA), are elicited by a stimulus (discussed elsewhere). The same differences are applied in the production of speech in which one kind of speech is spontaneous and controlled from the supplementary motor area whereas the other kind is repetitive and controlled from the APA.

Instinctive Behavior Inhibition—Disinhibition

Human beings also have a share of instinctive behavior, which is not learnt but expressed as response to specific stimuli, from a genetic repertoire. Maternal instincts, sexual instincts, and survival instincts are some of them. These appear in animals and human being without social learning and have been called the phenomenon of imprinting (Keeton, Gould

1986), and human beings can interfere with their expressions and modify them only by strong volitional efforts (Maslow 1987). Expression of some of these instincts is considered to be under the control of Orbitofrontal cortex. The Orbitofrontal cortex has direct efferent connections to hypothalamus, amygdala, and brainstem biogenic amine nuclei. The Orbitofrontal cortex mediates instinctive behavior through this connectivity. Disruption of the frontal control of the subcortical areas results in hyperactivation of the instincts. Hypersexuality, hyperphagia, and aggressive outbursts are some of the clinical examples of such disinhibition, seen in these patients (Starkstein, Robinson 1997).

Intellectual and Sensory Inhibition—Disinhibition

The Orbitofrontal-Basotemporal cortex has connections to dorsal temporal and parietal areas. Both visual and auditory input areas have connectivity with the frontal lobes. The connectivity of the Wernicke's auditory speech receptive area is with the Broca's area in the left frontal cortex, required for expressive speech which allows the receptive area monitors both inner (thoughts) and expressed speech producing awareness of speech created and recreated (Mukundan 1998, 1999, 2007a). Hallucinations as a release phenomenon (Cogan 1973) can be attributed to the release of controls exerted by a control center on the controlled system because of lesion either in the control center or network which are used for the control of the latter areas. In other terms the hyperactivity of the controlled system is the resultant of the inhibitory control of the controlling station. Release of the controlled areas from inhibition of ventral frontal and temporal areas may lead to intellectual and sensory inhibition. Grandiose and paranoid ideas, flight of ideas are examples of such intellectual disinhibition. Visual and auditory hallucinations are examples of sensory disinhibition.

Several single case reports of post-lesion cases have implicated presence of lesion mainly in the temporal lobes and then the frontal lobes as the reason for hallucinations and delusions (Braun et al. 2003; Andermann et al. 1999; Burke et al. 1999; Filley, Kleinschmidt 1995; Price, Mesulam 1995; Mace,

Trimble 1991; Savard et al. 1991; Stevens 1990). Dierks et al. (1999) reported in 3 schizophrenic patients with auditory hallucinations in whom the fMRI activation was localized maximally in the transverse temporal gyrus of the dominant hemisphere, and to lesser levels in the posterior superior temporal gyrus, middle temporal gyrus, frontoparietal operculum, and even in hippocampus, amygdala and sensorimotor cortex. However, the activation was the combined effect of auditory hallucination and motor pressing task they used in the study. Shergill et al. (2000) using fMRI showed in 6 schizophrenic patients had maximum activation in the right inferior colliculus, right and left insula, left parahippocampal gyrus, right temporal gyrus, right thalamus, middle frontal and anterior cingulate gyri, and right inferior and superior temporal lobe during auditory hallucinations. They concluded that auditory hallucination may be part of defective monitoring of inner speech as the same areas are involved in the production of inner speech. The loss of connectivity between the Wernicke's and Broca's area has been implicated as the cause of auditory hallucinations in schizophrenic patients in other reports also (Oyebode 2008; Frith 2005; McGuire et al. 1996a, b; Lawrie et al. 2002; Cleghorn et al. 1992). Lesion in the connecting pathways between the listening centers and talking centers of brain disables the ability to monitor the source of self-generated speech in thinking making the patient believe that the thoughts or speech have come from outside. Braun et al. (2003) suggests that lesions of the right hemisphere rather of the left hemisphere may be the cause for the production of visual hallucination in schizophrenic patients.

The neural disinhibition model of visual hallucinations is not as clear as that of the auditory model, in which the lesion is hypothesized primarily in the frontal and temporal connectivity circuit. In remembrance, presence of visual imageries produces neural activation in the primary visual cortex and visual secondary association cortical areas, which are to be monitored by the frontal cortex, which help one to know that the imageries are part of a process of remembrance and hence self-initiated. A frontal pathology can render such monitoring difficult or impossible, and the affected person would consider that the imageries are produced by real sensory inputs.

Emotional Inhibition—Disinhibition

The paralimbic areas are under the inhibitive control of the Orbitofrontal and Basotemporal cortex. Loss of inhibitive control in this system may lead to emotional disinhibition. The brain structures associated with emotions are several, which shows the complex nature of emotional experiences and expressions, and regulation of emotions. The structures closely associated with emotions are Amygdala and Hippocampus, Fornix and Parahippocampal gyrus (both are connecting pathways), Thalamus and Hypothalamus, Ventral Tegmental Area, Septum and the Brainstem, the Cingulate gyrus and Orbitofrontal cortex (prefrontal). All these structures are also associated with several other independent functions and additionally they play a role in emotions. Paul MacLean (1990) puts forth the "Triune Brain" theory, and has placed the "limbic brain" as the second brain structure, which developed according to evolutionary needs of life. This was followed by the "neocortex" that developed mainly in mammals, especially in human beings. Accordingly there are three brains put together in the human brain of which brain structure called the "Reptilian brain complex", consisting of the Basal Ganglia, Brainstem and the Cerebellum form the first structural brain complex. This brain took control essential of physical survival as it controls vital functions and "flight or fight" responses. The second brain, the "Limbic system" consists of mainly the Amygdala and the Hippocampus. Human emotions have passed through extended developments because of interpretive possibilities of the external stimuli. Cognitive interpretations run parallel to the physiological expressions of emotional states and together they form complex experiences and expressions of emotions. The Orbitofrontal cortex plays most significant role in such interpretations and controls, which receive inputs from the entire sensory cortex of the brain. These interpretations and control stake emotional responses beyond the territories of "flight or fight". As the controlling centers and the controlled centers normally function in great harmony, losing the controls because of lesion anywhere in the neocortex and more specifically in the Orbitofrontal cortex would naturally take away those immense cognitive features of human emotions. The affected patient may express more of the "reptilian emotions", and the disinhibitive effects may be seen as euphoria, elation, irritability, flight, or fight responses.

Executive Functions

4

The concept of Executive Function was developed by Lezak (1982, 1995). Luria (1966a, b, 1969) and Pribram (1973) had observed executive deficits in behavior in frontal lobe lesions in detail and discussed the nature of the deficits, and the role of the frontal lobes in executive skills. Luria (1966a, b) and Teuber (1963, 1964) are the contemporary stalwarts, whose original works contributed to the identification of the function, which could be later developed into a wholesome of concept of executive function. The concepts of "controlled" processing (Broadbent 1958), "selective attention" (Shiffrin, Schneider 1977), "cognitive control" (Posner, Snyder 1975; Posner, Petersen 1990; Posner et al. 1998), and of the "supervisory system" (Shallice 1988) have further contributed to the development of the concept of executive function. The concept of "central executive" developed by Baddeley (1986) as part of working memory cannot be considered to have a different executive functional role, though the working memory operations may be purely mental or mental problem-solving combined action execution. Executive controls encompass components knowledge of purpose of actions, volition, planning and setting specific goals, and regulated execution. Volition starts with the perception of a need state and drive/motivation to initiate actions for the satiation of the need state, development of an action plan from experience or as an original idea, setting goals, awareness of one's ability to achieve the goal, initiation of relevant actions in their sequences, and regulating the ongoing motor act/behavior using the actual and anticipated outcome of action at every stage. Executive function is therefore a complex mental process involving emotional arousal and planning, cognitive processing and controlled execution dependent on both emotional needs and cognitive feedbacks. Miller and Cohen (2001) have postulated that exercising cognitive controls may be considered the most important function of the prefrontal cortex. Cognitive controls are required not only for mental problem-solving but also for the execution of voluntary activities. Cognitive controls may be employed with intense awareness or almost automatically when the controls employed are already familiar and often practiced. Executive controls therefore, have extensive representation in the prefrontal cortex. The Orbitofrontal cortex has to accelerate the Anterior Cingulate cortex for release of the necessary drive to act, monitor the sensory inputs and motor outputs, link them with the drive state, and activate the dorsolateral Prefrontal cortex for goal directed planned execution of actions, a pattern of functional interaction shown present in the brain, in patients with frontal lesions by Luria (1966a, b, 1969, 1973). Banich (2009) calls it a 'cascade of controls' in the frontal cortex. Continuous monitoring of sensory-motor effects is required for updating the processing as per the requirements generated from own judgments, and preferentially inhibit and select components for action are important aspects of executive function (Miyaki et al. 2000).

Executive function is not called for hardly any voluntary act or mental activity. It is currently used as a conceptual system controlling a chain of online cognitive processes (Elliott 2003; Monsell 2003; Alvarez et al. 2006; Chan et al. 2008; Banich 2009). Its multiple components are planning, working memory, direction of attention, problem-solving using all forms of verbal reasoning, inhibition of selected activity, switching across blocks of information and action plans, and lastly initiation and monitoring of actions. Executive function is needed for all mental activities requiring control of temporal sequence and multitasking. The sequencing and multitasking nature of executive function reflects the need for a wide range of involvement of the brain areas. It requires the involvement of the different functional circuits of the frontal lobes, each functional system engaging to carry out a specific task demand. The logistic of the executive function could be explained using the model of working memory. Working memory task may employ the different functional capabilities in a complex chain of processing in a planned sequence. Working memory is required to understand or speak a logical sentence and to tackle a complex logical or strategic problem. It is needed for us to carry out the several things that we are currently engaged in as well as to start automatically the next course of actions just after completing the present engagements. The dual role of the frontal cortex in emotional regulation and working memory brings the two processes constantly in interaction with each other. Undue increase in emotional arousal has dampening effect on the efficiency of executive function. During overwhelming emotional arousal, processing related to working memory is inhibited, and effectiveness in planning, thinking, and decision-making is impeded along with narrowing of ability for attention and consciously supervise information intake and their processing. For example, "If you are thirsty while working in your room, you would wish to have a glass of water. You know from experience that you need to drink water to quench the thirst. Your experience may also reveal that drinking water is available in the adjacent room. Remembrance of these pieces of information helps to draw an action plan or repeat executing an earlier executed action plan, already known as it was rewarded. The action plan involves strategies to leave the work midway at a convenient point, get up from your seat, and walk out of the door and go into the next room. This is possible only if you have the necessary visual information of the location and distance of a door that would let you out of the room and into the next room. Since you have done this several times before, you hardly need complete details of the spatial positions of the door and the other objects in and outside the room. You would walk out automatically hardly looking around. If not, you will need lot of visual inputs so that you move out in the right direction without banging into other furniture and persons and walk out of the door. The movements are regulated by the relevant visual sensory information. The visual information of the location of the door and its distance help to walk in that direction. However, until one has walked through the door, the visual information of the door is only a hypothesis, which has a probability to be wrong. Walking through the door is the reality verification of information gathered from the sensory-motor effects. Once you have a glass of water in front of you on the table, you need to have further visual information of the location of the glass on the table and its distance from you. These pieces of information regulate your extension of the hand towards the glass and its termination before the fingers reach the glass. The next task is to lift the glass from the table. Even before the glass is lifted, you approach it with all the fingers of your right or left hand. How will you do this if you were to lift a piece of paper or a heavy book from the table? In the case of the paper, you will try to lift it with your index finger and the thumb, while you may use both the hands to lift a book or heavier object. Even before lifting them, you anticipate the weight of the objects and plan your actions in anticipation. Why would not we try to lift the glass with either hands, or just two fingers? It is the anticipation of the weight of the object that helps to presume a motor set even before the actual execution is on its way. Anticipation is based on your experience, which is readily made available to the frontal cortex so that it could be used to regulate the motor act. The anticipation is verified only when you carry out the act itself. It may often happen that you lift an object and find its weight is a lot more than what you anticipated. Motor regulation therefore takes place on actual outcome as well as anticipated effects of an intended act." A frontal lobe patient may struggle to carry out these acts, as we have noted several times and the struggle to lift increases with the location and extent of the lesion.

Wakefulness, Arousal and Attention

5

Traditionally, both sleep and wakefulness have been considered distinct aspects of consciousness, even though the brain interacts with the outside world only during wakeful state. Cortical arousal and wakefulness are induced by subcortical centers in the brain. Wakefulness is the condition when the brain can receive and interpret stimuli from the external world, as well as respond to them. Human brain carries out several important cognitive tasks during wakeful states. Ascending Reticular Activating System (ARAS) is a part of the brain stem and its main function is to maintain wakefulness and alertness in the individual. The role of ARAS in the production of the wakeful states of arousal has been identified from the original works of Morruzi and Magoun (1949). One major issue debated earlier was about the nature of interaction between cerebral cortex and the reticular system, whether the cortex or the reticular system aroused/inhibited the other. Current findings show that there are two subsystems originating in the ascending reticular activating system and each system is populated by discrete cells and neurotransmitters (Saper et al. 2001). The first system functions as the relay system responsible for thalamocortical connections of sensory information (Hallanger et al. 1987). The second system projects into lateral hypothalamus, basal forebrain, and the cerebral cortex (Jones 2003; Saper et al. 2005a, b). The pathways representing cholinergic, noradrenergic, dopaminergic, and histaminergic neurons are engaged in facilitating cortical arousal (Jonathan, Schwartz 2008; Saper et al. 2005a, b, 2001; Gallopin et al. 2000; Lu et al. 2000; McGinty, Szymusiak 2000; Sherin et al. 1996). The activity in the ascending reticular pathways centered in the hypothalamus interacts with the ventrolateral preoptic (VLPO) nucleus to affect the sleep-awake states.

When the ARAS is inhibited, the cerebral cortex is released from the positive activation effect of ARAS, and it is called the sleeping state of the cortex. During wakeful states, the Reticular Nucleus of the Thalamus (RNT) is activated into a 'transport mode' (Detari 1998) throwing the gates of the cortex open to the external world, for reception and processing of sensory signals (Steriade 2006; Faw 2006; Steriade & McCarley 1990; Parvizi & Damasio 2001). The ARAS starts from the brainstem area adjacent to junction of pones and midbrain and moving upwards into two branches. The ARAS also receives inputs from the thalamus, whenever the thalamus receives sensory signals from receptor organs. The ARAS in turn sends signals to the frontal cortex, and alters the frontal cortex and maintains the alertness whenever it receives the sensory input. The alertness induced helps the frontal cortex to attend to the sensory signals received in the primary cortical area via the thalamus. The activation of RNT therefore, serves the basic "gating" function and helps in selective perception or attending to selected stimulus (LaBerge et al. 2000). The ARAS gets inhibited periodically causing the sleep-wakefulness cycle in the individual.

There are 5 major neurotransmitter pathways present in the brainstem-cortical circuits, which controls sleep-wake states and play crucial roles in the maintenance and intake of sensory signals and their processing in the brain, and they form the acetylcholine, dopamine, norepinephrine, serotonin, glutamate and endorphins, hypothalamus histamine projection systems, which are directly and indirectly involved in the sleep-wakefulness states of the brain (Hobson 2005; Jonathan, Schwartz 2008; Hobson et al. 2000; Faw 2006). The basal forebrain anterior to the hypothalamus plays very important role in arousing the cortex and the maintenance of wakefulness (Schiff 2004; Jones 1998; Dringenberg 1998; Sarter & Bruno 1998). Wakefulness is not a uniform state of arousal. There are states of being quite aroused, being prepared and then finally releasing oneself into activity. Even states of meditation and hypnotic trance are to be considered as altered wakeful states. Being aroused and being released into action are different. Norepinephrine and serotonin activation are considered to be associated with the "go" state of arousal (Spiegel 2004; John et al. 2004) required for the initiation of actions in the wakeful states. The arousal-wakefulness system is complex biological machinery with several cognitive processing functions emerging from it, all of which need to be explored further for understanding the dynamic state of human mind that has emerged from it.

Consciousness

Consciousness has been considered the most fundamental functional state of the human brain. Philosophically consciousness is postulated as an independent and absolute entity of the universe, which exists within and outside the brain. There is absolutely no way such an independent existence can be attributed to consciousness within the neuroscience. Within neuroscience, consciousness is used most as a medical state, as injuries, lesions, diseases in the brain can take away the conscious state of the brain, when the brain is supposed to become unconscious. Anesthesia is introduced as a routine medical requirement for various forms of surgery, when the patient is either unconscious or does not have sensations of pain in the organs surgically manipulated. There are specific and clear parameters of physical and mental changes and responses, which indicate the degree of restoration of consciousness. When wakeful, consciousness on the one hand, indicates the capacity of the brain to monitor its own sensory and motor processing and use the information for controlling the sensory and motor effects, which brings the brain in contact with the physical realities of the world. On the other hand, consciousness is a state providing ability to monitor the cognitive and emotive processes taking place within, and use the information to semantically create or recreate new relationships. We presume consciousness occurs at different levels in each individual and a current level determines the qualitative attributes and the effectiveness with which the external world and internal processes are monitored and processed. There are independent scientific methods to measure the monitoring abilities and the effectiveness of using the monitored information for altering and adjusting the ongoing processes, and hence consciousness is used as a concept to refer to these complex and dynamic processes. Wakefulness and sleep are the most strikingly different phases of consciousness. We know that sleep is an essential state that should follow hours of wakefulness and processing takes place in the brain during both the states, though the nature of processing differs in the two states. Recognition of external stimuli and internal or proprioceptive physical changes do not occur during sleep and therefore the individual is considered to be in a temporary non-conscious state in sleep. During wakeful conditions, the cerebral cortex passes through two phases, which may overlap or remain independent. One phase is that of sensory-motor interactions with the external world, whereas in the other phase, the brain may remain partly or fully (?) independent of these interactions, but may engage in internal processing of retrieved information and creating new information. Internal processing may range from very active and focused states of problem-solving or states with minimal to nil processing. One learns to engage in processing of both external and internal signals and the processing efficiency may be determined by the relative importance allotted to the two domains by the individual.

Religiously and philosophically, consciousness was often postulated as an independent entity, considered to exist within and outside the brain. The consciousness that we speak about within neuroscience, is indeed different from this. Brain is indeed the instrument or the organ that embodies this property; it grows within the brain and perishes with the brain. Behaviorally and clinically, consciousness is only a state of processing; being conscious is accompanied by specific features, which may alone be considered the phenomenology of consciousness. Consciousness can only be considered an essential feature of a processing or functional state in the brain. There is no evidence of it being an entity dwelling inside the body-brain, though such a proposition was considered in philosophy and religion. When an individual perceives the contents of a sensory registration and recognizes the external stimulus, he is considered to be in a conscious state. He may or not respond to the stimulus, internally, behaviorally or verbally, based on the need as well as availability of motor faculties. The individual has to be in a conscious state for responding or intentionally not responding or responding to the stimulus. Attending to stimulus, recognizing, and responding to it are considered to indicate a clinically significant normal conscious state. Recognition is the process of identifying an internal image or memory trace, which matches with the sensory image produced by a stimulus. This is a process, which may be accomplished rapidly because of the frequent comparisons made, which result in familiarity. When internal models are not available, there is need to develop new internal models. The comparisons may be spontaneous or involve critical judgments. Hence, the state in which recognition can take place is considered conscious state. When it is not critically accomplished, the process is said to be subjective and the process may easily be affected by suggestive factors and the knowledge base, which one has acquired. Clinically significant conditions occur when recognition leads to abnormal recognitions resulting in derealization and depersonalization, considered parts of dissociative symptoms in psychiatric and neurological disorders. Source memory related to time and place of occurrences of episodes, allows one to remember the sequences and continuity of experiences. Loss of related information in these domains, while remembering may isolate the episodes. The frontal localization of source memory and critical thinking are discussed elsewhere. Interruption of these processing capabilities can be caused through suggestive inputs, which could block and alter processes of recognition, as shown in hypnotic suggestions. Critical processing ability is almost continuously required in each individual, unless one is recognizing and further processing confirmed familiar entities and changes.

Aspects of Attention

1. Passive attention
2. Active attention
3. Spontaneous arousal of attention-orienting response
4. Habituation of orienting response

5. Detection of stimulus change, novelty, and familiarity
6. Span of attention
7. Speed of detection
8. Divided attention and Channel capacity of the brain
9. Attending to relevant and irrelevant stimulus
10. Drive and attention
11. Attentional blink.

Attending is a state, which facilitates flow of sensory inputs from an external source into the brain through the receptors and the source is recognized by the brain. There cannot be attention directed to nothing. Attention is also required for selecting stimuli from within and processing them. When input from a specific source is selected, it is considered that the said source is selectively attended. Selection of a stimulus takes place intentionally within the brain or because of the intrusive effects of a sensation in the brain. When stream of sensations from a source are intentionally selected, attention is considered selectively focused on the source. Selection of a stream of sensory input from arrays of streams is selective attention. There is no focusing or selection of attention without reception and recognition of the sensory inputs. There is anticipation of sensation and the concerned receptors can be turned in the direction of the expected inflow of sensory inputs. The system in the brain, which controls this function must direct the sensory receptors intentionally or automatically to the spatial location of the source of sensory event, and prepares the brain to receive and process the flow of sensory signals. It may involve postural adjustments as well as readiness to receive the signals and process them. When this happens, the brain is considered attentive to the effects produced in the brain. As a selective process, attention has to be directed intentionally or by habit. Stimulus selection can occur because of the intrusive effects of a sensory input from the external world or because of the proprioceptive effects from within. Attending is a prerequisite for normal perception and further processing initiated from perception. One attends not only to external sensory inputs, but also to internal speech or thoughts created and retrieved information. Retrieved information may be purely conceptual information or autobiographical episodes. One may recreate sensory and motor imageries as part of remembrance and they too are selectively attended to so that the brain processes of recognition are carried out or when one becomes aware of the presence of the imageries. However, we use several of the retrieved information automatically, without attending to them. For example, during recognition of a person or object, the name is retrieved and may be used automatically. As a selective process, attention controls the inputs into and the outputs from the brain. Verbal awareness of one recognizing and responding to the particular stimulus may not be always online present, as one may not transcode the processing. Nonverbally awareness and recognition are considered the same. Responding to fear evoking stimulus may take place even without its recognition, which is discussed in detail elsewhere. Being attentive is a state of exercising such controls. Attention may need to be switched from one feature to another for intake of the details, or attend simultaneously to different aspects of a stimulus or external event. When attention is directed to a specific mental processing, it would involve the same shift of focus from one aspect to another for a sequential as well as holistic evaluation and understanding of the outcome of the mental processing. This may include retrieval of information consisting of remembrance of autobiographic episodes and other details of the knowledge base one has acquired. Attention is not cognitive processing, but gives direction to it, and cognitive processing is not possible without attending to the signal arrays or information units that are being retrieved or held online and processed. Attending and the cognitive processing that follows may be conscious or automatic by habit. Attention is an important requirement for one to become aware of a processing carried out, whether it is recognition or problem-solving. Continuous and directed attention with shift from one detail to the next in the time domain is necessary when the task involves sequential processing. Attentional shifts may also take place to units of information encoded across different points in time, for evolving a meaningful relationship across them.

Vision allows us to recognize objects and persons and reach out to them if we wish or intend. Recognition is a conscious process as it allows one to interpret and know a stimulus using own knowledge bank, whereas the controls used for online actions may not be consciously processed always. It has been well demonstrated that the ventral frontal system is involved in recognition whereas the dorsal system is associated with the use of sensory information for the controls required for actions (Milner et al. 1991, 1999; Franz et al. 2000; Norman, 2002; Glover 2004; Liu et al. 2008). This has been well demonstrated with regard to visual system (Norman 2002), with the ventral system involved in visual recognition and the dorsal system using visual information for motor controls. The important processes that take place in the brain, which lead to recognition of a stimulus are sensory registration, arousal of attention, followed by interpretation or identification, which involves comparisons of the external sensory model with internal models and identifying a matching internal model in the memory traces.

Sensory Registration

Visual, auditory, olfactory, gustatory, and somatosensory receptors in the body receive signals from external sources and streams of signals are passed on through the sensory pathways and registered in mode specific primary sensory areas in the brain. Sensations of taste and touch require intimate inputs, whereas auditory and visual sources could be far or near the receptors. Smell can travel across distances but has no comparison with auditory and visual signals. Of these, touch is experientially most significant as it allows direct experiential contact with reality, other than proprioceptive sensations accounting for muscle, postural and joint positions, and facial movements and expressions. The registration in the primary visual cortex (Brodmann's area 17) takes about 100 milliseconds after the signals are received in the retina of the eyes. In the auditory mode, the registration takes place (Brodmann's area 41) in primary auditory cortex about 70 milliseconds after reception of auditory signals in the cochlea of the ear. Brodmann's areas 1, 2, and 3 serve as the primary somatosensory cortical areas for registration of tactual and kinesthetic sensory signals. Taste sensations are picked up by taste buds on the tongue and received in the Anterior Insula/Frontal Operculum of the Gustatory cortex (Pritchard et al. 1999; Masayuki 2006). The Insular Cortex is part of the cerebral cortex that remains folded within the lateral sulcus, which separates the temporal lobe anteriorly from the frontal cortex and posteriorly from the parietal cortex. Smell signals are received from the olfactory receptor neurons inside the nose by the olfactory bulbs in the inferior part of the human brain.

Of the different sensations, the visual, auditory, and somatosensory sensations are of special interest in our discussions. The interesting feature of sound and smell signals is that their source of origin may be anywhere away from the human body, but they can directly reach the receptors (the ears and the nose). A sound may be produced somewhere behind the body or thousands of miles away from the ears, but the signals directly reach the ears and the sound is detected. Sound is produced by the reverberation of a medium and it needs a medium to spread. Electromagnetic radiation of certain frequency range is received by the eyes and this energy is called light. Light does not require a medium to travel through, as it can travel through even vacuum, but it travels through only transparent matter. Its propagation is always straightforward, and hence we consider it a ray of light, but bends when it moves from one transparent medium to another. The brain can make judgment of approximate location of the origin of the sound signals, wherever it may originate. On the other hand, a visual stimulus must be present in the left or right fields of vision to produce a retinal image and for the stimulus to be seen. We cannot see the visual changes that take place behind or anywhere outside the field of vision. Once the visual stimulus is not seen, it is not recognized and the brain has no knowledge of encountering the visual stimulus. If a stimulus produces sound, then the brain looks towards the source of the sound to know if it can see the stimulus. One may turn the head or turn oneself towards the sound source and searches for the visual inputs. Thus, we turn the head or turn ourselves around and look at a person who spoke from the sides or behind. Similarly, we may turn around to see what caused a strange sound behind us. The source of the visual signals needs to be searched out, as one must turn the eyes and look at the source of the signals. As auditory stimuli are used for normal communication, they have special importance in gating the movements needed for visual search. The auditory or olfactory signals are received directly in the brain, wherever their origin may be, while the brain has to search out a visual stimulus for its recognition. One may look out anticipating or expecting to see a stimulus and the anticipation therefore, plays a major role in visual search. It is indeed difficult or may be impossible to filter out irrelevant auditory or olfactory stimuli, but we can always filter out irrelevant visual stimulus by looking away from them. We can only cut of irrelevant auditory inputs, which we may call noise either by external filtering or by cutting of the flow of the sound. The retina of the eyes must receive the visual signals for the brain to process and recognize their source. The movement of the eyes may be saccadic for searching a visual field or they may be smooth pursuit movements, which help to track or follow a moving object. When the two eyes move in opposite direction for maintaining single binocular vision, it is called vergence. The eyes must rotate around a vertical axis for maintaining binocular vision. The rotation of eyes converges to look at close objects, while they diverge to look at objects farther away.

Orienting to an auditory, tactile, and olfactory stimulus can take place as a reflex response as the stimulus arrives in the brain on its own. On the other hand, visual stimulus can arrive only if the stimulus happens to be present in the visual fields. Even in the visual fields, it may get adequate registration only if the stimulus is strong and attracts the attention of the person or if the person is searching for the stimulus. Recognition of a stimulus can take place only after it is registered. Orienting to the stimulus is therefore an important aspect of attention. All brain lesions appear to have deleterious effect on orienting to a stimulus and it appears to be more acute if the stimulus is visual. Even a subtle change in the auditory stimulus quality may therefore be automatically detected. On the other hand, a change in the visual stimulus may be recognized only if it is in the intensity and/or any other conspicuous physical characteristics, rather than in content. Other processing functions can follow, only after the initial recognition of the stimulus take place. All neuropsychological assessments and understanding of the deficits are carried out from the responses made by a patient to various stimuli presented, which may require specific processing methods. Patients with cortical lesions have immense difficulty in visual search tests, and this difficulty is maximum in severity, when the lesion or damage is in the Frontal cortex. The Dorsolateral, Orbitofrontal and Anterior Cingulate functional systems have received maximum attention in neuropsychological, clinical and research investigations, as these systems directly control cognitive functions and behavior. The motor cortex, especially the Supplementary Motor Area indeed play a great role in motor and speech programming, though this function has not been well integrated into the knowledge system of neurocognitive controls that shape personality and achievement of the individual. The frontal eye field has received even less attention; despite the fact this function serves core capability of visual search of the external world and binding with visual stimuli.

Brodmann's area 8 in the Frontal lobe serves the functional role of controlling eye movements and hence Frontal eye fields. The speed of eye movements determine the speed of visual search and how fast one recognized the stimuli when they are in an array and how fast one recognizes the different features of an object or visual field. Somatosensory signals are the most important of all for establishing reality contacts by the self (body-brain-mind) and subjective verification of the reality. All other forms of sensations indeed facilitate and reinforce such verifications. Somatosensory sensations directly cause pain or pleasure and hence they have both survival values, as well as help create and establish new realities.

Broadbent (1958) proposed in his filter theory that sensory stimuli were selectively filtered using their physical properties before they are recognized. This helps to filter out irrelevant stimuli, which need not be recognized, and makes the processing task meaningful and easy for the brain. However, such filtering is achieved by physically directing the sensory receptors to a source, which may also receive signals partly from other sources and one may recognize them too. This was explained by 'late selection' position proposed by Deutsch and Deutsch (1963) and Norman (1968). One would not know the context of reception of such signals, though they too are recognized by the brain. Recognition of the source of signals takes place only after the signals are registered. The interpretation or recognizing system of the brain needs to be notified of the registration of the signals so that it can interpret or recognize the external source of the signals. Once the external source is recognized, it may be necessary to direct the sensory receptors towards the source of the new signals to facilitate further intake of the signals, which in turn may require withdrawal of the sensory receptors from other sources. Attention is a state needed for reception of signals from outside or from within for further processing. The receptive state may be developed (a) intentionally, or (b) may be because of the intrusive effects of the signals penetrating the sensory receptors. The signals generated may be from external sources or internal sources. One may intentionally recreate imageries, thoughts, and emotions or they may be recreated in an intrusive and automatic manner because of their personal significance to the individual. When attention is directed intentionally, it is referred as active attention. The state of attention, when there is no intention to attend to any particular source or mental task, is called passive attention.

The three important components of attention are spontaneous arousal of attention, direction of attention towards a specific source, and remaining focused at the new stimulus. One may direct the sensory receptors in anticipation of receiving signals and detecting an external source. Attention may be directed intentionally in anticipation or the receptors may be turned towards a stimulus, as the brain considers the stimulus significant or the signal intrusive. Spontaneous arousal of attention is accompanied by widespread physiological responses, often called the Pavlovian 'Orienting Reflex' or 'orienting response' (Sokolov 1960, 1963). The brain may adjudge a stimulus intrusive because it may be unexpected, or too strong and threatening. Attention may involve postural adjustments for facilitating the reception of the selected signals for their recognition. Recognition of the attended stimulus is the next stage. The stimulus appraisal takes place at two levels, one at the first signal system level, evaluating the physical properties of the source, and then at the second signal system level, which involves evaluation and expansion of the meaning of the stimulus. Signal processing at the second system leads to recognition of the stimulus. Activity in the sensory registration areas is therefore an important requirement for generation of attentiveness. The other area required is the arousal modulation system so that the signals registered can be selected or attended to for further processing. The orienting response refers to the physiological activation present, which in turn directs sensory receptors to the reception of signals from a stimulus. Selective attention refers to the selection of one source of stimulation over the others present in the same spatial and temporal domains. Mesulam (1981) and Posner and Petersen (1990) have postulated ARAS based models of attentional arousal. Posner and Petersen suggested the role of anterior cingulate for stimulus detection, whereas Corbetta et al. (1991) found significant activation in the lateral orbitofrontal cortex and in right superior frontal cortex in another study (Corbetta et al. 1993). Findings were affected by the nature of the stimuli, whether the tasks were spatial or non-spatial ones. Corbetta et al. (1995) found right superior parietal activation with spatial tasks, whereas Rees et al. (1997) found right prefrontal activation with non-spatial tasks. Coull et al. (1998a, 1997, 1996) observed activation of right dorsolateral prefrontal cortex and anterior cingulate using selective attention tasks. Coull et al. (1998b) concluded that attention is mainly localized in right frontal and parietal cortices and thalamus and that the attention generators in these areas send feedback to sensory association areas for selective processing.

Attending to mental tasks is important requirement for their fruitful processing. The major difference between attending to an external source and to a mental task is the direction of attending. Attention is directed outward when external stimuli are to be attended whereas attention is directed inward or to within the self for attending to own mental tasks. There may be occasions when one has to shift between the two when mental processing needs to be time locked to recognition of external events and their processing. One has to attend to what is being processed in the working memory or the imageries recreated in the brain (Theeuwes 1991; Posner, Petersen 1990; Posner, Rothbart 1998; Mukundan 2007a; Wright, Ward 2008). This endogenous type of attention is a core requirement for mental executions for problem-solving, mentally executed working memory tasks, as well as controls needed for execution of sequence of movements, speech and harmonizing the motor outputs or actions. Action synchronization and sequencing is normally carried out by the frontal cortex and supplementary motor area (SMA) (Nachev et al. 2008; Goldberg 1985). The important outcome of attending to mental tasks is the development of awareness of the tasks being carried out mentally. Recognizing and responding to external sources can be carried out without awareness, whereas awareness of the tasks is a certain outcome of attending to mental processing.

Awareness is a self-reflection of the sensory-motor processes, by which one knows what one is processing viz., thinking (encoding and transcoding) using words and symbols, applying reasoning skills, creating or recreation different sensory and motor imageries, and repeat experience of the emotional states created or recreated in a given context. There is no equivalent example that could be cited to explain what awareness is, except it is similar to the mirror reflection of a physical entity. Awareness is as real as the mirror reflection, but can be seen only in the brain which is engaged in the processing. Awareness is the self-reflection of possession of specific information, of processing information mentally, or of sensory-motor engagements by mutual monitoring. Awareness could also be that of remembering an autobiographic episode and having the mental sensory-motor imageries recreated. One becomes aware of the thoughts created or recreated during encoding or transcoding (discussed elsewhere). Both share the same knowledge base for understanding and controls. Such reflection is possible because the sensory system has the feedback of the motor outputs and *vice versa*. Retrieval from knowledge bank is required for even simple recognition. A self-reflection is a reality only as long as the memory trace causing reflection is activated in the brain and only to the extent that it tells about the presence and contents of the memory trace. Awareness is as real as a mirror reflection is. The mirror reflection is seen by the same sensory system, by which one sees its source, because of which we call it a self-image.

The amazing aspect, which cannot be explained by any neurobiological-neurochemical processes, is the fact that stimuli need to be recognized or a meaning created purely based on subjective interpretations and experiences of the individual. This cannot be automatically accomplished based on the permutations and combinations of the physical properties of the neurobiological processing entities in the brain. What one recognizes and the idea created could be unique and what the system has never experienced before. The process of attaching or learning a meaning is done in a physically and chemically determined manner, but the meaning itself is self-created. Such evaluations may lead to the production of responses or behavior, which may be beyond the natural survival needs. If a repeatedly occurring stimulus has no value or meaning to the perceiver at the second signal system level, and if the stimulus has no intrusive effects, the process of attending to the stimulus is withdrawn and the orienting responses produced by the registration of the irrelevant stimulus is habituated. One learns to ignore to take note of such stimulus, though it may be registered in the brain, as one may not be in a position to avoid or block its registration itself. Brain has knowledge of a stimulus only after the neural signals from the source are registered in the brain. Stimulus registration always takes place in the modality specific sensory cortical area, which we call the primary sensory cortex. Attention therefore, is the process of receiving or getting notified about specific arrays of sensory neural signals already registered in the brain, for its evaluation and recognition. All normal responses to stimuli occur after their perception or development of awareness of perception. However, the brain has the capacity to detect certain types of stimuli and respond to them even without its perception and awareness. This detection without perception occurs before sensory registration takes place or at a preattentive state and is responsible for emotional responses or some of the fear evoking responses, which are called preattentive emotions (discussed elsewhere).

Spontaneous Arousal of Attention-Orienting Response

When a stimulus in the environment becomes strong enough to make a significant registration in the brain through the receptors, it is notified in the frontal cortex, giving rise to spontaneous arousal of attention. The individual attends to the source of stimulus and recognizes it. This could be called automatic arousal of attention as the arousal of attention occurs because of the intrusive effect of the stimulus. The individual's attention is directed towards the source of stimulation and causing postural changes, which facilitate reception of the stimulus. This is called the orienting response or reflex. The orienting response is accompanied by changes in the neural processing, the effect of which can be detected at the neurophysiological and electrophysiological levels. For example, attending to the stimulus may be accompanied by changes in the electrical activity of the brain and autonomic functioning viz., heart rate, blood volume flow into extremities, pulse rate, respiration rate, galvanic skin resistance responses. If the same stimulus is repeated without any need for response, as it has no value in the second signal system to the individual, these responses will subside fully or partly, which is called habituation of the orienting response, except registration of the array of original sensory signals. Sensory registration takes place in the modality specific primary sensory cortex. Sensory registration is accompanied by the production of a positive evoked response called the P1 followed by a negative response called N1. In this N1 is considered associated with arousal of attention. If the same stimulus is repeatedly presented, another positive response called the P2 appears on the scalp surface. The P1-N1-P2 complex peaks at 100 ms, 140 ms, and 200 ms in the visual mode and at 70 ms, 100 ms, and 180 ms in the auditory mode respectively, in routine laboratory test procedures. Arousal of attention may take place intentionally, when the individual is in the process of searching for a stimulus.

Span of Attention

The quantum of stimuli or signals from a stimulus that can be simultaneous held on for further processing is called the *span of attention*. Span is indeed a function of quantum or units of information as well as the span of time over which they are received. Greater the quantity or the number of units of information that can be attended for processing at a given time, larger the span of attention is said to be. In other words, span is an estimate of the quantum of information that one can mentally hold on to at a time for mentally processing or using it. In a most commonly used clinical test is digits forward or backward presented at slow regular speed, in which it is estimated how many digits or numbers one can simultaneously and correctly hold on and report. The digits are read out as independent digits at short intervals and the subject who is tested must correctly reproduce the digits in the same order. Once these units of information are used, one shifts attention to new units of information. The best example of shift in attention is seen when one reads a book. Most of the good readers fix their gaze at two, three, or more equidistant points in a printed line, depending on the length of the printed line, one after the other and read the prints on both the sides of the gaze. Once reading one line is finished, the gaze is shifted to the second line and the same movements are executed. One, who is a competent reader, may fix the gaze in the middle of a printed line and read/recognize all the words on either side. Reducing the number of gaze fixations one requires for reading a line is the best way to increase speed of reading. Continuously attending to stimuli facilitates intake of signals continuously and their continuous conversion to information, though the individual always thinks what he has heard or seen are what he has recognized. Normally one has no idea that his brain has converted signals into information. This is realized only when one sees or hears what one cannot recognize. Span of attention can be enhanced through retraining programs thereby enhancing the quality of cognitive processing in a normal individual.

Directed and continuous attention was found to be a function of right frontal lobes in several studies (Salmaso, Denes 1982; Wilkins, Sallice, McCarthy 1987; Denes 1982; Richer et al. 1993; Rueckert, Grafman 1996). Continuous attention therefore, would mean acquisition of blocks of information by moving from one block to another of attention, and linking the blocks of information received in every span of attention. Recreating the meaning of a long complex sentence would mean quick retrieval of the meanings of each word heard or read and recreating a meaning by creating or assigning meanings created by sets of words. Recreation of meaning of large number of words is faster and easier, if one can anticipate a meaning. Using anticipation, one would recreate a meaning even before all the words are heard or read. The anticipated meaning may be or not the actual meaning, which the original speaker or writer wanted to convey. The observer or listener who recreates the meaning may not realize the faults unless makes effort to compare and verify the meanings. Encoding is the process of creating meaning as in thinking and recreating meaning as in comprehension. When experiences are verbalized using words and recreating meaning referring to the experience, the process is called transcoding.

Divided Attention

One may attend to groups of signals in independent clusters so that the different clusters can be processed separately. This has the effect of dividing attention so that one can multitask. Dividing attention across different sensory modalities is a common strategy one uses for processing different tasks at a time. Thus, one may read newspaper, listen to the news, drink a cup of tea, and also talk on the phone. One may divide attention in the same modality but for processing different issues. For example think over two or more independent issues almost simultaneously. Dividing attention is often a common need to meet the ever changing work exigencies. Attention may be divided for attending to information in different spheres which require different types of processing strategies. However, as one divides attention for the sake of processing information in different spheres, the ability to focus and process deeply and extensively in one sphere may be indeed affected. Such division of attention is useful when one is dealing with familiar pieces of information. Dividing attention may also help to selectively process information from different sources, provided they are familiar and do not pose cognitive challenges. This ability is also called multitasking. Diving attention for processing different spheres of information will lower the processing ability, if information in one sphere is challenging, complex and unfamiliar. Therefore, problem-solving may often require intense and focused processing and all the attentional resources one can command. Brain has limited channel capacity at any given time, and there is no way one can overload or exceed this capacity without losing information and their processing. However, it is indeed possible to raise the channel capacity to certain extent through right type of brain exercises.

Attention in Stimulus Selection and Response Selection

Attention needs to be directed to external stimulus, internal events which produce proprioceptive effects and the effects of externally directed actions and responses. Distractibility of attention has therefore, its effect on both stimulus and response selection. Stimulus selection enables the individual to focus processing on a selected stimulus, while action selection enables selective control of a certain action component. Selective visual attention is controlled by posterior parietal, anterior cingulate and prefrontal areas in conjunction with the striate areas, which have already discussed elsewhere in this chapter. The right frontal dominance seen with respect to visual attention warrants greater visual attention deficit in right prefrontal lesion than in left prefrontal lesions, which was seen in studies using unilateral frontal lesion patients (Weintraub, Mesulam 1987; Dwivedi, Mukundan 1993; Aron et al. 2003). However, attentional selection of response is concerned; the exact frontal lobe involvement is debated. The involvement of Anterior Cingulate Cortex (Turken, Swick 1999), Medial Frontal Cortical regions

(Suskauer et al. 2008) and Ventro Frontoparietal regions (Corbetta et al. 2002) shown are examples of the complexity of response selection and the need for participation of multiple frontal regions in response selection process. The conflict-monitoring hypothesis states that the ACC detects the conflict in the information processing carried out in the brain and pass on the conflict to the dorsolateral prefrontal cortex (DLPFC) to resolve the conflict (Liston et al. 2006; Mansouri et al. 2009; Pastötter et al. 2010).

Comparison of the performance of the frontal lobe patients with the Huntington's disease showed that the prefrontal patients made significantly more errors of commission by over responding to a target, while the HD patients made more errors of missing to respond to the target. It has been postulated that Alzheimer's patients show distractibility because of a deficit in voluntarily initiating a process of inhibition needed not to initiate a response as in the "go - no - go" paradigm (Simone, Baylis 1997; Tipper et al. 2000). This is different from the process of "lateral inhibition" (Tipper et al. 2000) in which neurons working in different directions would inhibit each other. This is different from the neurons working in the same direction would excite each other. The latter would bring about a facilitation of target reaching response while the opposite effect will be seen with regard to the former type of inhibition. Lateral inhibition will therefore, result in a type of distractibility by the nonrecruitment or selection of action components.

Attentional Blink

Attending to a visual event can lead to functional blindness for other events in the visual field. Attentional blink is the transient blindness developed to features and events in the visual domain while the brain is selectively attending to one target or set of events (Jolicoeur 1998, 1999; Raymond et al. 1992). Brain fails to detect other events in the visual domain for a transient period. The channel capacity of the brain is severely affected by attentional blink. If there are two or more targets for visual examination and if the brain is attending to one of the targets, the brain may become functionally blind to other targets. This would mean that if the brain turns to a second target, there may be functional blindness for a short duration during which it fails to visually recognize or detect the second target. The functional blindness may last for about 500-1200 ms. A second visual event may be perceived only after this interval, when one moves the search from the first to the second visual event. Attentional blink has a special effect on visual perception and this effect may be a matter of concern especially for those who continuously monitor visual displays on computer monitors. It has the effect of lowering the channel capacity for intake of visual information and the resultant loss of time when irrelevant visual displays are examined. Frontal and parietal brain areas are found to be involved in the manifestation of attentional blink (Marois, Chun 2000).

Attention Deficits

6

Close observation and examination of a patient is of paramount importance for deciding about the presence of behaviorally significant deficits and for estimating the nature and severity of deficits. The deficits manifested are generally dependent on the premorbid level of functioning, which have to be estimated most often from the interviews with the patient, his records, and his informants. A clinical assessment of cognitive and behavioral deficit, in this respect, must be considered different from a disability assessment of brain lesion patients using psychometric tests for their rehabilitation and financial compensations.

1. As clinical assessment of a patient and assessment of presence of different focal signs, indicating impairment and the level of impairment caused by defective processing methods cannot be decided only in terms of comparison with normative data.
2. Astute observation of the patient, his gestures and actions, style and content of talking, ability to anticipate reactions from the examiner and respond to it and attentional strategy deployed are important aspects of a clinical observation.
3. The observations of the patterns of attitudes and behavior of the patient are extremely important for deriving a sharp picture of the effects of brain pathology.
4. Equally important is to arrive at a useful and accurate profile of the premorbid functional patterns and levels of efficiency of a patient.

5. Interview of the informants—close relatives, is important to obtain a clear picture of the premorbid patterns of functioning of the patient. This will help to obtain relevant details of how and when those who live and work with the patient started noticing changes in his behavior.

Premorbid Cognitive Processing Levels and Functional Patterns

Different strategies are to be used for patients if they are children and adults and studying, have started working, and have been already working for many years, nature, and responsibilities of employment, or have retired from work. One must also keep in mind during of the current illness, before making decisions on the premorbid functioning. Special preferences in work, lifestyle, and hobbies may reveal relative merits of verbal and nonverbal interests, as well as abstract thinking styles of a patient. Disorders like epilepsy, focal lesions of the brain, space occupying and vascular lesions, degenerative disorders, traumatic brain injuries may produce characteristic differences in the symptom profiles. Individual variations across patients coming from rural and urban areas were very significant in the earlier years, and the typical differences that used to exist have almost disappeared in the current times. Effects of economic background can still produce some changes in the living styles of individuals, but these may not influence intellectual and academic achievements as they used to in earlier years. If the assessment of the patient is done for the purposes of detecting current functional efficiency on a test and its interpretation in terms of impairment, it has to be done by comparing the scores of the patient with normative data collected from socioculturally and educationally comparable normal individuals. If the aim of the assessment is to determine specific changes and deficits, which have appeared as sequel to brain pathology, mere comparison with normative data does not help. Comparison with normative data is indeed important to show the level of efficiency—disability a patient have subsequent to the brain pathology. The first type of assessment is important for clinical understanding and monitoring of the neuropsychological profile of the patient.

Observation of the Patient

Keen observation of a patient's behavior is the primary step in neuropsychological examination. Observations of how the patient is kempt, the pattern of walking, moving around, using limbs, posture, the manner in which he scans the environment, looks at the examiner(s), attends to speech, manner of speaking, facial expressions, emotional responses, etc. are very important to arrive at significant understanding of current status of the patient.

Appearance of the patient

While meeting a patient for the first time, it may not be possible to know if the patient had dressed himself or he has been helped by relatives or attendants. A patient may appear immaculately dressed even if he has helped himself; or may appear physically clean but not wearing clean clothes and appear unkempt. It is necessary to note down the appearance of the patient and emotional responsiveness of the patient. The personal appearance, especially when disturbed, is generally an important indicator of the mental state of a person. When a patient has been deteriorating as in the case of dementia or is having an episode of depression or psychosis, personal appearance and cleanliness are often neglected.

Locomotion and use of limbs

The ease and freedom, with which the patient may walk in to meet the examiner, will depend on the gait, muscular conditions of the lower limbs, etc. unless the patient is brought in wheel chair or support. Difficulty in walking and using limbs may be because of impairment of associated muscle controls or indicate presence of rigidity, akinesis, apraxia, etc. The presence of motor deficits, its degree and nature is evaluated as part of the physical examination. However, this may not always be available to the neuropsychologist and therefore, it is necessary for him to look out for any significant deficit that may be conspicuously present, especially those features, which the patient must intentionally take care. These deficits may directly affect the performance on various performance tests involving psychomotor functions.

Activity level of a person may be affected in both psychiatric and neurological diseases. Lesions of the Orbitofrontal and Dorsolateral areas of the brain have significant direct and indirect effects on psychomotor activity level of a patient. Reduced emotionality and motivation could be the basis for lowering of activity level in orbitofrontal patients. Dorsolateral lesions, on the other hand may affect psychomotor performance directly, as they could produce impairment of visuomotor coordination, persistence in performance, kinetic melody, bimanual use, etc. Increased psychomotor activity, described as hyperactivity and restlessness are also the result of frontal involvement. Reduction in psychomotor speed and activity are generally associated with subcortical and medial frontal lesions, whereas increase in activity is often associated with disinhibition may be seen in orbitofrontal disorders.

Impairment of Attention

Impairment of attention produces wide spectrum of disabilities, which can render all types of cognitive processing difficult for a patient. Attentional impairment is a major symptom in psychosis especially schizophrenia. Attention deficit is an important deficit associated with hyperactivity in children as well as adults. Different types of attention deficits are seen in lesions in different frontal cortical areas, and in traumatic brain injury affecting the frontal lobes. Attention deficits can be the outcome of anxiety and other emotional disturbances. Since attention is not focalized function of the brain. The best of attentional control is possible only when the entire functional system of the brain is intact and functions optimally. Lesions of Orbitofrontal cortex, Anterior Cingulate cortex and Dorsolateral Frontal cortex have differential effects on the various aspects of attentional controls. Detection of attentional deficits is the first step of a clinical neuropsychological examination of patient. Evidence for some of the attentional deficits can be observed while interviewing the patient. Further indications can be seen while examining the patient. Need to find evidence for subtle impairment of attention would often require careful testing of the patient, especially when the patient himself complains that there is deterioration of attentional ability compared to his premorbid levels of functioning.

Impairment of Visual Attention

Being attentive or attention being aroused is the most preliminary state of the brain that facilitates recognition of the external world. Deployment of the motor functions of the body facilitates such attention arousal as well as for responding and navigating in the external world. Extensive valuable information is available in clinical lesion studies about the functional role of different areas of the brain in attending to the world. These findings help to understand the intricate steps and processes involved in attending to a stimulus. Results of some of the 'paper-pencil cancellation tests' used for detecting attentional impairment, are discussed below. These results are from patients with focal lesions, which caused minimal to moderate clinical severity. Tests used for the detection of presence of attention impairment are all visually presented except the digits forward and backward tests, and the two serial subtraction tests. The results presented here are from studies reported by Mukundan et al. (1991), Mukundan (1996), and Dwivedi and Mukundan (1993) using various visual search tests, viz., visual search of (a) figures, (b) Number Scanning (20 and 50 numbers), and repetition of numbers, (c) Trail Making Test, and (d) visual field inattention test adopted from the test of Weintraub and Mesulam (1987). In visual tests 'a, b, and c', the patient was allowed to move eyes laterally and vertically for scanning the visual field, whereas in test 'd', the patient was to detect the targets printed on the right and left fields of a sheet of paper, using a central gaze fixation. In the number scanning tests, the patient was instructed to mark the numbers printed randomly on a paper sheet, sequentially, with a pencil and the total time taken for the completion of the test and the errors committed were measured. There were no distractors along with the sequence of numbers in tests 'a' and 'b'. The Trail Making tests—Form A and B, were also used, though only the results of Form B are presented her for discussion. As there were illiterate patients, a visual test 'a' with small figures of objects printed on a sheet were used with instructions to scan and identify the figures one by one. They were to verbalize and mark on each picture, and the time taken for completion of each presentation was recorded. Another visual test was the adaptation of the Wechsler's (1981) Digit Symbol Substitution test. The tests were not administered as time limited test. The subject was given as much time as he wanted to perform the tests continuously. The performance of the patients with lesions in the left Frontal lobe (n = 32), right Frontal lobe (n = 32), bilateral Frontal lobes with the lesion dominantly either on the right or left side (n = 10 each), in the non-Frontal (temporal and parietal) left and right sides (n = 10 each) were compared with that of age and education matched normal control group (n = 30). Further performance of groups of patients with lesion in the left and right Dorsolateral Frontal cortex, Anterior Medial Frontal, Posterior Medial Frontal areas, and Basal Frontal Lesion patients were compared with that of normal controls. The performance of the different groups of brain lesion patients groups in each test was compared with that of an age and education matched normal control group. All the tests discussed here employ visual search based on response set or need state instructed by the examiner. The instructions on each test required the patient to visually search for a specific stimulus in a sequence in a limited space and respond to the detection by marking each stimulus. Visual search strategy employed by each was not studied. Only the total time taken for completing each task and the errors committed were noted for further analyses and comparisons. Impairment in visual search was inferred by comparing the performance of patient groups with different brain lesions with that of normal control participants.

Stimulus Flow into the Brain

The patients groups with different cortical lesions performed very slowly on all visual search tests. High intragroup variability

Table 1: Mean (X) and SD values of time (in seconds) taken by FI, NFL and NC groups on tests of (a) Visual Search Test, and (b) Number Scanning Test (NST) from the NIMHANS Neuropsychological Battery by the Left Frontal (LF), Right Frontal (RF), Bifrontal Lesion with predominant Left lesion (BFL) and predominant Right lesion (BFR), Left Non-frontal (LNF), Right Non-frontal (RNF) and Normal Control (NC) groups and the F values

Site of Lesion	n		Visual Search Test Secs	Number Scanning Test (NST) Seconds		NST CR in 2 Min	Trail Making Test (TMT) Form B		Digit Symbol Substitution Test	
			Figs.	20 Nos.	50 Nos.	20 Nos.	Form B	Err	Time	Err
Left Frontal	32	X	55.8	96.5	443.8	9.5	319.8	8.4	570.6	6.6
		SD	34.9	100.6	259.3	3.8	193.5	5.6	291.0	5.48
Right Frontal	32	X	48.8	86.7	467.7	8.9	328.9	6.7	756.3	10.3
		SD	25.4	51.6	193.0	4.5	165.1	5.8	383.1	12.1
Bifrontal Left Frontal	10	X	52.6	86.4	460.3	9.4	610.8	6.4	574.4	6.0
dominant		SD	21.8	59.7	150.7	4.2	256.7	5.0	258.4	4.4
Bifrontal Rt Frontal	10	X	59.1	81.8	462.6	8.5	699.0	10.4	596.5	10.2
Dominant		SD	27.4	35.2	152.0	5.1	312.5	8.8	414.3	10.6
Left Non-Frontal	11	X	33.0	66.4	297.0	13.3	187.3	3.2	344.2	4.8
		SD	19.0	52.2	149.5	4.0	60.5	7.6	154.8	11.3
Right Non-Frontal	11	X	42.2	50.9	285.0	11.2	190.7	1.2	524.5	4.6
		SD	18.7	24.8	138.8	4.2	89.6	2.1	242.9	5.2
Normal Controls	30	X	22.0	35.7	200.3	14.6	125.7	1.6	185.6	2.8
		SD	8.7	13.5	49.6	2.2	40.6	0.6	65.6	1.5

X = Mean, SD = Standard deviation, CR = Correct Response, Err = Error

Table 2: Mean and SD values of time (in seconds) taken by Intra-frontal (IFI) and Non-frontal (NF) lesion groups on tests of visual scanning

Site of Lesion	n		Visual Search Test Secs	Number Scanning Test (NST) Seconds		NST CR in 2 Min	Trail Making Test – Form B		Digit Symbol Substitution Test	
			Figs.	20 Nos.	50 Nos.	20 Nos.	Sec.	Err	Time	Err
Dorsolateral Frontal	18	X	45.8	84.6	392.4	10.4	276	5.9	576	3.8
		SD	22.1	76.0	158.3	4.8	113	4.5	187	5.7
Anterior Medial – AM	14	X	48.9	89.0	467.9	7.9	375	9.7	633	10.0
		SD	26.9	61.1	169.1	3.5	193	6.6	78	11.9
Posterior Medial – PM	17	X	60.9	99.7	509.4	8.8	387	8.1	768	13.0
		SD	39.6	59.5	240.7	4.2	207	4.8	439	11.6
Orbito-Frontal – Basal	11	X	49.9	75.2	427.2	9.0	226	8.1	709	10
		SD	26.6	41.0	140.3	5.0	79	8.5	337	8.3
Left DLF	9	X	53.1	91.1	370.3	10.7	287	4.3	508	3.1
		SD	25.0	97.5	163.6	4.9	85	3.0	184	6.5
Right DLF	9	X	38.4	78.1	414.4	10.1	265	4.3	644	4.6
		SD	17.0	51.5	159.4	4.9	115	3.0	184	5.1
Left AM	7	X	47.4	70.0	371.6	8.9	104	7.9	440	4.1
		SD	28.8	43.3	108.0	2.9	145	8.4	259	7.4
Right AM	7	X	50.4	108.0	564.3	6.9	446	12	825	16.7
		SD	27.0	73.2	168.9	4.0	218	6.7	435	13.3
Left PM	8	X	63.1	111.5	562.4	9.5	418	9.3	776	11.5
		SD	50.6	72.7	33.5	3.8	244	2.9	401	10.5
Right PM	9	X	58.9	89.1	462.2	8.1	359	7.2	761	13.9
		SD	29.5	46.7	122.2	4.6	177	5.8	435	13.0

Table 3: Comparison of Mean Scores of Right and Left Lesion Groups

Comparison of Groups Mean Differences	VST	NST 20	NST 50	NST CR	TMT		DGST	
		Sec	Sec		Sec	Err	Sec	Err
Right Frontal vs. Normal	SD	SD	SD	SD	SD	SD	SD	SD
Left Frontal vs. Normal	SD	SD	SD	SD	SD	SD	SD	SD
Bifrontal LD vs. Normal	SD	SD	SD	SD	SD	SD	SD	SD
Bifrontal RD vs. Normal	SD	SD	SD	SD	SD	SD	SD	SD
Left Non-Frontal vs. Normal	SD	SD	SD	NS	NS	SD	SD	SD
Right Non-Frontal vs. Normal	SD	SD	SD	NS	NS	SD	SD	SD
Left Frontal vs. Right Frontal	NS	NS	NS	NS	NS	NS	SD	SD
Left & Right Bifrontal	NS	NS	NS	NS	NS	SD	NS	SD
Left & Right Non-frontal	NS	NS	NS	NS	NS	NS	SD	NS
Left Frontal vs. Left Non-Frontal	SD	NS	SD	SD	SD	NS	SD	NS
Right Frontal vs. Right Non-Frontal	NS	SD	SD	NS	SD	SD	SD	SD

SD - Significant Difference, NS – Non Significant

was found in all visual search tests. No attempt was made to understand if any relationship existed between test performance (slow visual search) and severity of the lesion in each group. Each test required application of visual search skills of scanning the sheet of paper by continuously shifting the gaze, which helped to recognize figures and numbers. In the figure recognition test, the subject had to report verbally the figures seen in the plate, whereas in the visual search of numbers, they had to cancel the numbers in serial order or mark numbers that were repeated. When normal participants took a meantime of 22 seconds, the patients with lesions in different sites took 33 to 59 seconds for completing a visual task of searching the figures. There was no indication of anterior—posterior (frontal—non-frontal) differentiation in the performance pattern. All focal lesions consistently affected the performance on the tests. In the 50 numbers scanning test, the normal group completed the search in 200 seconds, the patient groups took minimum of mean 285 seconds and maximum of 468 seconds for completion of the test. In TMP, the minimum and maximum mean times for completion were 187 and 699 seconds, while the normal participants completed the task in a mean duration of 125 seconds. The variability of performance as indicated by the standard deviations was very high in the patient groups. All brain lesion groups showed significant slowness in visual search on all the tests compared to that of normal group. Only the left and right non-frontal (temporal and parietal lesion patients) groups showed performance comparable with the normal group on the Correct Response scores of Number Scanning test, and the time taken on the Trail Making Test. Both left and right Frontal lesion groups performed equally slow on the Visual Search, Number Scanning, TMT, except on the DSST, on which the right Frontal lesion group took significantly greater time for completion. Successful completion DSST needed working memory ability along with visual search ability for its successful completion. Absence of lateralization effect in the right and left frontal lesion patient was seen in another earlier study (Shailaja, Mukundan 1989) also. The Bi-frontal right dominant lesion group made significantly greater number of errors on the TMT and DSST compared to the left Bi-frontal left dominant lesion group. The left Frontal lesion group required significantly greater time for visual search on Number Scanning test and TMT than left non-Frontal lesion group. Similarly, the right Frontal lesion group took significantly greater time than the right non-Frontal lesion group for visual search in the tests of Number Scanning, TMT, and DSST. The brain lesions considered in the study had differential effects on tests of visual and verbal learning memory, and visual scanning (Mukundan et al. 1987, 1991; Mukundan 1996). The primary involvement of the Frontal lobes, whether left or right, has been strongly supported in visual search tasks, by the above findings.

Visual searching and becoming stimulus bound have no parallels in other sensory modalities. Becoming visual stimulus bound or focusing on a visual stimulus means a lot more than moving the eyes looking into the visual space. It has been a common experience with TBI and other frontal lesion cases, that they have difficulty to recognize a visually presented single stimulus like an alphabet or a number (Christina et al. 2009; Mukundan 2012), if the stimulus is presented for short exposure time. It is common observation with many of these patients need a single number or alphabet needs to be presented for more than 3 seconds or occasionally even longer on a computer monitor, for their recognition, after recovering from a TBI of moderate severity. Two to three weeks of regular cognitive retraining using these simple visual recognition tasks bring down the exposure time considerably, enabling them recognize numbers and alphabets with 2 to 4 digits, when they are presented for 300–500 milliseconds. Their performance on other working memory, visual comparison, word detection, and reading speed, presented visually, starts improving only when the visual search and detection reach near normal levels. Gaze fixation and shifting gaze are important for all visual search tasks including reading. Children in their early years of reading from printed textbooks start with fixing gaze on each word and then change the gaze to the next word for reading. Faster reading occurs when gaze fixation becomes less in number in each line and when the child learns to shift the gaze to the next point faster. This is a difficulty often seen in TBI and other brain lesion cases. On the other hand, this difficulty is not seen with auditory inputs. Even when patients perform well on some of the verbal learning and memory tasks, they show difficulty in visual search and working memory tasks. This is discussed further in a later section.

The results presented in the Table 3 above show that visual search is impaired in all Frontal lesion groups. Time taken for completion of the visual search is significantly longer in all the tasks used. The limitation of the test was that it did not measure the stimuli detected in the left and right visual fields of the subject. The subject was allowed to move the head and eyes across as well as up and down in search of the stimuli. The mental task in each was to hold on to a number and then search for the next serially increasing number. Since the number already marked continued in the visual field, the true task was that of searching the next ascending number. These patients did not have difficulty either in number recitations or in simple mental arithmetical calculations. In the absence of dyslexia, the increased time taken for completion of each task must be considered to indicate only slow visual search. All brain lesions, which included left and right Frontal and non-Frontal lesions, caused significant slowness in visual search tasks, indicating that a lesion anywhere in the cortical areas of the cerebral hemispheres could delay visual search. There was no differential effect between the left and right Frontal lesions. Bifrontal lesion patients with the lesion predominantly on the right side and left side also did not show any differential effects on visual search. Similarly, both right and left non-Frontal lesions show the same effects on slowing the visual search in the different tasks. The left and right Frontal lesion groups showed significant increase in visual search time on six of the eight variables measured in comparison with the performance of the respective non-Frontal lesion groups. It is evident that the Frontal cortex plays most crucial role in visual search and for being visually stimulus bound, which are core components of visual attention, which leads to visual perception, though all stimuli perceived may not be recognized. Visual focusing may last as long as one requires examining the stimulus or the visual field. However, once the gaze is fixed, there appears to be a left visual field preference. This was demonstrated in several earlier studies (Damasio, 1979; Salmaso, Denes, 1982; Weintraub, Mesulam 1987; Posner, Petersen, 1990; Dwivedi, Mukundan 1993), which indicate a stimulus in the left visual field is detected and responded faster than stimuli in the right visual field, demonstrating right hemisphere superiority for visual attention and recognition.

In the second visual recognition task, which was adapted from the original work of Weintraub and Mesulam (1987), the subject was to look at a middle vertical line on a sheet of paper kept horizontally in front of him, and look for the targets on either side (in the left and right visual fields) without changing the gaze and mark them. This helped to find the visual recognition ability of stimuli in the constant left and right visual fields, as well as presence of hemi-inattention, if present in the patients. Since the targets are well defined, the subject could search for the targets ignoring the non-target stimuli. It is interesting to note that if competing stimuli are present while attending to auditory stimulus, the noise cannot be filtered out, as one can ignore irrelevant visual stimuli. With regard to visuals stimulus, most of the noise produced by competing visual stimuli can be voluntarily blocked to facilitate the flow of the signal arrays from the selected or desired visual stimuli, present in any visual field at a given time. Maintenance of the direction of the eyes is an important regulator for remaining focused at selected visual stimulus.

A top-down view of the brain functioning considers a need for visual search and several factors that could influence the process. Visual inattention is a comprehensively studied aspect, in this respect. Several studies have shown the right hemispheric dominance in visual attention, which has been considered to indicate a right hemisphere dominance in visual processing. Visual processing requires simultaneous consideration of several visual input cues, which do not happen with auditory inputs. In auditory inputs, the individual has to hold on to the information encoded and mentally connect the new incoming inputs to the information held or being created in the working memory. On the other hand, several visual input signals can be simultaneously attended to as they continuously present in the visual domain and one can change gaze across them as many times as one wants, in most of the real life situations, except when there is a change or movement in the visual field. For example, one can keep looking at the same picture or page in a book or keep looking at the same person. Even if this may involve gaze changes, gaze can be directed to the same feature of the stimulus repeatedly. This is a core difference in the sensory fields available to the brain. A wholesome profile or gestalt can be built online from the visual inputs, whereas it can only be inferred from the inputs in other sensory modalities, especially auditory inputs. One has to make an inference or prediction that a certain friend is coming in, after listening to and recognizing his voice or footsteps, whereas the whole person presents himself visually. Predictions are also made about an object, person, or field by looking at part of the stimulus. Visual movements are also monitored as they occur. Visual inputs therefore attain much higher value for establishing contact with reality and their verification. Visual stimulation plays immensely greater role in shaping the functional development of a developing brain. Visual inputs are received and processed by both the right and left hemispheres. However, the right hemisphere appears to specialize in gestalt processing while the left hemisphere specializes in sequential processing, or at least the left and right brains perform these two functions more efficiently when information is processed separately by each cerebral hemisphere. Gestalt processing effect cannot be achieved when the stimuli are auditory, as they are not simultaneously recognized. However, the brain is able to hold on to the auditory stimulus elements received across time and relate them to create meaning. Such sequential processing capability in the auditory mode has indeed resulted in relating events across time. The preceding event is often taken as the cause and the antecedent event as the effect, as we presume that the second state has emerged from the first, in such sequential changes of events. The sequential and simultaneous processing required for auditory or visual inputs respectively into the brain has emerged as the two major basic information-processing capabilities of the brain. These two information-processing methods, which have their basic origin because of the mode of signal inputs into the brain, have indeed developed into paradigms that are more complex.

A bottom-up view of the brain starts with sensory inputs to the brain. There are such drastic differences in the sensory input patterns into the brain, especially in the auditory and visual modes. In the auditory mode, signals are input into the brain in temporal sequence, one after the other. If it is speech inputs, the brain hears word by word, often less than a word, in the form of phonemic blocks. The brain has to accumulate them sequentially for interpreting and creating a meaning or predict a meaning with parts of the speech heard. Sequential flow is the characteristic feature of auditory stimuli. Once the signal is received and processed, it cannot be gone over again, unless the process is repeated. Quick mental repetition of a few words heard for the first time is possible, if the individual has practised and trained himself in such repetitions. The whole sequence of words could indeed be written into memory through practice. We have overcome the difficulty by creating systems, which can store the flow of sound, which can replay the recorded sound any number of times. While speaking, meaning is created by forward sequential arrangement of words. On the other hand, a cluster or array of visual signals can be attended to continuously and simultaneously, and continuous intake reflects the changes that may occur in the source, which are continuously monitored by the brain. The eyes must be moved across the visual field or the stimulus and the different visual components must be arranged to produce a meaningful visual profile of the object. Spatial locations, orientation, and comparative size estimation of the visual components are some of the most important features that allow organizing a visual profile of an object or stimulus, whereas it is the sequential placement of notes and words that contribute to a meaning, which are to be considered when auditory signals are composed. Somatosensory inputs can also be continuous and one can keep receiving the inputs by making continuous physical contact with the stimulus. As the somatosensory contact can often be voluntarily maintained for long durations and the body contact can establish a comprehensive contact with the entity outside the body, we accept it as the highest level of experiential verified contact of reality. We can establish such experientially verified contacts only with a tiny spectrum of entities in one's surrounding. Similarly, smell and taste too have high experiential value as they help establish contact with reality. However, they too vanish, as the medium carrying the sensory signals may have limited physical presence. Such continuous contacts cannot be established in the auditory mode. Sound signals are energy signals, which need to be produced by a source, and they last for varying temporal segments. The receptors receive them for the same duration. On the other hand, vision is an extraordinary sensory process. The source does not produce any energy or signals, on its own. There are special visual receptors, which can receive the visual image if light falling on a source is reflected into a receptor. What is produced in the receptors is only a reflective image, which is recognized by the brain. The reflective image can last as long as the receptors are directed to the source and the reflected light from the source is received by the source. The reflective image may represent changes that occur in the physical image of the source. The reflective image of a source can be received, as long as the receptors keep receiving the images. Sensory signals of all modalities, except the visual, can intrude into the body forcefully and register in the respective receptors. Visual images from a source can be received passively if the receptors are open and directed to the source; otherwise, the images need to be received intentionally.

The sources of auditory and visual signals, which are received and processed in the brain, have always slipped into the past, by the time the signals are processed and the sources are recognized in the brain. Auditory signals take time, may be milliseconds to seconds, minutes, or more, to travel from its source of generation to the receiving centres, wherever they are present. Visual signals indeed travel fastest and one may never be able to know experientially the time elapsed for the reflected images to reach the receptors. By the time signals are processed and recognized, the outside sources of signals—the world outside, has either ceased to exist or changed. The changes may or not be recognized, when they are subtle, and the individual has the experience of constancy of the entity. In the auditory and visual modes, the signals recognized in the brain have obviously left their sources before a certain span of time, though the brain believes that it is online monitoring the source. It is always a mystery for children when they watch a bright lightening in the sky and have to wait to hear the thunder several seconds after the visual effect is seen. In experiential terms, one can never keep listening to the same sound, once it is heard and recognized as a word, a musical note, the barking of a dog, or the sound of an object falling on the floor and so on. In short, the source of auditory stimulus that may continue existing is not what created the stimulus a moment ago. The time elapsed between the point signals leave the source of stimulations and they are recognized in the brain, is indeed maximal in the case of auditory stimulation. Somatosensory signals help to produce continuous recognition of the images of the source in the brain, whereas one has to believe that the words heard were spoken by another. Somatosensory sensations establish direct contacts with external reality, whereas visual sensations only produce a reflected image of the external reality. There is nothing like a physical auditory contact with external reality. The differences in the nature of different sensory inputs indeed have differential effects in the processing strategies of the associated signals and for deriving meaning from them.

On the other hand, we experience looking at the same object continuously, whether the object goes through changes or remains without any change, it moves, or remains stationary. Array of visual signals from the different regions of the visual field/source arrive in the brain and they can be simultaneously processed. On the other hand, auditory signals arrive in the brain in sequence of blocks, one after the other, and the only way to process them is to interpret them in a sequential manner creating a meaning. The drastically different signal input patterns have cultivated different processing patterns in the brain. Auditory signals, which are received in sequence, are processed sequentially, whereas reception of simultaneous visual signals allows their simultaneous processing. Serial and parallel processing capabilities are therefore the outcome of the differences in the signal input patterns into the brain. The purpose of signal processing is essentially for assigning meanings to the received signals, whether it is recognition of a word presented in auditory or orthographic modes, or recognition of an object, animal, or person. With regard to word recognition, the processing has developed into a complex pattern, as meaning needs to be retrieved for each word, using which a meaning needs to be created or recreated for the combination of words received in sequential order. Interestingly, one hemisphere has cultivated superior capability for sequential processing whereas the other hemisphere has cultivated similar capability for simultaneous or parallel processing. Sequential processing would involve identification of words from the phonemic pattern of the sounds heard, retrieving the meaning of the word and finally interpreting the meanings of different words into a complex idea or meaning. Simultaneous or parallel processing allows creating a meaning from the total pattern of the signals seen, which we have always called the gestalt perception. Choice of processing is therefore the result of the pattern of sensory inputs. However, the differences in the sensory inputs lead to choice of a processing type, though one can intentionally process signals serially or parallely provided they satisfy the processing requirements. Creation of meaning from verbal inputs has been called encoding, whereas creation of meaning from visual inputs require gestalt processing, which allow the meaning to be inferred from the combination of inputs.

Meaning could be a mere "recognition", or it could be the verbalization of the relationship between two objects or entities. The meaning or the idea created may refer to a new state or change of state, it may be a concept, or mere narration of the sequence of events taking place from one moment to another, etc. Meanings could be infinite, in the sense, it is for the brain to create a meaning, and it is limited only by the knowledge base used for creation of the idea. The meanings are mentally assigned and understood by each brain. Meanings are most easily carried by auditory and orthographic expressions. Meanings may be assigned by visuomotorcreations like paintings and sculptures. Meanings may also be symbolically represented. Every experience has a meaning to the experiencing person. The new meanings created may be expressions of expectations, navigational plans of actions, and expressions conveying what the outcome is and what it means to self and others. The neural tissues in the brain endow their signals with meanings form the structural basis of what we have always called the mind. The meanings—recognitions, ideas, and concepts created by the brain form the mind. In short the mind is created by the brain. Human mind is indeed not a structure, and not a phenomenon or epiphenomenon. It is a unique and unparalleled composition of ideas created and meanings assigned for physiological arousal, activities, which we have learnt to call emotions. They interact with each other, grow, and influence the functioning of the brain and the body. The mind can influence or activate the brain to initiate movements, which are deployed for several independent and interrelated bodily needs, as well as the needs mentally created. The relationship between the brain and its product mind is therefore reciprocal, which creates the unique brain-mind platform. Emotions provide the body with drive to be used as fuel to carry out the actions required for survival as well as for the satisfaction/gratification of the needs created by the brain-mind, which we call the mental products. When, the necessities are that of the body, we call them biological, when they are for fulfilling the mental needs, we call them psychological. The needs may be simultaneously for the body and the mind. When the body needs food for survival, it can be fed while walking, sitting in a field, under a tree, inside a house, in an office, ordinary restaurant, or a three-star or seven-star hotel. The body's need is food, and food is what is given to it in all these places, but each experience is different for the mind, as these places are the choices and creations of the mind. Brain has boundaries decided by physical realities, but no boundaries may exist for the mind. The boundaries, if any present are made only by the limitations of mental imagination.

The human beings have always had a huge problem with the use of the word "self", whether to use it for identifying the body or the 'mind', and if 'self' can be used as a scientifically acceptable entity at all. However, all use the word 'self', as a practice in all languages, for referring to own body, emotions and thoughts. It has been consistently used by all, in all the times, as conceptual reference to "own" body and the mind. One may use the 'self' to refer more often to the body and less to the mind or the other way. The self becomes a reflection of own body and mind in own thoughts and communication with others. Once the mind becomes established as the self, any harm to the body may not be considered to harm the self, as it becomes a reflection of the values and the ideas of an individual, which may not perish or disappear. An idea may be expressed by words and symbols, lines and colors as in painting or sculpture, or through chemical and physical interactions. If one identifies oneself with the mind and its values, the ideas may be preserved across generations; one may consider the self to be preserved even after death. All those who entertain similar ideas and values, which they cherish and adore, share and move forward referring themselves to the same self. The question then is if the body or the idea is more important or man can attain a body-idea existence. The brain must first create ideas with values, which represent the mind and consider them truly valuable for it to be carried through its span of life. If the self is not identified with ideas, and represents only the body, the self disappears as the body perishes. Otherwise, even if the body perishes, the mind need not perish.

The sleeping brain creates dreams, and the wakeful brain creates the mind.

Distractibility and Spontaneous Arousal of Attention

Patients with Orbitofrontal lesions show spontaneous arousal of attention to all stimuli around and they have difficulty to withdraw or show habituation to irrelevant stimuli. This is expressed as distractibility while they are engaged in a relevant task, which may include even talking to the examiner. This could be very acute rendering it impossible for the patient to being interviewed or carry out even simple instructions in clinical examination. The severity of the deficit is related to the severity of the lesion and other clinical symptoms present in the patient. This has been generally Attention of the patient is easily distracted by almost any stimulus occurring in the immediate surroundings. Distractibility could be so acute and frequent, the patient is unable to attend continuously to any task to perform, or even be interviewed. These patients show not only distractibility but also respond to the irrelevant stimuli. Impairment in response inhibition could often have effects that are deleterious during dealing with the environmental demands. Response inhibition deficit is a major dysfunction associated with Orbitofrontal lesions in patients.

Lesions in the Anterior Cingulate cortex, on the other hand, block spontaneous arousal of attention and leave the patients without attentional arousal to attend to stimuli. In these patients, attention may not be aroused by even a strong and pain evoking intrusive stimulus. In the normal cognitive processing situations, a subject tries to withdraw from attending to intrusive irrelevant stimuli so that attention can be directed to the stimulus or problem otherwise being attended. This is not. It is normally not mere distractibility alone seen, in many frontal lesion patients, but the patient responds to the irrelevant stimuli. This indicates the effects of an extensive frontal lesion. Impairment in response inhibition to the irrelevant stimuli is more impairing than mere distractibility.

The early demonstration of the role of Orbitofrontal cortex in spontaneous arousal of attention was by Kluver (1933) in a monkey with frontal lobe lesion. The monkey dropped the grape that it was eating, when another grape was offered and it started eating the second one. Every time a new grape was offered, it dropped the grape it was already eating. Several later studies showed the significant roles of the dorsolateral and medial parts of the prefrontal cortex in the control and regulation of attention (Luria 1966, 1973; Fuster, Alexander 1971; Heilman, Valenstein 1972a, 1972b; Damasio et al. 1980). Interestingly Laplane et al. (1981) observed that limbic lesions have greater effects on attentional impairment and suggested that lesions of Cingulate Cortex along with that of frontal lobes could produce more severe effects of attentional impairment than frontal lobe lesions alone. Cingulate cortical lesion studies showed that limbic lesions easily produced distractibility, hypermotility, and impaired goal directed behavior (LeMoal et al. 1975; Stinus et al. 1978). Lesions of Dorsolateral prefrontal lesions were reported to affect attention to novel stimuli, by Daffner et al. (2000a, b), who stated that frontal lobe lesions affect novelty seeking ability and ability to direct and focus attention to novel stimuli. According to Daffner et al. (2000a, b), these lesions produce emotional apathy, which in turn affects attentional arousal and response to stimuli.

Increasing attention to a stimulus or mental process online would mean increased withdrawal from processing any other information to enable intake of greater amount of signals from the stimulus. This happens whenever one makes a decision of increased and complex task demands. Attending to relevant tasks is enhanced by withdrawing from processing irrelevant signals and thereby withdrawing attending to them. These could be alternate mental tasks or external stimuli. It is also necessary that one withdraws from responding to irrelevant stimuli and mental tasks so that the intake and output channels are occupied by only relevant inputs and task demand respectively. However, withdrawal from irrelevant processing and stimuli alone will not enhance attentional inputs to a selected stimulus. The quantum of signals that one can convert to information is indeed an important aspect of attentional efficiency. Emotional arousal caused by unrelated life events and preoccupation with other unrelated tasks can reduce this ability to increase attention to a given task demand and lower the total efficiency in brain performance. Ability to increase attention to a relevant task at any given time and to withdraw attending to irrelevant tasks must be cultivated through self-controlled training in the early years of life. Ability to inhibit responding to irrelevant stimuli is very important to enhance or facilitate attention to relevant task demands. Ability to suppress responding or ignore responding is a condition that one should develop. Cultivation of tuning attention must take place during play as well as studies in the early years of life. Absence of such self-induced training can make a person always perform at average or below average levels of performance efficiency, as one would not have learnt to deploy own cognitive resources fully. Attention training may help such individuals provided the training is carried out systematically and in controlled manner.

Speed of detection of external stimulus is indeed an important feature of the cognitive processing ability of the brain. Fast detection enables one to fill the processing channels faster with signal arrays for their quick processing and responding. Once processing of one task is completed, signals from newer stimuli can be acquired for further processing. Both stimulus detection and processing speed are significantly affected in various brain-damaged conditions. An effect overtly not apparent is that of the emotional arousal or drive. If emotional arousal or drive is positive and optimal, it facilitates the intake of stimuli as well as cognitive processing. Excessive drive or negative emotional arousal has deleterious effects on attention and signal intake, as well as cognitive processing. Impairment may be present if there is emotional overload or excess anxiety in the individual, which may get the person fixated on a specific theme or aspect, without allowing flexibility to inspect various blocks of information, which can be easily seen in the clinical interviews of these patients.

Attention is aroused in a spontaneous way by a novel stimulus or a change in the stimulus characteristics or the stimulus field. Arousal of attention has a general and specific factor. The general arousal of attention could be achieved by any type of stimulus and a special interest if it has personal significance, novelty effect, or intrusive value. Such attentional arousal may bc immediately followed by behavioral, postural adjustments, and anticipation of the new or novel stimulus or change in the stimulus field. Arousal of attention may happen while the individual is in a passive state. The novelty effect of a stimulus plays an important role in the passive state. When vigilant, the individual may get into a search mode, and expect to detect newer interesting or novel stimuli.

Lateralization of Visual and Auditory Attention

Both the cerebral hemispheres are involved in visual and auditory perception and recognition. However, hemisphere specific superiority in certain aspects of perceptual processing has been shown to exist. Right hemisphere superiority in visual attention was supported by several workers (Damasio 1979; Salmaso, Denes, 1982; Weintraub, Mesulam 1987; Posner, Petersen 1990; Dwivedi, Mukundan 1993). Greater distractibility in the form of interference effect was seen in right frontal patients than in left frontal patients in studies (Weintraub, Mesulam 1987; Dwivedi, Mukundan 1993). These studies demonstrated left visual field dominance, and found that lesions of right hemisphere and frontal lobes lead to greater deficits of visual attention or inattention. Tests of visual exploration described by them showed visual inattention and neglect in both right and left visual have in right lesions patients. On the other hand, left hemisphere lesions produced visual inattention only in the left visual half. In the case of auditory attention, right ear dominance with left hemisphere specialization of speech processing has been well established, even though right hemisphere does have important roles in certain aspects of verbal processing. Maintenance of attention (sustained attention) is yet another important aspect of attention. Maintenance requires clear aim or purpose so that attention can be intentionally directed for signal detection and processing unless attention is drawn because of the novelty effects or intrusive effects on the perceiver.

With regard to auditory lateralization, the findings are still more interesting. Left hemisphere auditory cortex and speech areas predominantly and more accurately mediate acoustic processing of speech (Belin et al. 1998; Liégeois-Chauvel et al. 1999; Zatorre and Belin 2001; Zatorre et al. 2002; Zaehle et al. 2004; Meyer et al. 2005). The left hemisphere speech areas process phonological processing of speech more effectively (Scott et al. 2000; Liebenthal et al. 2005; Obleser et al. 2007). Left hemisphere dominance of semantic processing is also reported clinically as well as in other studies (Wagner et al. 2001; Rodd et al. 2005). Interestingly, there is another factor reported to be based on the rate of signal input, that determines auditory lateralization (Poeppel 2003). Slow non-speech acoustic stimuli at the rate 3-5 Hz are processed more efficiently by the right hemisphere (Boemio et al. 2005), whereas the left hemisphere speech areas processes acoustic stimuli in the 20-50 Hz range (Zatorre and Belin 2001; Zaehle et al. 2004; Schonwiesner et al. 2005) more effectively. Abrams et al. (2008) have shown that right hemisphere neurons are better specialized than left hemisphere neurons to decompose auditory signals of speech syllables and recognizing them in terms of their temporal features.

The neuropsychological examination of patients for the detection of impairment of attention focuses on the following aspects:

1. Evidence of absence of spontaneous arousal of attention.
2. Distractibility of attention.
3. Excessive narrowing or broadening of attention.
4. Fatigability of attention.
5. Attention needs to be aroused with repeated commands.
6. Difficulty to shift attention when a novel stimulus or change in the stimulus field occurs.

7. Impairment in continuous, directed, and focused attention.
8. Reduced span of attention.

Attention is not a highly localized function in the frontal cortex. Attention is influenced and controlled by several other factors and some of them are arousal level and emotional state, purposiveness, goal directedness, volitional state. Emotional state may vary from natural curiosity and anticipated effects of anxiety and fear. Other than these attention control is a highly cultivated ability, which can bc impaired in all types of frontal lobe lesions, whether it is diffused or focal. Inferences and clinical decision of presence of attentional impairment can be made only after careful observation of a patient during interview and testing. Spontaneous arousal of attention is the first component that may be considered for evaluation. Spontaneous attention may be considered adequate when the patient looks up in anticipation during demonstration and presentation of instructions for tests. Absence of spontaneous arousal of attention and the need to arouse attention by repeated instructions are associated with lesion of the mediobasal areas of the frontal cortex. On the other hand, the opposite profile may be found in lesions of the Orbitofrontal cortex. In this case attention is easily aroused and the patient responds to even irrelevant stimuli around him, which interferes with sustenance of attention. An impairment of ability to broaden or expand attentional span may result in increased narrowing of attention and the patient will be unable to attend simultaneously to several aspects of an object, stimulus field, and task demands. A right Orbitofrontal lesion may result in distractibility. Therefore, there are three major aspects of attention viz., spontaneous arousal of attention, responding to irrelevant stimuli or distractibility, and ability for focused and sustained attention, to be judged. Impaired attention will have a significant adverse effect on all other performance tests. Therefore, an accurate understanding of attentional process in the patient is essential before commenting on performance on other tests.

Absence of spontaneous arousal of attention has been found to be present in mediobasal-anterior cingulate lesions, whereas distractibility and other deficits are present in orbitofrontal and dorsolateral prefrontal lesions. A spontaneous arousal of attention is called the orienting reflex/orienting response. Extensive physiological changes are seen within the brain and in the autonomic nervous system during the occurrence of the orienting response. The orienting response is elicited primarily by the meaning of a stimulus rather than its mere physical attributes. A knock on the door arouses attention in this manner and it is accompanied by not only physiological changes but also postural changes. One looks up in the direction of the door anticipating someone is attempting to come in. The anticipatory effect comes from interpretation of the stimulus based on experience. If this comparison is not available, the intruding stimulus will arouse a novelty or surprise effect. The orienting response also interrupts the current attention process, as attention is redirected partially or fully to the new stimulus. If the intruding stimulus does not have any meaning, and if it is repeated, the orienting response becomes weak and ultimately habituated. The process of habituation is critical for selective attention as it helps to suppress attentional arousal to irrelevant stimuli so that attention can be directed to relevant stimulus. Deficits of attention seen in frontal lesions are deficits in arousal of attention, selectivity, directed attention, its maintenance, and distractibility, difficulty in shifting mental set and neglect or hemi-inattention.

In clinical situation, a frontal patient will be seen to respond to and/or comment upon things and people around him, while engaged in performing a task given by the examiner. Continuous performance is interrupted by distractibility. Distraction is primarily caused by irrelevant external stimuli. Deficits in this function may also manifest as slowness of performance and errors due to poor strategy and neglect. A frontal involvement may be the basis for both types of difficulties. The disruptive effect may be so severe that the patient has to be repeatedly reminded of the task he is performing and task instructions have to be often repeated. The need for repeated instruction is more frequently encountered when patient has difficulty to maintain the purpose of the task. If distractibility is caused because of attending to irrelevant external stimuli alone, the patient is likely to get back to the task on his own.

Visual attention involves the need to scan the visual space. Scanning involves shift of the gaze, which may be carried out in a systematic, and directed (Lezak 1995) or random manner by a person, and involves selection, comparison, analysis, and integration of visual stimuli (Weintraub, Mesulam 1987). The most important factor to be considered before administering any visual scanning test is to understand the intactness of the visual field of the individual. Field defects are caused by lesions in visual system (retina, pathways and the occipital lobes). Mukundan et al. (1996) have shown that visual scanning is maximally impaired in dorsolateral prefrontal lesions; deficit is also seen in right parietal lobes lesion. No frontal lateralization effect was noticed in these studies. The complex nature of the components involved in attention is indicative of an extensive frontal involvement, which will include dorsolateral areas, orbitofrontal, orbitobasal, and premotor areas. The distinct effect of anterior cingulate lesions on attention is discussed elsewhere.

Attention selects stimulus as well as actions. Distractibility of attention has therefore, its effect on both stimulus and response selection. Stimulus selection enables the individual to focus processing on a selected stimulus, while action selection enables selective control of a certain action component. Selective visual attention is controlled by posterior parietal, anterior cingulate and prefrontal areas in conjunction with the striate areas, which have already discussed elsewhere in this chapter. The right frontal dominance seen about visual attention presupposes the possibility of greater visual attention deficit in right prefrontal lesion than in left prefrontal lesions, which was seen in studies using unilateral frontal lesion patients (Weintraub, Mesulam 1987; Dwivedi, Mukundan 1993; Aron et al. 2003). However, as far as attention selection of actions is concerned, the middle frontal gyrus has been seen to found to have a greater role than orbitofrontal or medial frontal areas. Comparison of the performance of the frontal lobe patients with the Huntington's disease patients showed that the prefrontal patients made significantly more errors of commission by over responding to a target, while the HD patients made more errors of missing to respond to the target. It has been postulated that Alzheimer's patients show distractibility because of a deficit in voluntarily initiating a process of inhibition needed not to initiate a response as in the "go - no - go" paradigm (Simone, Baylis 1997). This is different from the process of "lateral inhibition" (Tipper et al. 2000) in which neurons working in different directions would inhibit each other. This is different from the neurons working in the same direction would excite each other. The latter would bring about a facilitation of target reaching response while the opposite effect will be seen with regard to the former type of inhibition. Lateral inhibition will therefore, result in a type of distractibility by the nonrecruitment or selection of action components.

Visual Search [visual exploration]

Ability to visually search is an important aspect of visual attention. Difficulty in visual search can be detected while interviewing the patient and instructing to take note of and describe objects placed on a table or on the wall and in the examination room. Further testing can be carried out if the examiner has doubts about presence of visual search difficulty using simple test procedures. Serial scanning of numbers printed at random on a paper allows observation of the smoothness and rapidity with which the individual can systematically search a given visual space. Firstly, a slow shifting of the gaze leads to slow scanning. Secondly, tardy exploration of the visual space because of absence of a spatial plan and difficulty in serially looking for numbers can affect the speed and accuracy of visual search. Testing the presence of difficulty in shifting gaze fixation can be tested by observing gaze shifts in a patient while cancelling numbers printed on piece of paper or a computer monitor. The patient is instructed to cancel numbers from 1 to 20 printed in a space of 4 cm × 15 cm on a piece of paper. Testing visual exploration needs serial cancellation of numbers from 1 to 60 and printed in a larger space of 12 cm × 15 cm. The third item has 12 numbers out of 36 repeating twice or more and the subject is expected to score out all the repeated numbers one by one. The total time taken to scan each number series and the errors are recorded. The test of visual scanning of figures was normally used for illiterate patients, who could not read numbers, though there was none in the studies reported here. A picture with 5-6 distinctly visible items can be used for this. It is very important for the examiner to consider that the purpose of the test is to detect the presence of difficulty or impairment in visual search and not to test how good the patient can carry out the test. The patient may be already disturbed, anxious, and may have neuropsychological deficits affecting his performance. These would render his performance slow and a forced one, and the examiner cannot expect the patient to do his best for comparison with others. However, if the purpose of examination is to report disability, then it is important to compare patient's score with normative data. Identification of printed objects is not as sensitive as number search and cancellations. If a patient has difficulty to identify the items in the picture spontaneously, it could be an indication of a visual scanning difficulty or visual agnosia. The visual exploration test described by Weintraub and Mesulam (1987) in which subject has to choose targets from non-targets and cancel them in the right and left spatial halves on a paper placed in front is an effective test to demonstrate lateralized spatial search difficulty. Presence of lateralized visual attentional deficit was further demonstrated by a repeat study on Indian patients by Dwivedi and Mukundan (1993). These studies have shown a normal preference of the left half of the visual field over the right, and significantly greater deficit or visual neglect of contralateral visual field by right frontal lesion patients on scanning both the halves compared to left lesion patients.

Visual search is a function of visual attention and hence it has to be evaluated along with attention. However, the localized effects or impairment of visual attention cannot be drawn if visual recognition itself is affected because of involvement of primary visual and secondary visual association areas. A conclusive formulation of visual attention deficit can be made only after verification of the absence of other sensory and perceptual impairments in a patient.

Attention Retraining

Attention retraining is an important need in many brain lesion/disease conditions. Attention retraining may seldom be attempted in typical brain lesion cases. However, conditions like ADHD may require isolated attention retraining until the clinician wants to incorporate other forms of cognitive retraining. Computerized attention retraining has the advantages of selection of several parameters like intensity, size, spatial location, complexity, exposure time, inter-trial intervals, etc. whereas these facilities are not generally possible for noncomputer based retraining programs. However, computer friendliness of the patient may be an important factor to be considered when a task is selected. The different aspects of attention that need retraining are the ability to spontaneously attend to the presence of stimuli in the environment, reduce distractibility while increasing ability to focus on a stimulus or a processing.

Perception: Recognition

7

Perception of a stimulus takes place only after it is registered in the sensory cortex. However, before perception the brain must attend to the stimulus, which is a process of mediation carried out by the frontal cortex. This mediation causes further delay for recognition and the process that is called arousal attention. In the visual modality, the attentional arousal takes place about 140 milliseconds after the reception of the stimulus in the retina and in the auditory mode it takes place about 100 milliseconds after the reception. Perception follows attentional arousal and it may be followed by awareness that one has perceived the stimulus. These neural processing stages are seen clearly in the electrical evoked potentials of the brain, which can be recorded by repeated presentation of a stimulus at intervals. During registration of the signal a positive electrical potential called P1 is elicited from the brain and during attentional arousal, a negative evoked potential response called N1 is elicited. P1 and N1 are at 100 ms and 140 ms respectively in the visual modalities and at 70 ms and 100 ms in the auditory modalities. There have been hundreds of research studies of the potentials in normal and patients with neuropsychiatric and neurological involvements. When the same stimulus is repeatedly presented another positive potential called the P2 emerges indicating focused attention. P2 occurs at about 200 ms and 160 ms after the stimulus onset in the visual and auditory modes respectively (Mukundan 1986b, e). The figures below show the presence of P1, N1 and P2 responses in a normal subject. The presence and the delay of the potentials can be affected by pathological conditions of the concerned brain areas and hence they are routinely used as diagnostic indicators of brain lesion.

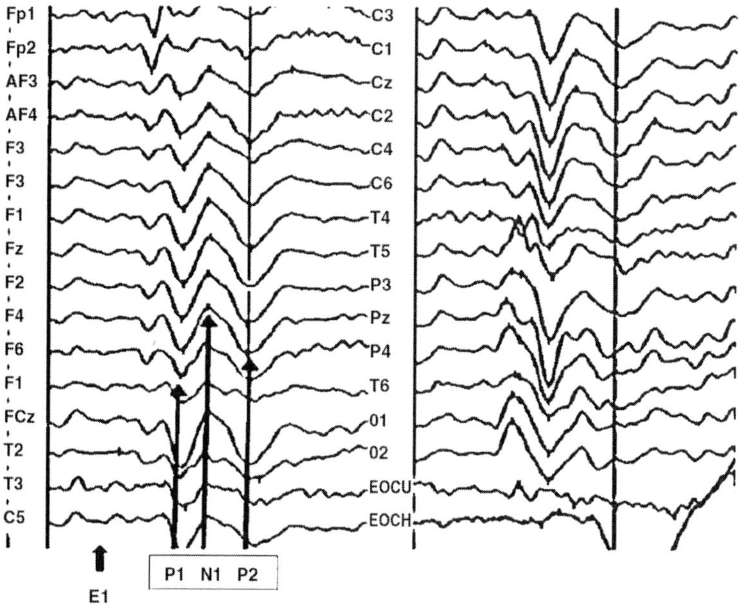

Fig. 5: Showing the timeline of occurrence of stimulus (duration 100 ms) and the Event Related Potentials in the brain. If the stimulus has no novelty effect or meaning to the subject, only Sensory Registration and the closely related process (P1-N1-P2) take place in the brain and the processing phase is over within 250 ms in the visual mode. In auditory mode, P1-N1-P2 components occur earlier. If recognition of novelty or meaningful aspect is involved in the detection of the stimulus, its processing may last as long as 250-650 ms

Attending to a stimulus or stimulus field in the environment, to a thought being created or to a mental process, is an important step towards their perception and for the development of their awareness. It is recognition and its awareness that lead to higher cognitive processes required for problem-solving and decision-making. Perception is an important requirement for responding to a stimulus or navigation. However, response from the brain can be elicited by a stimulus even without its perception and awareness.

Recognition

Perception is a neural processing of interpreting signals received in the brain using the knowledge bank already available in the brain, leading to its recognition or identification of the source of the sensory signals. Recognition or identification of the source would mean that the source is already known and relevant information is already present in the brain of the perceiver. The neural model of perception describes the following processes:

1. Formation of an external model based on the sensory signals representing the physical characteristics of the entity received in the primary sensory projection area of the brain.
2. Retrieval of existing internal models (engrams or memory traces) of entities, which would match with the external model.
3. Identification of the engram, which matches with the external model.
4. Recognition of the entity/object, which is the source of the external model as the object or entity in the internal model or associated with the engram.
5. Recognition includes remembrance of knowing the entity recognized, which gives rise to familiarity. This may or not be accompanied by remembrance of awareness of earlier recognition.

Entities perceived may be external to the individual, existing as part of the external world, or internal body conditions. The internal conditions perceived or proprioceptive perception may be that of pain, and physiological states related to respiration, heart rate, pulse, gastrointestinal conditions, etc. All internal conditions are not obviously perceived. Only those movements within the body, which reach a certain physical magnitude, may be perceived by the individual.

Perception is a process of recognition, in which a trace of memory or engram is retrieved for matching with the sensory image produced by the external stimulus. This would mean that the engram has been acquired earlier and stored in the brain. This acquisition could have taken place any time in life. For example as we recognize an object as a "pen", it is necessary the engram of the pen is retrieved in the brain. The memory trace of the image of a "pen" could have been acquired or learnt in the very early years when one was a 3-6 months old child. The internal model in neural trace would have been modified and enriched over years. If no memory trace representing an internal model exists, which matches with an external model, it would mean that one has to learn and create a new internal model. Learning could be a time-consuming process, as a new internal model needs to be created. If the memory is not accessible because of a brain lesion, it is called "agnosia" in the clinical parlor. Even if the external object is not recognized, one forms an external model of the object or entity from its physical attributes, which one recognizes, and this part of the process is perception. Recognition can only follow perception, which is the primary processing that takes place within the brain. For example, one perceives a language one cannot recognize or understand. Recognition cannot take place without having an adequate knowledge base, which can provide information for matching the external model. Recognition would therefore demand an internal judgment or acceptance of the internal model as the matching external model. When familiar objects are routinely recognized, this may happen in an automatic manner. However, if it is not a routine recognition of familiar entities, such internal acceptance may be required, whether it is consciously accepted or not. Recognition using minimal information may indeed need such decision-making, as it is a predictive decision. Studies using hypnotic suggestions indicate that the origin of such judgment or decision is from the Frontal lobes (Mukundan et al. 2013, 1999c), indicating a direct Frontal involvement in recognition, when there is conflict or uncertainty in recognition. Hypnotic suggestion can alter recognition of the intensity of a stimulus or even block its recognition (Figs. 8 and 9) even though sensory registration of the stimulus remains unaffected. Interestingly the source of perception is not merely the entities of the external world. These suggestions induce variety of meaning at the second signal system level, which individuals may readily accept without further verification. Experiential interpretations pose even greater intellectual and emotional threats/challenges, as they are readily accepted as reality verified. Individuals may strongly believe in them, unless alternate explanation or meaning is imposed or voluntarily accepted. One recognizes processes taking place within the body if they produce sensations, which can be monitored by the same sensory receptors, which we call proprioceptive perception. Yet another important process that takes place within the brain is creation of words using sound and orthographic designs, which are monitored by the same brain and recognized. Such recognition produces verbal awareness, as all other forms recognition produces awareness of the entities as received by the sensory system singularly and in combination. Verbal awareness needs special discussion as it is an internal and self-directed process.

Predictive Recognition

What we do not know is the actual process used for retrieving a memory trace from the database of the brain. Comparison of the external model is made with the internal model after retrieval of the internal model by locating it in the database using part information of the external model. However, this would require the individual to identify the 'familiar' part-information of the external model, using the part-information of the internal model, and then retrieve the whole block of information. How localization of a familiar part from several thousands of memory traces (?) stored in the brain is still not understood. The best we can use for understanding this is a computer analogy of recognition. Familiarity of a part may arise from a few frequent use or encounter of the stimulus. One may identify the familiar part straightaway, if it has occurred in an expected source context. One may develop familiarity with more than one part, and the presence of any of those parts in the external world has the potentiality to initiate retrieval of the specific blocks of information containing the familiar part. Perception invariably is a prediction, as one does not wait to receive complete signals from the different features of the source before its Gestalt is arrived and recognition is made. This was first proposed by Biederman (1987, 2001), who postulated that the brain predicts the total or the Gestalt of the external source using only minimal information from the gestalt. This makes recognition or knowing the external world fast so that one can deal with the changes and the demands of the external world swiftly. Biederman (1987) called this the Component Theory of Perception. According to this theory, we recognize objects by its parts, called 'geons'. Once a geon or a few of them are identified, we predict the object from the geons. Thus we could identify a person, just by identifying part of the face viz., the eyes, the forehead, the lips, or the hairstyle. Total examination of an object may obviously consume time and perception can become a slow process. Recognition by components becomes a fast process, though the outcome is predicted. Recognition is therefore a process of anticipation until it is verified. The predicted recognition may most often go through reality verification. However, if it fails in reality verification, one readily accepts the mistake and makes efforts to re-recognize the same. Reality verification is always experiential unless one resorts to experimentation. Experiencing is the only subjective method of reality verification, which helps establishing contact with reality in the perceiver. Thus, one can perceive a door and verify the perception of the door by walking through door. One can perceive another person in the same room; verify his or her presence by going near the person and shaking hands with the person or hugging the person, and thereby verifying the presence. Normally perception is taken for granted for the presence of the entity. Predicted perceptions are invariably correct, unless it is a hallucination, which may happen in a psychotic condition. The source memory may play a part in prompt recognition, as one expects to identify the familiar components readily in a particular context, space and time.

We manage to recognize the entities and changes in their environment fast and deal with them efficiently. We learn to believe in our own recognitions even without reality verification. Such predicted perceptions have become the normal pattern of brain functioning in several familiar life situations, including work situations. However, one learns to be prudent and verify the perceptions, if one is in unfamiliar situations. Prediction is present in all sensory modalities, which is also conspicuous in the auditory modality. During a conversation, we often listen to part of the sentences spoken by another person and seem to readily understand or comprehend what the other person intends to convey, and respond to it even before fully listening to the speech. However, we recreate the meaning from the words we listen, by anticipating the words, and take it for granted that it is the same idea that the other person wants to convey. The talker may anticipate that the listener has already understood what he wanted to say and may continue with the conversation. This has been referred to 'intellectual empathy' and is an important factor that controls communication among people. Predictive recognition is possible only when one perceives familiar objects or speech. Speed of perception thereby depends on the speed with which the significant component(s) is recognized by a person and how quickly a prediction is made. Mindset of the viewer or listener, and what he expects to perceive are important factors that control prediction. The word perception is also used for referring to the recognition and understanding a point of view or idea. Perceiving the relevant stimulus, cue, theme, or points of view are important for understanding the ideas of others and fast comprehension and resolution of the problems stated by others. What one does not want to miss is the perception of an important change in the environment or in the expected sensory inputs. Such perception would depend on how fast one recognizes familiar features and how fast an unfamiliar feature is detected.

Awareness of Recognition

Recognition is a process of identification of a known entity, object, person by the brain, when sensory signals from the source arrive in the brain. Recognition may lead to its awareness, i.e. the brain has identified it in the external world, a process different from mere identification. The issue of awareness of recognition has been of immense philosophical value and it has been discussed in details. What is that follows recognition as awareness? Awareness of recognition may be defined as the knowledge one develops when one has recognized a certain entity, which can be stated as 'awareness of recognition'. There is no problem in understanding this as long as this awareness is verbal awareness. One may readily verbally transcode recognized object or entity, most often naming the entity. We know this happens when we have difficulty to access or remember the name, when we struggle to state what is that we have recognized. When the transcoding takes place and one has a ready verbal label for the recognized entity, one automatically uses the name to identify the recognized entity. The speech receiving centers readily monitors the speech expressions or thoughts. As one knows the source of the speech expression or thought as the same brain, one monitor the thought created in another center in the brain, as own thoughts, which we call verbal awareness. For example, one recognizes an object, calls it a 'pen' and monitors the name 'pen' being used, and reports that one is seeing a 'pen'. Even if one does not know the name 'pen', one is able to verbalize the act of recognizing an object. This is knowledge of the internal processing that takes place, i.e. one is in the process of seeing or recognizing a pen. The process or the act of recognition is different from the outcome of recognition. The verbal awareness of recognizing is indeed different from recognition. There is no evidence to state that there is a nonverbal awareness different from recognition. The verbal awareness one develops through transcoding of nonverbal processing may be said to be a bonus or advantage that the brain has. Such awareness allows verification of the process of recognition instead of unquestioned acceptance of recognition. It is the awareness of recognizing, which allows one to accept the recognition and even to make judgmental decisions based on the act of recognition. Matching the external model with internal model and accepting the external model as the entity in the internal model can be automatically carried out by the brain. There can be only total or partial acceptance of the two models (external and internal) matching. A prediction of the external model based on its part recognition can take place automatically. During the process of the brain receiving sensory signals from an external source or making movements of some body parts, the brain has the option to carry out sensory monitoring of the motor effects. This can happen when the sensory signals are not intrusive (unconditioned), already conditioned or fear evoking stimuli, and the motor effects are neither unconditioned nor already conditioned responses. This may allow opportunity and time for the brain to know that it has recognized an external source or is making some specific movements with body parts. Such online monitoring of the sensory and motor processes is a capability, which needs to be cultivated by the brain. This allows time for engaging in online transcoding, which results in the further development of verbal awareness of the processes taking place.

Matching the external model with the internal model is a subjective process, in which one could make mistakes by totally wrong to approximate matching and identification. Selection of an internal model for matching with the external model may have personal biases affecting the accuracy of selection and decision on the matching effects. The knowledge base one has acquired indeed is the most important factor that would affect recognition. The idiosyncrasies of the knowledge base each person has acquired and carries in the brain significantly affect the quality and accuracy of recognition, unless one makes critical efforts to filter out such effects. One may create meanings and values and attach them to persons, external entities, and objects that are recognized. One would believe them and accept them as self-verified realities, and use the same to explain experiences of one's own and others. The quality and accuracy of recognition may therefore vary from person to person, though recognition serves as the reality verifying method used by each brain. One makes interpretations and judgments within a context, which may be known and accept as a condition for encrypting the same meaning, or may not be known and hence not accepted. The relationships and ideas one uses may have been acquired as part of socialization and created from own experiences. The acceptability of recognized meaning and values to other individuals, who may not share the same personal contexts, will be decided by the meticulous and objective manner in which one would interpret the relationships.

Matching the internal models with external model is required for recognition in all sensory modalities. Accuracy of recognition depends on the correctness of the matching internal model accepted. When recognition is that of understanding the meanings or ideas expressed verbally by others, what we normally call comprehension, such matching becomes critically important. For comprehension, one has to recreate the meaning conveyed by others and believes that one has succeeded in recreating or comprehending the same meaning. The possibilities of over, under, and defective encoding may be considered in this context, which result in incorrect meanings being recognized or understood. One may carry out such incorrect or defective identifications of meaning without awareness and it can become the source or genesis of abnormal behavior. This can be repaired only through cognitive restructuring (Ellis 1994, 2004; Taylor et al. 1997; Pull 2007; Hope et al. 2010). There may also be delays between retrieval of the modality specific engram and the transcoding efforts, especially identifying names, as the names (lexical details) are stored elsewhere in the brain (Damasio et al. 1996; Damasio 2001). If the verbal details are not retrieved, the individual may recognize the entity but will not be able to name it.

Consistency in recognition across individuals can occur only if all agree on the presence of commonly accepted factors, which contribute to assessing a stimulus pattern. For example, a square must have four equal straight sides and two adjacent sides must be at right angle. There are several thousands of such perceptions, which have commonly defined equations, and all recognize the same stimulus, whereas we may not share such consistent values for estimating values and meaning of behavior of others as well as those of the self. A visual stimulus of 100 milliseconds and an auditory stimulus of 50 milliseconds duration are registered in the respective primary sensory cortex after 100 and 70 milliseconds respectively after the presentation of the stimuli (Mukundan 1986b, e) in normal wakeful condition of an individual. The stimulus should last this long or more so that the retinal or cochlear image can reach the primary sensory cortex, and the 'sensory registration' is made. Though the stimulus has physically stopped to exist, its neural activation effect continues even after its cessation. A repetitive stimulus is recognized only well after 140 - 100 milliseconds after they have ceased to be present. A difference in the stimulus characteristic, i.e., a novel effect or a personal significance is recognized almost 300 milliseconds or more after the sensory registration, i.e. 300 milliseconds after the cessation of the stimulus. The P300 event related potential is the marker of such recognition and the Figs. 6 and 7 show the different types of paradigms in which P300 has been elicited. There is indeed a time delay between external realities and their recognition within the brain. The brain engages processing those recognized entities of the world, ideas and concepts created from them and about them, even if it is not encountering those realities. As mentioned earlier, this recognition takes place automatically or can be influenced by suggestive components. This has been amply proven in studies of individuals under hypnotic trance and suggestions. Mukundan et al. (1999, 2012) report the effect of hypnotic suggestions on the amplitude of P300 event related potential in normal individuals (Figs. 8 and 9). Hypnotic suggestions could block the occurrence of the P300 potential to the infrequent stimulus in an oddball paradigm, even though the infrequent stimulus was registered and attentional arousal took place as evident by the presence of P1-N1-P2 complex. Similarly hypnotic suggestions that the subject would hear loud tones, could enhance significantly the amplitude the P300 potential (Fig. 9) even though the tones were of half the intensity of the earlier experiment. The low intensity tones could hardly elicit P1 potentials by normal amplification used for eliciting other related signals, indicating low levels of sensory registration with the 40 dB intensity auditory stimulus, though significant N1 and P2 components of lesser amplitudes were elicited. Recognition is an important experiential method of making contact with reality by the brain. The sensory signals are interpreted using subjective and experiential values. The role of the Frontal cortex in interpretations of sensory inputs based on suggestive inputs has been discussed elsewhere in the book. However, there is no alternative for an experiential verification of moment-to-moment contacts with reality, which embodies the essence of living.

If the object or entity at the source of sensation does not trigger retrieval of an engram, then it is most likely that a matching engram is not present in the knowledge base and the individual fails to recognize the object or the entity. Perception is then that of unrecognizable entity and there is need and scope for individual to learn/develop a new engram. However, this

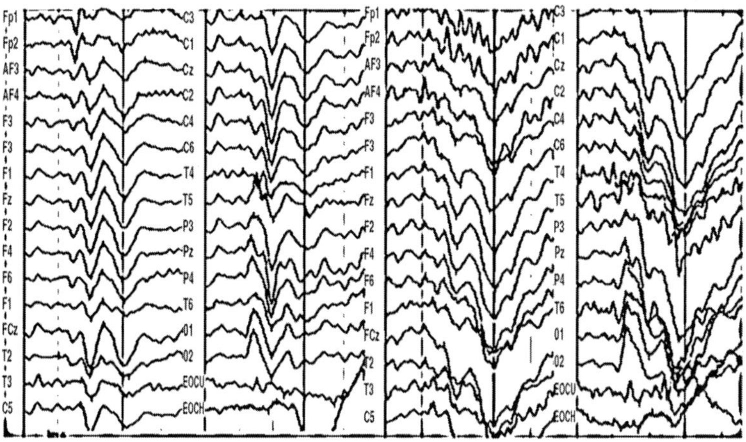

(A) (B)

Fig. 6: (A) showing P1-N1-P2 produced by frequent visual stimulus (horizontal rectangle) and (B) showing the P300 produced by an infrequent vertical rectangle

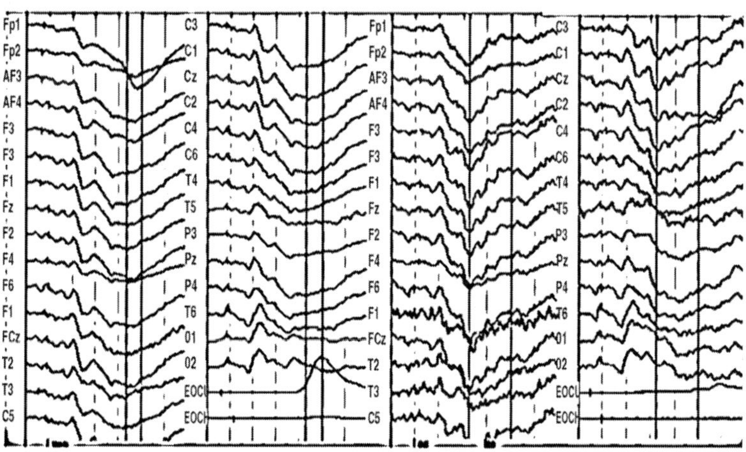

(A) (B)

Fig. 7: P300 in '1 = n' back test. (A) shows the P300 produced by different geometric patterns presented on the computer monitor and (B) shows the P300 produced by immediate repetition of a pattern infrequently. Epoch length 1000 ms

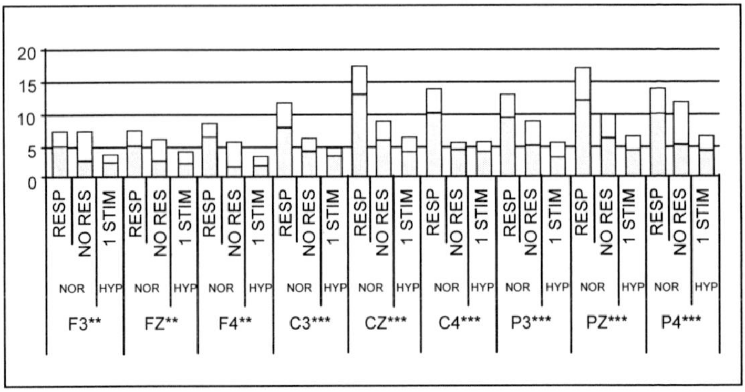

Fig. 8 (P300 in Hypnosis): Mean amplitudes in microvolt and SDs of P300 component in the Oddball paradigm, in (A) Normal Wakeful condition (NOR) with (RESP) and without (NO RES) responses and in (B) Hypnotic state with suggestion (HYP) that the participant will hear only the frequent tone (1 STIM) at 80dB intensity, and the results of comparison of the P300 amplitudes (microvolt) between the two conditions (A) and (B).*** P < 0.001, **P < 0.01

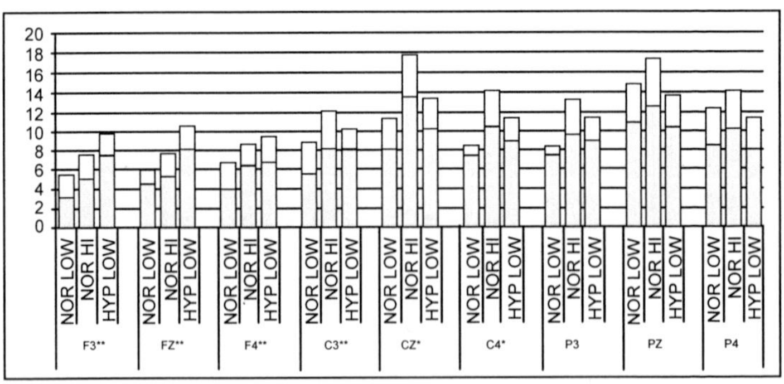

Fig. 9 (P300 in Hypnosis): Mean Amplitudes in microvolt and SDs of P300 in (1) Low intensity (LI = 40 db) stimulation in Normal state, (2) High intensity (HI = 80db) stimulation in Normal state, (3) Low intensity (LI = 40db) stimulation in hypnotic trance with suggestion that loud tones would be heard. Comparison between Mean P300 amplitudes produced by Low intensity stimuli in Normal and under Hypnotic suggestion as loud tone - ** - P < 0.01,* - P < 0.05

may be a slow process and developing a new engram is a process of new learning. It is a common error that a brain uses a nearest matching engram for matching with the external model and recognizes the object as its content. This is highly possible as recognition may have been made using only minimal information, and the perception may not be reality verified. This error can result in perceiving aspects of the object, which is not present, or not perceiving aspects, which are indeed there, because the engram, which one accepts as matching is not a complete one, or does not have those aspects. Such errors could be more pronounced and misleading with regard to auditory perception especially that of speech perception. It might be possible to avoid these errors if one is aware of the possibility of making such errors and remains vigilant.

Stimulus from Past to Future: Continued Neural Activation in Perception

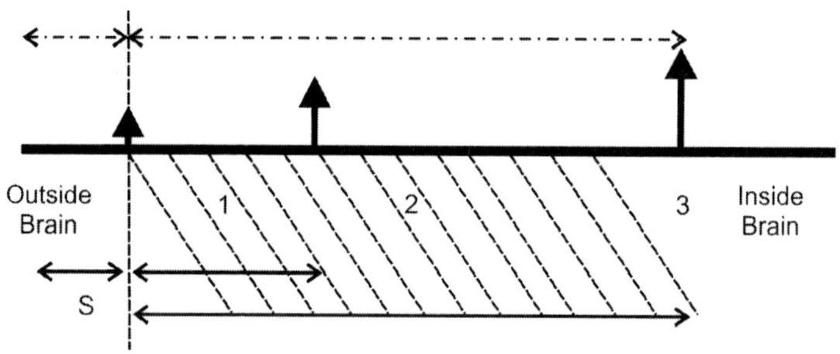

0 - 1 - Stimulus(S) presented for fixed duration outside the brain. Stimulus received by the receptor cells.

1 - 2 - Stimulus ceased to be present outside the brain. Stimulus induced signals are carried across and registered inside the brain.

2 - 3 - The signals are interpreted or readily recognized and the interpreted details or the occurrence of perception may be stored and the concept used in future processing. In visual mode, signals reflected from the same source may keep flowing in. In real time in auditory mode, the source exists transiently as it is flow of energy.

The stimulus recognition is influenced or determined by information already available in the personal knowledge bank, which needs to be retrieved first before it is used for deciding the stimulus characteristics seen or heard. A decision regarding the relevance of the stored information, which matches with the sensory image formed in the brain needs to be performed by the perceiver before or during the process of recognition. This decision is always subjective though it could be critical, habitual, or induced one. For example, the recognized entity could be a stranger (person), or one's love—the loved one. The brain could engage itself in processing a stored stimulus of the past, and interpret the stimulus characteristics and recreate its imagery. Processing the past is the current job of the brain at any point in time. In other terms, the past continues its presence in the brain even after it has ceased to exist as part of the real world. The brain is engaged in interpreting the stimulus received and it may continue as long as the brain needs to perform the processing. If the stimulation continues to be present as in visual and somatosensory modes, the sensation is continuously recognized at different points in times. The brain can be trained to hold on to the neural image of the stimulus for its further processing or interpretations for longer periods, even after it has ceased to exist. This can be done without storing and retrieving the stimulus and the continuous presence of stimulus imagery is described as holding the stimulus. The processing of the stimulus needs not be for its recognition, when it has been already been recognized. What is important is the fact the stimulus related information is available in the brain for longer periods, almost as long as (?) one may hold on mentally to it, if its presence is not interfered with the presence of other blocks of information. One has to practice and develop this ability. The brain continues to process and interpret the meaning from the present to the future. Holding the stimulus for its recognition and further processing contributes to its lingering awareness. Blocks of awareness or knowing of several stimuli occurring one after the other give the notion of a continuity of awareness of the mental world.

Processing of a stimulus, entity, or condition of the external world, detected by the brain, does not normally end with its mere recognition. Perception could be the beginning of a long process of learning through encoding/transcoding for determining relationships resulting in extensive explanations of various physical and systems related relationships. These relationships created using words and symbol as ideas and concepts are parts of the mental world representing the external realities, which each brain creates for itself. This may also involve creation of new concepts. Processing started with recognition may thus continue and the ideas created using words and symbols contribute to a stream of verbal awareness in the individual. The brain has the option to make this world in agreement with the realities, or create a world of own using choice imaginations, departing from realities, to the extent one chooses. The brain also has the option to believe in those imaginary concepts and to recognize and explain the realities using the same concepts and ideas. The mental world collapses gradually or instantly when the brain cannot stage such drama any more.

Gestalt Principles of Visual Perception

Perception of a physical entity depends on the presence of some important principles, which help configure the perceived physical form or the pattern of the object or the entity. According to Gestalt theory, "The whole is greater than the sum of the parts" (Hothersall 2004; Carlson et al. 2010; Bruce et al. 1996) and the ability to perceive the visual world as a whole rather than in parts is an important ability of the human brain. It is physically evident with regard to visual inputs, as these inputs occur simultaneously, unlike auditory inputs, which are always sequentially received in the brain and real time interpretations need to be evolved by relating the sequentially received pieces of information. These are called Gestalt principles of perception, named so by the early German psychologists (Humphrey 1924), who discovered the principles. Gestalt means that the total perception is not merely sum of the perceived parts. We call what we see as a cat, though what we truly see are the parts viz., the eyes, ears, the nose, the face, the legs, the body, the tail, etc. of the cat. Together we call the entity a cat, which has these body parts. Consideration of several factors that are simultaneously present in the visual inputs is important feature of visual perception, as several factors concurrently present in this mode contribute to the visual form of the entity. The appearance of a cat is different from that of a dog, as the appearance of its body parts differ. Cats are different from one another in appearance, size, etc., but we perceive them all as cats. We see hundreds of trees around, though each tree is different in the physical appearance of its branches, leaves, height, shape, etc. The appearance of a figure or form is always affected by the background in which it is presented or seen.

The following visual relationships of the part of an object or the characteristics of the stimulus and the visual field contribute to a Gestalt view of the visually perceived object. These principles are related to the figure and its background and the figure-ground relationships determine the visual perception of the object in the brain. These are the Gestalt Principles or visual organizations of physical reality that affect visual perception in the human brain.

1. Principle of Proximity: Objects and features, which are close to one another are perceived together.
2. Principle of Similarity in Color: Objects, which have the same color, shade, or appearance are grouped and perceived together.
3. Principle of Similarity in Size: Objects, which are similar in size are grouped and perceived together.
4. Principle of Common Fate (change or fall away from group): When a group formation is disrupted, it is detected easily.
5. Principle of Good Continuation: Tendency to perceive continuity, if discrete objects are presented continuously.
6. Principle of Closure: If gaps are present, they are compensated and a total is perceived. If two objects overlap, the overlap is easily detected at the cost of the originals and one perceives the overlapped figures as single.

7. Principle of Area and Symmetry: Principle of Area denotes when two large figures overlap, the smaller portion of the overlapping figures is perceived as a separate figure.
8. Principle of Figure Ground Relationship: What one perceives may be decided by the figure or the background. However, one perceives either the figure or the background at a time in these figures.

Not all the above Gestalt principles may be present in all visual exposures in everyday life. However, continuous inputs from several adjoining spatial locations in the objects and their visual field are rules, which determine visual perception. Inputs from several spatial locations need to be processed in synchrony and together for the visual recognition of all entities. The meaning or the interpretations used in recognition may change based on the background in which the source is perceived. The normal strategy used by the brain in visual perception is to combine several effects present in the visual field, which contribute to stationary and movement effects and to recognize the total effects produced by the object and its background. The simultaneous presence of neural signals representing the various components in the brain facilitates such a perceptual strategy, instead of relating the blocks of signals received in sequence in the brain, as in the audio mode. Information processing using the two modes provides different results, each has its unique unparalleled advantage, and they render the brain an unparalleled instrument of information processing. The origin of sequential processing and parallel processing in the brain is thus based on the differential sensory input formats available in the audio and visual modes. In the visual mode, there are several components simultaneously present and one can move the eyes or gaze and look at a large perspective of inputs. In the auditory mode, the stimuli occur in natural time domain, and the ears can listen to only one cluster of sounds and they are to be received only in sequence. This is the natural characteristic of the physical presence of auditory stimuli or sound in the universe. Understanding the differences between the physical properties of the visual and auditory streams of sensory inputs is extremely important for understanding the differences and versatility of the two processing methods developed in the brain, which has been already discussed elsewhere.

Some of the important principles that determine visual perception are the following:

1. Principle of Proximity

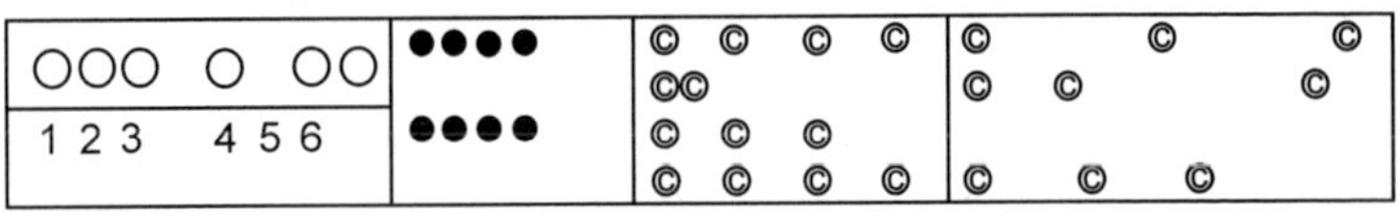

Objects and features, which are close to one another are seen together.

2. Principle of Similarity in Color

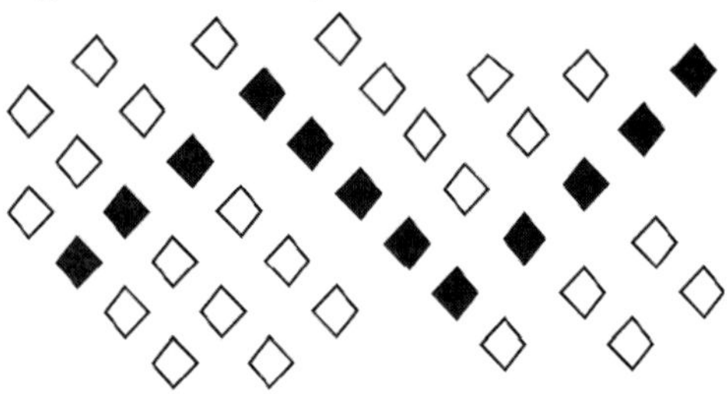

Objects which are in the same color are grouped seen together.

3. Principle of Similarity in Size

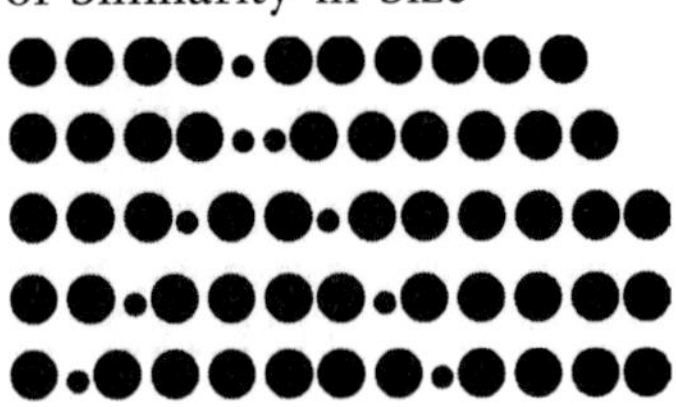

Objects which are similar in size are grouped seen together.

4. Principle of Common Fate (change or fall away from group)

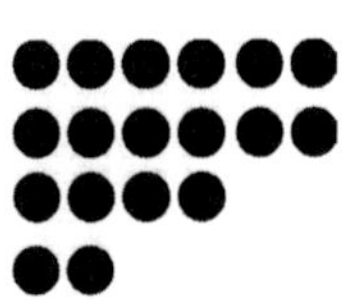

When a group is disrupted, it is detected easily.

5. Principle of Good Continuation

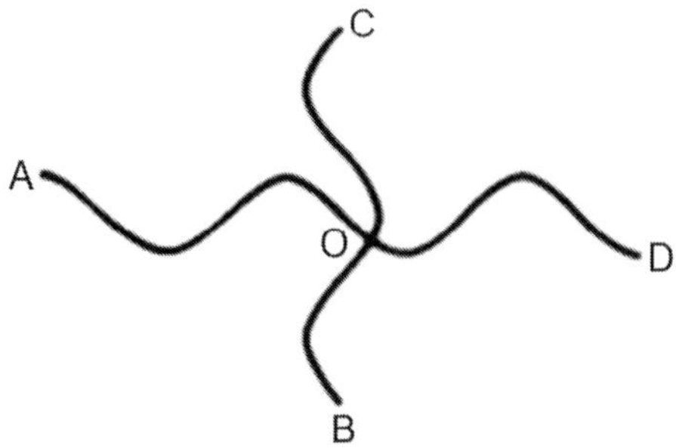

A - O and O - D are two lines

C - O and O - B are two lines

The four lines appear as crossed lines

Tendency to see continuity if discrete objects are presented continuously.

6. Principle of Closure

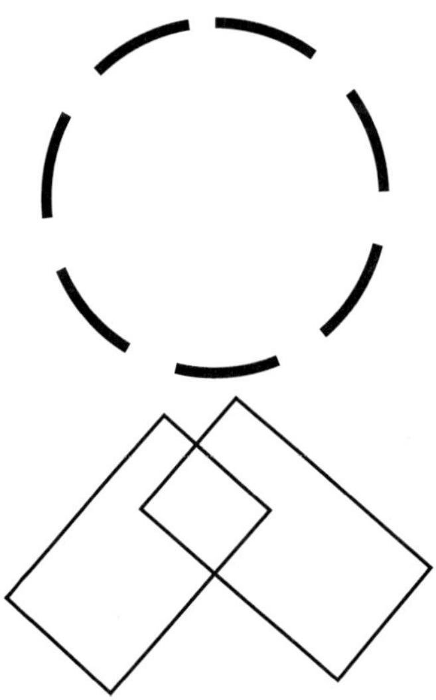

If gaps are present, they are compensated and a total is seen.

If two objects overlap, the overlap is easily detected at the cost of the originals.

7. Principle of Area and Symmetry

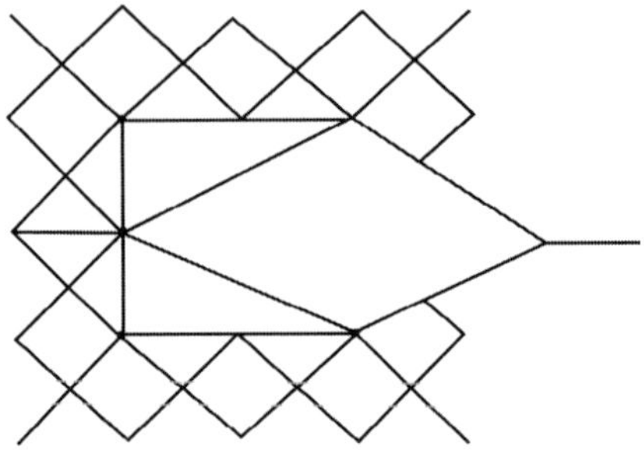

Principle of Area denotes when two large figures overlap, the smaller portion of the overlapping figures is perceived as a separate figure.

Principle of asymmetry explains that the whole of a figure may be seen rather than the individual parts, which constitute the whole figure.

8. Figure Ground Principle

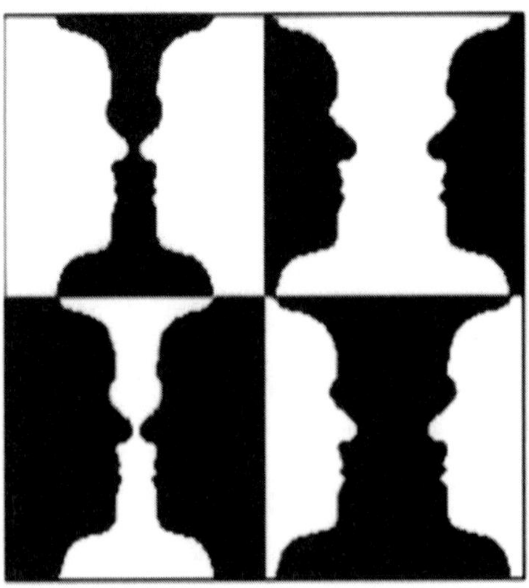

What one perceives may be decided by the figure or the background. However, one perceives either the figure or the background at a time in these figures. These configuration principles are not applicable in the auditory mode of sensory inputs, in which sequence is the only rule that contributes to creation of meaning.

Perceptual Constancy

Perceptual constancy is the tendency to perceive familiar objects as constant in size despite the fact they may have changes in shape, size, color, or location, etc., in size constancy of the image developed within the retina and the brain. One perceives the object as of the same size despite the fact distance of the object from the perceiver may vary, which visibly affects size estimation. Size constancy allows for the compensation of the size seen at various distances. For example, it helps us see buildings and other constructions on the land below, seen from a flying plane as of real size even though they look very small in reality. Perceptual constancy allows for compensation for the effect of distance on the size of the retinal image, and the object is perceived as total and of original size irrespective of the reduction in the visual image created in the brain.

Perception of Illusions

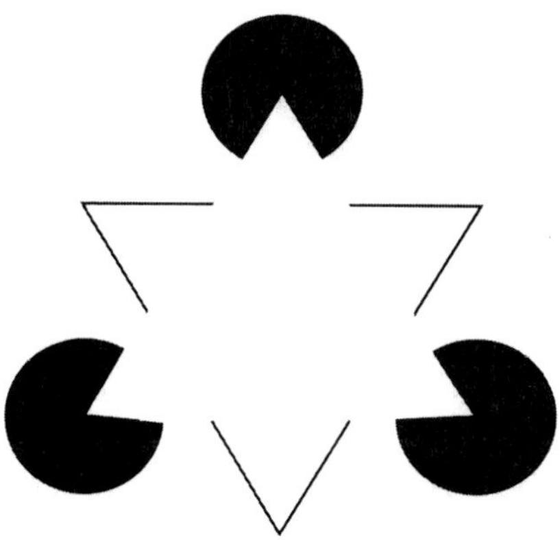

Illusionary Contours

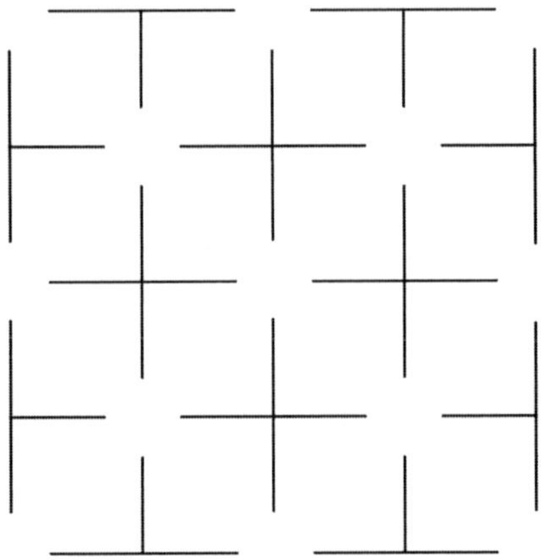

Ehrenstein Effect

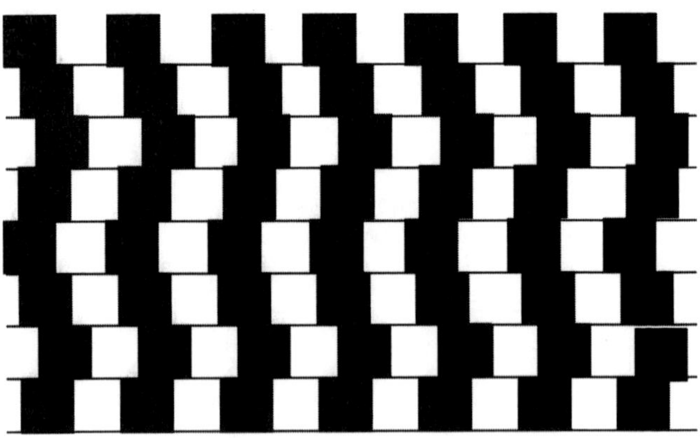

Are the horizontal lines parallel?

Visual Dominance: Colavita Effect

The Colavita visual dominance effect was first shown by Colavita (1974) when he found that one chooses a visual stimulus for recognition, if visual, auditory, or audiovisual stimuli are presented together. The preference of a visual stimulus to an auditory may be as much as 98%. This has been further demonstrated in several other studies (Posner et al. 1976; Koppen, Spence 2007a, b; Koppen et al. 2008; Spence

2009; Hartcher-O'Brien et al. 2010). The preference of significantly larger amount of visual signals received and processed in the brain may be considered an indication of the dominance of the visual system over the auditory systems especially when information formation and communication are primary goals of the sensory inputs. The preference of visual stimulus over the others enables the brain to transcode information mainly from the visual signals rather than any other. Information extracted from visual signals significantly exceeds the information drawn from signals in other modalities. Even auditory information is stored and presented in visual mode (orthographically) than in auditory form. Maximum visual dominance is seen in most of the people even over touch for determining shape, and proprioception for knowing own limb position (Hartcher-O'Brien et al. 2010).

Visual domain has the potentiality to offer enormously larger extent of sensory inputs to the brain than it can accommodate. Even after selective search of the visual domains, the signals could be much higher than the eyes can receive. Man is often called a visual animal because of the preponderant use of visual signals for encoding, transcoding, and documentation using orthographic skills. Even though, information can be stored and presented orthographically, processing of the information in the brain need to be carried out sequentially all over again. Word recognition can indeed be carried out directly from the orthographic representation, instead of identifying the words from their phonemic presentations. Amongst the signals received, in different sensory modalities, those signals in the visual modality are more persistent, and one can easily revisit signals in the visual domain, compared to any other sensory domain. For example, one can read a book, article several times, or watch a movie or video any number of times. The most important aspect is the perception of sensory organization and gestalt effects of vast range of sensory inputs of external reality. One moves, in time along with the external realities, and can still revisit many of the known realities repeatedly and almost continuously. The visual world moves with time, which includes personal time. Other than receiving new auditory inputs, most of the auditory information is retrieved from the storage created in the past, which can be recreated in the brain or reproduced externally. There is no way to revisit the same live (identical) auditory stimulus source twice, as one can do a stationary visual stimulus or reality, except to listen to recorded signals all over again. The visual reality can stay on for long durations, whereas the auditory reality must be recorded, stored, and retrieved. However, reality undergoes changes across time and affects the visual appearance. One can repeatedly listen to the same audio record, as modern technology has made revisiting audio signals very easy. In terms of sensory inputs, the time locked brain cannot revisit the past inputs, except to recall the same from memory. On the other hand, the same time clocked brain can revisit the same space at another point in time, and repeatedly recognize the visual signals, which he had accomplished earlier. One can go over the same orthographic representations (written sentences) any number of times and even mentally rehearse the same. One can stare at a visual stimulus including their pictures or photographs over hours or days and get back to the same any number of times, even though the revisiting is always at a different points in the time domain. An auditory presentation whether a conversation or speech is over once it is completed, and one has to record the same and replay it for repeat listening. Even during repeat listening, the auditory presentation lasts for a preset duration and it has to be repeatedly played if one wants to listen to the same all over again. When words are uttered as an expression of ideas with emotional overtones experiences and expressed, one may never be able to reproduce it in the same format and in the same experiential context, in another point in time. It is not exaggeration that we receive most of important information through reading and watching than listening. Writing skills are indeed scientifically more significant and exacting than speech skills. Further, the brain can receive multiples of visual stimuli continuously, which would produce continuous neural activation in the concerned brain areas. Visual stimuli may be considered to produce lasting effects on the brain compared to transient auditory stimuli. Somatosensory stimuli, especially related to touch, have a greater personal or experiential value in terms of establishing reality contacts, whereas such contacts are only presumed to be true with regard to visual and auditory stimuli. It is true that one can wear an ornament for e.g., a ring on a finger and have the touch sensation of a special personal relationship continuously. However, such experiences are indeed rare and they do not generally contribute to any other valuable information to the individual.

Auditory inputs to the brain have been the foundation for language development.

Amodal Perception

The word perception is also used in an amodal sense, for referring to detection of an idea or a mental process. Perception in this context refers to becoming aware of ideas, concepts, or relationship across words, sentences, etc. Perception of a relationship or meaning may be important step towards problem-solving and creative thinking.

Engrams and Neural Binding

An engram or memory trace is considered to contain neural signals representing specific information of a perceived object or an idea. The engrams contain signals representing the visual structure of an object, details of its applications, and user's specific preferences of its application, all of which may be represented in different locations in the brain. Retrieval of one set of information may automatically trigger the retrieval of other applications from the different centers in the brain, unless one intentionally blocks the follow of a set of information. As the knowledge of an object, person, or entity may gradually increase, the additional units of information are stored in additional neurons recruited through new synaptic connections. Hebb (1949) called a group of these neurons representing a set of information a "cell assembly". For example, there may be a 'cell assembly' representing neural representation of information related to the physical appearance, another cell assembly representing the functional properties, yet another cell assembly representing experience with the concerned entity. Different engrams are represented by different cell assemblies. The entire knowledge base of the brain is therefore, considered to be represented in such cell assemblies. Cell assembly is still a conceptual model as we have little knowledge of the structural basis of such assembled storage. Cell assemblies may keep increasing/expanding as more information related to what is already stored is further acquired. There may be more than one cell assembly, which may contain related but independent units of information and all the cell assemblies may be activated during activation or retrieval of one specific unit of knowledge. The cell assemblies may be activated together or in quick sequence during recall, based on the retrieval requirements in a given situation. For example, one may retrieve an engram, which helps to recognize another person, and the process continues as one remembers the activities in which they participated together, the food habits, and other personal habits of the other person. As activation of cell assemblies may be selective and strategic, a frontal regulation of the same is implicated in selecting remembering the pertinent pieces of information.

Neural binding enhances the quality of information processing both at the acquisition and retrieval levels. Integration of the functional attributes along with the information acquired over time produce superior levels of understanding. Neural binding of the cell assemblies is an important neurocognitive functional capability. Neural binding helps activation of one cell assembly to activate other cell assemblies so that one can retrieve and integrate all relevant blocks of information stored in different cell assemblies. It helps to integrate the independent sensory-motor events with emotions and the relevant knowledge base for experiencing and remembering the total experience, in a given situation. Neural binding facilitates and enhances comprehensiveness of any cognitive task engaged by the brain as it helps to consider different variables in their different perspectives and their varying effects, as stored over time in the brain.

The concept of neural binding was developed by von der Malsburg (von der Malsburg 1996) as an essential neural process in cognitive processing. Three types of cognitive binding effects have been reported. They are three neural binding principles, viz., binding by convergence, by assembly, and binding by synchrony (Tanaka 1993; Singer 1996).

- Binding by convergence refers to the propensity of the cell assemblies to respond selectively to particular objects.
- Binding by assembly is the propensity of cell assemblies indifferent areas in the brain to contribute different features of an object.
- Binding by synchrony is the propensity of cell assemblies to converge information acquired over sequence of time (Joliot et al. 1994; Gray 1999; Rodriguez et al. 1999, 2004).

Neural binding has been considered an important cognitive strategy used for integrating several components of information. These may otherwise be independently processed in object recognition, attention, writing into and retrieving from memory, motor synchronizations and controls, language processing and extraction of logical inferences (Hummel, Biederman 1992; Niebur et al. 1993; Damasio 1990; Murthy, Fetz 1992; Roelfsema et al. 1996; Pulvermüller 1999; Shastri, Ajjanagadde 1993). Temporal binding allows synchronization of (a) several related aspects of information attended to and in recognition, (b) information written and retrieved from memory. The process of binding needs to be applied in visual and verbal modes of information processing. Additionally, logical processing of information involves simultaneous consideration of several independent components of information so that possible logical interrelationships and effects can be considered as well extracted. Engel and Singer (2001) proposed that sequential binding over time within the range of milliseconds is necessary to engage in continuous conscious processing. Mashour et al. (2005, 2004a, b) considered that cognitive binding is the method of achieving simultaneity of conscious understanding from different neural processes. Neural binding of cell assemblies within milliseconds of activation is expected to lead to their conscious processing affecting arousal, attentional selection, perception, and working memory. Different functional centers of the brain are recruited for contribution to the processing culminating in the final processing results in perception, remembrance, etc. However there are limitations of processing ability as there are conditions when opposite effects cannot be combined and simultaneously perceived as in the case of 'vase and faces' and 'Necker's cube' figures.

Deficits of Perception

8

Perceptual tests used for clinical neuropsychological testing are mainly visual and auditory in mode. The visual tests are visuospatial drawing and construction tests. Auditory tests are part of speech reception and expression abilities. Both clinical examination and assessment by neuropsychological tests are needed to detect the presence and assess the disability levels of perceptual disorders that may be present in a patient. Clinical neuropsychological examination of a patient may be conducted first and then only assess him using the various neuropsychological tests for estimating the magnitude of disability. Visuospatial tests are used to test impairment in visual analysis and synthesis. The specific features of impairment looked for in the clinical assessment are the following:

1. Size estimation (Micrographia and Macrographia)
2. Impairment in Verticality and Horizontality
3. Fragmentation while drawing
4. Distortions
5. Impairment in perpendicularity, angularity, curviness, etc.
6. Visual extinction
7. Unilateral neglect in perception
8. Hemi-inattention
9. Constructional Apraxia
10. Perseveration
11. Impairment in visual integrative ability
12. Visual illusions

The above focal deficits seen are specific to fronto-parietal and occipital lobe lesions, and cannot be compared to any normative data. Comparison with normative data is important when one wants to assess the current potentiality level of the patient in specific functional areas for determining disability caused by the disorder. This is indeed important if the disability is caused by a neural disease, or brain injury. Detection of specific types of impairments including focal signs is important not only for diagnosis, especially lesion location, but also for monitoring the progress of the disease or condition. Continued presence of such deficits is also very important indicators of the functional capability of a patient, even if he has recovered to a significant level. A narrative description of the details of the focal deficit is important for one to obtain a comprehensive understanding of a deficit and its effects in the daily activities of life of the patient.

Table 4: Patients showing various Visuospatial Dysfunctions in BGT and Visual Learning & Memory Functions (Trial V) test

Visuospatial Deficits n (Patients)	LF 32	RF 32	BFLD 10	BFRD 10	LNF 11	RNF 11
Total number of patients with one or more of visuospatial deficits.	14 44%	26 81%	3 30%	10 100%	5 45%	11 100%
Micrographia	4 13%	3 9%	0	0	2 18%	0
Macrographia	2 6%	5 16%	0	1 10%	1 9%	5 46%
Distortions	5 16%	4 13%	1 20%	1 10%	2 18%	5 46%
Perseveration	4 13%	4 13%	5 50%	5 50%	1 9%	1 9%
Overdrawing	1 3%	5 16%	0	1 10%	0	1 9%
Fragmentation	0	1 3%	0	2 20%	0	4 36%
Spatial neglect	0	1 3%	0	1 10%	0	3 27%
Hemineglect, missing features, loss of associations (proximity)	2 6%	7 22%	4 40%	4 60%	0	0

Clinical Assessment for Detection of Perceptual Anomalies

Assessment of deficits in visual Gestalt is an important requirement of Neuropsychological assessment. Drawing tests used are the Bender Gestalt and the Visual Learning and Memory Function Test. The second test uses drawing from memory as well as copying of a complex figure (Mukundan et al. 1979a, 1987, 1991).

Visuospatial drawing tests: None of the patients had constructional apraxia while drawing. Significantly greater number of right lesion patients showed perceptual deficits in drawing tests. Less than half of the left frontal and nonfrontal lesion had visuospatial dysfunction. Both the right frontal and nonfrontal lesions caused deficits, though it was more severe in the nonfrontal lesion cases. Distortions and micrographia were the main features of left hemisphere lesions whereas hemineglect, missing features, loss of perception of proximity, macrographia, overdrawing, distortions were the main features of dysfunction in right frontal and nonfrontal lesion patients. Certain aspects like drawing over what is already drawn, and inattention and related deficits are significantly more in the left frontal lesions patients. Distortions and perseverations were seen in both lesion groups. Perseveration was seen more frequently in bifrontal lesion patients than in unilateral lesion patients. A lesion on one side would indeed affect the processing of the other hemisphere also, especially if that contribution is needed for the total effects of the processing. Lesion on one side of the hemisphere therefore, causes specific functional deficits, which in turn affects the total functioning of the brain. In every cognitive processing there are specific processing needs, which contribute to the context specific requirements of the processing. Such context specific application may be considered the outcome of total processing by the brain. This is most apparent in language processing in which processing from both the hemispheres is needed for several types of high ended processing and problem-solving. It is well established that the one hemisphere, invariably the left, does sequential type of processing, whereas the other hemisphere's contributions are required for simultaneous or parallel and deductive processing. What is directly seen in a neuropsychological assessment is the nature and degree of different types of dysfunction and not the total outcome of positive contributions of the different functional attributes.

Dysfunction: Dysfunction was marked only when the patient displayed one of the predefined type of difficulties in the performance. On Block Design test dysfunction was noted when the patient arranged the blocks in a straight line, one over the other, or placed them apart. In Object Assembly test, these were identified when the patient totally failed to guess what the pieces placed together would form, and placing two or more pieces of the picture in incorrect positions. Number of patients who made more than one wrong comparisons in the Spatial Comparison Test were considered to have impairment in visuospatial comparison. Similarly, patients who made wrong sequences and failed to explain their own sequencing were considered to have dysfunction in understanding the sequence of events from the visual display of the sequence of events.

Visuospatial Construction

The purpose of giving the Block Design test was primarily to see if the patient could assemble or put together nine blocks of cubes as shown in the patterns presented to the patient. The patient was instructed to reconstruct the pattern displayed using the blocks. After giving a demonstration of the task, the patient was instructed to carry on his own, giving as much time as needed, unless the examiner wanted to terminate the testing, as patient was desperately making efforts, which were erroneous for carrying out the task. It was necessary to observe if the patient resorted to an explicit method in which he compared the design after completing one, or an implicit method in which he systematically built the pattern from a corner or side. He was shown five different patterns and the time taken for assembling each pattern correctly or unsuccessfully giving up the effort was recorded.

Interpretation: Spontaneous performance is of great significance and greater the time taken more is the possibility of impairment in a patient. It may also be noted that the patient's ability to assemble the blocks can be impaired by a more basic visuospatial impairment due to a Parietal Lobe lesion, and hence it may not be possible to comment on the integration

Table 5: Mean (X) and (SD) values of the Correct Responses and Time (in seconds) obtained by groups of patients with brain lesion and Normal Control group on Spatial Comparison Test (SCT); Block Design Test (BDT), Object Assembly Test (OBT), and Picture Arrangement Test (PA)

Groups	n		Block Design Test Total Items: 5			Object Assembly Test Total Items: 4			Spatial ComparisonTest Total Items: 6			PA Total Items: 6	
			CR	Time sec.	DF	CR	Time sec.	DF	CR	Time sec.	DF	CR	DF
Left Frontal	32	X	4.2	321	2	2.8	550	3	5.2	124	6	3.8	4
		SD	1.5	184	6%	1.4	174	9%	1.2	67	18%	1.1	12%
Right Frontal	32	X	3.8	330	26	2.8	652	28	3.8	157	25	2.2	25
		SD	1.8	218	81%	1.3	248	88%	1.7	71	78%	1.2	78%
Bi-frontal	10	X	4.2	256	2	3.1	548	2	5.3	145	1	3.9	2
Dominant Left		SD	1.5	265	20%	1.3	173	20%	1.0	62		1.0	20%
Bi-frontal	10	X	3.2	453	8	2.2	561	8	4.7	151	9	2.6	7
Dominant Right		SD	1.7	318	80%	1.6	162	80%	1.59	68	90%	1.4	70%
Left Non-	11	X	4.5	209	0	3.7	490	0	6.0	81	1	4.9	1
Frontal		SD	1.0	174		0.5	136			32		0.3	
Right Non-	11	X	3.7	351	8	2.2	684	9	3.7	124	10	3.0	7
Frontal		SD	1.5	217	73%	1.0	223	82%	1.5	67	91%	1.5	66%
Normal Control	30	X	5.0	185	0	4.0	450	0	6.0	75	0	5.5	0
		SD		95			111			25		0.3	

CR - Correct Responses; DF - Number of patients showing one or more features of procedural dysfunction during performance of the test. X - Mean Score. The time taken by the Normal Control Group is the (1) true mean time taken by the participants or (2) the maximum time when the patients were stopped by the examiner. The mean of all these are shown as Mean time in the different tests.

ability of the patient. The patient may fail to put the 4/9 blocks together to form a larger square, and they may keep the blocks in a row or put them together in a disassembled manner. The accuracy of the pattern built is the second aspect that is tested. If visuospatial analysis is impaired, the patient will not be able to compare the pattern of the design shown to him with the pattern that he may assemble. This dysfunction can be seen in various drawing tests. In the absence of such dysfunction, an inability to put the blocks together is an indication of integration difficulty, which can be considered an indication of right frontal-temporal lobe involvement. An implicit method will require a primary visuospatial analysis of the pattern and only then, it can be reconstructed using the blocks. This spatial analysis may be largely absent in the explicit approach and the patient often notices the discrepancies in the pattern that he has built only when he is made to take note of them by the examiner. The patient will otherwise sit back with an expression that he has correctly designed the blocks. Visuospatial analysis involves careful study of the pattern and analysis of the different components of the patterns and their shades. One has to look for fragmented models, closing-in phenomenon and rotation of the completed models, all of which may indicate a parietal lobe involvement. Presence of constructional apraxia can render the performance on this test impaired. In the absence of constructional apraxia of an executive type, the impairment seen on the Block Design Test can be attributed to either a right parietal or a right temporal lobe lesion. Number of patients who displayed typical processing difficulties during the performance was definitely largest in the right nonfrontal and frontal lesions groups. These were difficulties in assembling the cubes together because of one or more of the following difficulties viz., as they could not put all the cubes together, made wrong designs without recognizing the incorrectness, repeatedly used trial and error methods without learning a strategy despite the efforts of the examiner to help each patient take note of the mistakes, and perseverative tendencies during the assembly. These were rarely seen in the left lesion cases and they appeared to benefit when their attention was brought to specific mistakes.

Visual Integration

This was a jigsaw puzzle, a picture depicting the face of a person, or another body part cut carefully into several pieces and the patient must reassemble them into the original total. Using a sample test, the patient was shown how to assemble the parts so that they made the complete picture. The Object Assembly test is the ideal material for giving this task to a patient. To start with, the patient must examine the parts and the part of the picture on each piece and guess what the total picture could be. Using this information, he must assemble and join the parts so they formed the total picture. The patient was first asked to examine the parts and identify the object that he was to assemble. He was allowed to take the parts in his hand and examine them one by one. If the patient had difficulty to report what the assembled object was, he was assisted in gradually identifying the object from the various parts and this information was recorded. There was no time limit for the test, but the time taken for assembling each picture was recorded. The patient was first allowed to perform the task, on his own, and was informed positively when he completed the task correctly. The examiner gave cues or asked for comments if the patient totally failed to perform. The test had four items; each was given one after the other for assembly.

Interpretation: Object Assembly Test has concrete and familiar cues assembling the total whereas the cues are based on abstract designs presented in the Block Design Test. This test involves certain degree of abstraction, which is absent in the Block Design Test and in which the pattern to be constructed is kept in front of the subject. Further, the subject has to make use of visual imagery and an understanding of the position of parts is essential for object assembly. There is also spatial planning involved, as the subject has to decide from which part he has to proceed and which parts have to be assembled in a stepwise manner. There are different difficulties encountered by a patient on this test. Firstly, it may be difficult for the patient to guess what the object is. Examination of the parts may not give any clue about what they belong to and what form the assembled parts would take. This difficulty to identify the total from components indicates a Front-parietal involvement. These patients may also show impairment on other visuospatial tests used for eliciting Parietal dysfunction. However, in the absence of a definite visuospatial difficulty, the impairment may be considered due to an inability to anticipate the object and hence may be associated with the absence of Frontal lobe contribution. The whole process of putting the parts together in a meaningful way to compose a total effect is the integrative function, which is generally affected in right frontal and temporal lobe lesions. Therefore, impairment on this test reflects a Fronto-Parietal or Fronto-Temporal involvement or both. Positioning of body parts are spontaneously done by left lesion patients, whereas right lesion patients have difficulty to decide where each part must go during the assembly. They do this by trial and error and not by knowing the principle of spatial positioning of body parts. Presence of Constructional Apraxia can again confound the performance on this test and therefore interpretation has to be made with caution. It is necessary to exclude the presence of constructional apraxia in the patient before these tests are given.

The Spatial Comparison Test

This test has six plates and each plate has a target design on the central top position and six alternatives in two rows below the target. Five of choices closely resembled the target but were significantly different in some components. One of the six designs was the same as the target. The position of the correct design was different on each plate. The plates were given one by one to the subject for comparison of the target with the choice figures. The correct responses were recorded and the scores were statistically compared across the groups.

Interpretation: The patient is expected to point out the matching figure and verbally report the differences seen in the non-target figures on each plate. The test is useful when the patient has constructional apraxia or other psychomotor disabilities for drawing or carrying out construction tasks with hands. The responses of the patient help to differentiate if the deficits are due to impairment in visual perception or drawing/construction ability. The right Frontal and non-Frontal lesion patient groups have shown significant difficulty in spatial comparisons and their performances were significantly lower than that of normal control group and left lesion groups. The test performance was hardly affected in the left lesion patients. Their difficulty was found to be mainly in transcoding the design, which they tried to convey through gestures more efficiently. Otherwise, their performance was comparable with that of the normal controls, indicating a clear right frontal and non-frontal involvement in spatial comparisons. The test could not differentiate between the performances of right frontal and nonfrontal lesion groups.

Visual Sequence Arrangement

The test involves arranging 6 different pictures, each of which contributes to a theme presented in sequence of activities engaged by two persons depicted in the picture. The pictures are of (1) two persons carrying empty bags, (2) both walking down a road, (3) standing in front of a shopping complex, (4) buying things in the shop, (5) walking out of the shop with filled bags, and (6) walking down with filled bags on their shoulders. What is expected is that the patient must (a) verbalize the theme of the pictures, and (b) arrange them in sequence and explain the sequence to the examiner. Correct responses were the number of pictures arranged with correct sequence. The results presented above shows that both the right Frontal and non-Frontal lesion groups of patients have shown maximum difficulty, though the impairment is most severe in the right Frontal lesion group of patients. The left non-Frontal lesion group performed almost as good as the normal control group. The main difficulty seen in the patients with right hemisphere lesion was for arriving at or making out the theme of the picture and the component of the theme that separates a sequentially separated, though they had no problem in verbalizing or transcoding the picture.

Continuous and close observation of the patient, descriptive details of the moves made in performing the tests, nature of difficulties encountered by each patient, the way each attempted to overcome the difficulty, how persistently each made the attempt were recorded. If a patient completed the test successfully, no dysfunction was considered, expect recording the time taken to complete the test and any significant inference based on the speed of performance. Patients with neurological symptoms and disabilities generally took extra time to perform even if they had no other difficulty for performance.

Working Memory

9

The working memory processing was first introduced by Miller, Galanter, and Pribram (1960) and later developed by Atkinson, and Shiffrin, R.M. (1968). Baddeley and Hitch (1974) developed the conceptual model of working memory and explained it as a procedure of using short-term memory for a current cognitive processing. The working memory system was further developed by Baddeley (1986, 1992, 1998) for explaining the principles of using immediate memory for cognitive processing. They postulated immediate memory as part of larger memory system called the working memory, in which information is transiently stored. The information thus stored is employed for current planning and processing. They considered working memory to have buffer memory system, one for storing verbal and the other for visual information. A third component was called the Central Executive, which served the managerial function to manipulate and coordinate the information stored in the buffer areas for problem-solving as per the instructions received or self-planned intentions. The two "buffer memory" systems used for online storage of relevant blocks of information (Baddeley 1998) were called "visuospatial sketchpad" and "phonological loop". The phonological loop stores words, names, numbers required for online processing of information and execution of planned actions. The visuospatial sketchpad holds all visual and spatial information for processing. The Central Executive is modality nonspecific as it is involved in the processing of verbal and visual data received in any sensory mode. The left prefrontal activation demonstrated in verbal (Kapur et al. 1994a, Shallice et al. 1994, Tulving et al. 1994a, 1994b) and nonverbal (Haxby et al. 1996) processing clearly indicated a material nonspecific

CES role in encoding. The most significant aspect of the working memory was considered its transient nature. One can take up new assignments in the working memory as need arises to hold on to selected relevant information and process them according to plans of action which two is held in the working memory.

Baddeley (2000) later added a fourth component called the 'episodic buffer', which binds all other information in the working memory fold at a time, into an episode. However, this component has not been found to be equivalent to or have the source memory component, which is an essential requirement for autobiographic episodic memory retrieval. It is now well established that the whole frontal and nonfrontal cortical areas of the brain may be used as buffer memory and hence the most important component of the working memory is the Cental Executive. Working memory is sensory nonspecific and cannot be truly differentiated from the mental equivalent of complex motor programming. It is an online mental processing ability, which can be carried out only if one can hold on simultaneously to several units of information including executive plans. It indeed refers to several independent cognitive processes carried out online by a person. Studies by Paulesu et al. (1993), Shallice et al. (1994) and Salmon et al. (1996) have localized the seat of the expressive aspect of phonological loop in the lower left supramarginal gyrus with Broca's area being responsible for auditory rehearsal. Such consistent findings are not seen with respect to the visual sketchpad. The right hemisphere areas normally serve as the visuospatial sketchpad, especially the right fronto-temporal and parietal areas are engaged in holding visuospatial information related to shape, size, texture, color, position, location, etc., of objects and other entities. Extensive investigations have revealed the frontal localization of the Central Executive Systems (Chen et al. 2008; Alvarez et al. 2006; Lezak et al. 2004; Monsell 2003; Elliott 2003). Its applications are complex with several dynamic features. The central executive is the dynamic processing mechanism, which helps to hold on to the information (considered held in the short-term memory) and process the data according to the action plan that too held on by the individual. An important aspect of working memory operations is that it is a subjective mental processing and the problem-solving strategy and solutions remain known only to the person engaged in it until they are disclosed or expressed.

Working memory is an online information processing method and does not involve any long-term storage requirement. Processing skills are called in as per the requirements of the action plan and it may even require retrieval of information from long-term storage. The main difference between working memory and episodic/semantic type of memory is the direction of time in which the two processes take place. Working memory is an online forward processing method involving holding on to blocks of information and executive plans and processing. On the other hand, blocks of semantic or episodic information stored in the long-term memory are retrieved for a current use in semantic or episodic recall. Storage of information after working memory operation must take place intentionally or because of personal significance of the information processed. Holding on to blocks or units of information is a crucial mental process, as once the blocks of information have served their purpose in the mental processing they are removed from working memory. Another way to explain the process of holding on to block of information is to say that one remains aware of the blocks or units of information, it is said to be in working memory as one can readily access the information without retrieval. This would mean that either auditory or visual imagery of the blocks of information are held on in the brain until they are made use of or processed. One can shift attending to the units of information held on, or from one task to another, depending on the processing needs. Once the unit of information is not required for a current processing, one can remove the imagery or cease to be aware of the particular block of information. The significant aspect is that as long as one holds on to the units of information, there is no need for their retrieval as they are available online for processing. Having mental access or awareness of several units of information concurrently, helps one to understand and extract the relationships that may exist across the units sequentially or in parallel. Such simultaneous mental processing alone may give insight into unique relationship, which can help the person to extract the relationship in a methodical manner. However, there are limits for the number of units of information one can hold on. Greater the number of units that one can simultaneously hold on higher is the cognitive processing capability and the understanding that one may derive from their processing. Any unit of information held on thus can be used straightaway or for cognitive processing. Once the blocks of information are already used and if there is no further need for them, one can drop them from the working memory or cease to be aware of them. If one still wants to remember, it can be stored and retrieved from the short-term or consolidated memory. What is important is the fact that the working memory contents including the data need not be stored unless the processing system decides.

Utilization of working memory capabilities contribute to organization of performance in all streams of life, from early childhood until the end. This is all the more important when controls for personal organization need to come from within. Additionally working memory processing is essential for creative problem-solving and cognitive growth of the individual. Working memory capabilities need to be cultivated by practice. Working memory impairment is one of the chief cognitive processing deficits that occur in various types of brain disorders involving the frontal cortex. However, there is no indication that different types of working memory operational formats exist in the brain. A few of the important parameters that determine the excellence of working memory operations is the quantum of information that one can transiently hold on for processing. This includes blocks of information, which need processing as well as the executive plans for processing. The processing ability itself may depend on other abilities and skills of the individual, such as arithmetic skills, sequential reasoning ability, etc. Technically, one who has determination and resources, can depend on external aids instead of using own working memory, especially for organized execution of work schedules in life. Problem-solving too can be handled by external aids. However, there is no alternative for working memory use, when one wants to process information for understanding and creating new concepts and ideas.

Holding on to Information and Executive Plans

Phonological loop and visuospatial sketchpad are indeed important constructs that account for the mechanisms used for holding information in working memory operations. However, it is important to know how the brain achieves the capacity to hold on to information. There is no way the phonemic image of a word can be held for longer period than it truly lasts either in the brain or outside, unless images of words are recreated, which will help to reproduce the different time-frequency characteristics of the original inputs. Holding on is synonymous to a temporary storage, but different from the storage in consolidated memory with or without linkage to other units of information stored in the brain. 'Holding' is the commonly used word for referring to online accessing of blocks of information in mental processing. However, it does not mean that individual is continuously aware of all the blocks of information. The amount of information that one can hold on simultaneously is referred to the span of attention. It means that the individual can readily use any block of information held on in the span of attention for further processing. A working memory problem is usually verbally designed and presented, even though the words may refer to entities in other sensory modes, including the logistics of processing. The blocks of information may be visual too, when one has to hold on to the visual image(s). The individual is not simultaneously aware of all the blocks of information; he can verbally repeat the blocks of information and access them. As one can verbally repeat all the blocks, one is able to select the blocks required for processing in a sequential manner. Lots of sensory-motor experiences and information retrieved from these effects may have no further personal significance to the individual. Repeated recreation of words is what children and even grown ups learn through rote learning. Children learn arithmetic and periodic tables, nursery rhymes and prayers, rules/laws, and important statements in all subjects, including dialogues for dramatics and lyrics of songs, through rote learning. Even illiterate children learn prayers and songs through rote learning, though they have never learnt formal language. Quick repeat recreation of the auditory images provide opportunity for the brain to select the blocks of information repeated and process them according to the execution plans, which too are repeatedly recreated. On the other hand, visual information can be held on for longer periods without transcoding, even though reference to its use must be verbally made. If it is a past visual design or pattern that need to be used in the processing, it needs to be recreated as many times as one wants, or the individual must relocate and re-recognize it for further use. One may hold on to the transcoded information and select the visual design and other verbal information, and process them according to the executive design. It appears working memory operation is the processing of information made available through repeat recreation of their imageries. Such mental engagement is needed for creative thinking and problem-solving. There is indeed need to know more about the actual process used for 'holding' information for working memory executions.

The units of information that one can hold on in working memory operations may be a function of the type of executive strategy one may need to carry out. If the task is mere repetition of sequence of blocks of information, one can practice and learn to hold on to large spectrum of words. However if it involves in between processing too, then there may be limits for the quantum of information that one can hold on. Cowan (2001) and McElree (2001) found that there were set limits in their participants, beyond which they could not hold units of information. This may be the case with holding numbers and names in a list. Mukundan's (1979a, 1987, 1991) working memory test consists of several mental arithmetical problems presented one after the other to the patient. Each problem has three parts presented at a time. Part 1 and 2 have numbers requiring independent arithmetical solutions and the answers of the two parts sequentially obtained are to be used for another exercise. Individuals successfully handle these mental arithmetic problems, though Frontal lobe lesion patients have significant difficulty in holding and solving both the parts one after the other. They frequently ask for a repetition of the part problem, which they failed to hold on. On the other hand, even normal individuals have difficulty in crossing the number of digits (generally 3-4) in a digit backward test. Miller (1956) had proposed that one could hold on to and process maximum 7 units of information through chunking, whereas Cowan (2001) proposed that short-term memory can hold a maximum 4 blocks of information. One may never come across a normal subject with such capacity in a clinical situation. Another test commonly used for detection of planning ability as part of executive functioning in working memory is the Tower of London test originally devised by Shallice and its minor modifications (Phillips 1999, 2001).

Computer Analogy

Man has built computers using the model of the functional capability of his own brain, knowingly or unknowingly. One of the important aspects of a computer is the random access memory (RAM) for holding digital signals online and processing, according to the executive program accessed and deployed by the Central Processing Unit (CPU). The CPU may retrieve information online as per the preset commands, viz., the processing commands and any other additional information from the hard disk (long-term memory) or use the commands fed straight into the RAM from the keyboards or other inputs, for processing the data in the RAM. The program used for processing the data in the RAM is generally retrieved from the read only memory. It is like using the skills viz., arithmetic and other skills from memory, when they are needed. Once power supply is terminated to the computer, the information stored in RAM is lost. The Central Executive system is analogues to the CPU of the computer, which executes the steps of the algorithm on the data temporarily stored in the RAM. Similarly, when one becomes unaware of or when one has to switch awareness from one phase of a task to another, the details of which are held in the working memory, one learns to hold on to them and reuse them (Mukundan 2007a). If one fails to hold on to them, they are lost and the entire mental exercise is halted. For example, distraction can easily make one lose the last number from which the next serial subtraction has to be made. If the person is able to hold on to contextual or source memory details of what was being processed and the independent sets of information are still available in the span of attention-awareness, it will be possible to initiate the entire working memory operations all over again. The efficiency of the RAM device accounts for the complexity of the information that can be stored, whereas the efficiency of the CPU will decide the complexity of the problem that can be solved. Other forms of memory, for example, isolated and consolidated memories are available for storage of relevant information, and they will be lost or not accessible for storage, if the storage device itself is damaged. Working memory as online processing is only for holding various types of information for their timely processing or execution. However, a total computer analogy necessitates that there is a structural basis for the temporary storage of information, which would remain unoccupied or empty when not used. We only know that this function is carried out best by certain areas (dorsolateral prefrontal cortex) of the brain, which are also associated with several other processing requirements. Working memory operation may call for skills and abilities associated with all other areas in the brain. Therefore, it is only the control functions required for such mental processing, which needs to be localized within the frontal cortex.

A complex cognitive processing carried out mentally may involve large spectrum of information and executive plans divided into several sequential steps, needing solutions in different phases. This is a process of onward processing in time as any current processing takes place only in the present. In episodic and semantic types of memory, information stored in the past is called to the present. In contrast to this, working memory deals with holding information including execution plans, and allows processing the information sequentially. Any current processing may need consideration of several aspects of a problem simultaneously, and the different steps (aspects) are carried out in a forward direction. If one has to solve an arithmetical problem on a sheet of paper, each step could be written down and solved in a stepwise manner. It may involve referring to previous steps and/or switching across steps to take the process of solution forward, all of which can be recorded on the sheet. If the same is done mentally, results from various steps will have to be mentally held, while solving the problem in parts and making the progress. Working memory applications are deployed by each throughout the day for meeting various work related demands. These may be related to the schedules one has at the workplace and at home on each day as well as important programs or visits one may wish to make in the immediate future. Once the appointment is executed, there is no need for one to hold the schedule in working memory and one automatically ceases to be aware of it, except remembering the act. One holds on to important pieces of information and even their processing, while engaging oneself to other activities. Therefore, attending to those units of information and even their processing may be carried out by dividing attention or simultaneously attending to more than one mental tasks. The degree of attention allocated depends on the task complexity and the processing needs and their urgency. One may even hold on important responsibilities and life plans though one may not actively process them, until the opportune and appropriate time has come. The following is another example of working memory. Suppose you are reading a book and there are several issues to be noted for critically understanding the matter discussed in a certain part of the text. Normally, we would make mental notes of those points as well as may write down important aspects for consideration. Processing may involve understanding the significance of each unit of information and the critical comparison of the semantic implication of several such units of information. This would involve holding on to these pieces of information in awareness temporarily. Working memory uses concurrent awareness of two or more units of such information and switching between/among them for processing. The number of such units, which can be concurrently considered and processed, depends on the amount of information each unit contains as well as the ability of the individual to expand the span of working memory for holding as many units of information as possible at a given time. The entire processing carried out is also as per an action plan, which too is to be held in awareness along with the data. Working memory operations are required for even verbal comprehension and expression, in which encoding or transcoding is carried out by connecting words and creating meanings from them. Ericsson, Kintsch (1995) opined that large demands of working memory applications, because of the extensiveness of the data that need to be processed, may help shift storage of data into long-term memory and their swift retrieval into working memory whenever needed.

Signal Inflow into the Brain and its Processing

Working memory may be considered a capability that the brain develops because of the nature inputs of the auditory signals into the brain. Unlike visual inputs, which occur from the spatial domain and simultaneously from different locations in a visual field, the auditory inputs occur in the temporal domain. The auditory signals received are not accessible again as one can go over stationary visual signals. There is no need to hold on to stationary visual signals as they are continuously pouring into the brain, whereas most of the auditory signals present themselves for short duration and then stop making inputs into the brain. Processing such transient signals require a different strategy compared to that of visual signals. Even most of the somatosensory signals (except pain) are transient and they do not have second signal system values as most of the auditory signals have to the individual. If the inputs have meanings as in speech reception, the only way brain can process the inputs is by holding on to the inputs received over a certain time domain, and then extract meaning from the lot held. This process has to be carried out mentally, unless one writes them down as they are received. This basic characteristic of auditory inputs into the brain has contributed to the development of working memory capability. The auditory signals flowing into the brain in a stream need different processing methods from the array of visual signals arriving in the brain. The stream of sound needs to be processed in sequence in the time domain, whereas the array of visual signals needs to be simultaneously processed. This has been discussed in details in the earlier section on stimulus inflow into the brain. Working memory refers to the method of holding blocks of verbal information received over a span of time, along with execution plans verbally expressed, so that the blocks can be processed according to the execution plans. Holding on to information received one after the other, across a span of time, is the most important aspect of working memory operations, the actual execution or processing is carried out by the brain using the skills it has already acquired. There is no need for mentally holding visual signals if they are continuously present. Need to hold on to visual imagery arise only if its recurrent presence must evoke a motor response. What one may still need to hold on mentally are the verbal instructions, used for visual processing. The same can be done without mentally holding and switching, if one can process the same from a printed or written up document. It is important to know that several such executions in life are carried out mentally, even if they are documented. Such operation becomes critically important when one engages in creative thinking.

Central Executive System (CES)

The executive function within the context of working memory operations refers to the role played by the frontal areas in holding on to blocks of input information and processed information, switching across the blocks, and engaging the relevant skills for cognitive processing. The need to hold blocks of information and process them arises of a specific need or drive state. One can carry out working memory processing only if the drive is sufficiently strong to initiate and carry on with the task. The origin of all drives is the same; clinical lesion studies have shown ample evidence to indicate the role of the ACC in providing the drive, though its regulation and initiation may be carried out by the adjacent orbitofrontal areas. The actual mental activities related to holding and processing take place in the dorsolateral prefrontal cortex. These aspects have been already discussed in detail in the earlier sections, and some of them form core issues for discussion in the section on emotion.

A few of the major functional roles identified as part of the Central Executive operations are:

(1) Ability to hold on to one or several units of information simultaneously and action plan(s), and deploy the necessary cognitive skills for processing the information according to the action plan. This would mean that one must hold and switch across units of information and execution plans, and then deploy the necessary cognitive skill or ability for processing the block(s) of information. The CE does not process the data, but only deploys or engages the necessary skills or abilities for processing them. The skills may be applied in explicit or implicit manner. The cognitive skills or abilities are available in specific cortical centers of the brain.

(2) Data for processing may be received from the sensory inputs or may be retrieved partly or fully from memory. Material specific sensory inputs are recognized by the brain and if they require further processing, they are to be attended to as long as the processing demands. This function of attending to or holding on to selected pieces of information is another core functional feature of working memory application. When the individual remains aware of them, it is called a process of holding. It may also be necessary that one attends to an array of stimuli and selects and hold on only to a few in the array simultaneously for processing. Thus, the span of awareness or the amount of information held on changes according to the problem-solving requirements or executive plans.

(3) We presume, since the data and plans of action are held on for processing, the online process of holding—attending to must be identified as the major happening in the working memory capsule. Working memory is thus conceptualized as special function of the brain. Wanting to process is an imperative need, without which it does not take place. It is also important that one must cultivate the abilities for holding and switching. It is posited that early childhood training in rote learning

help to cultivate the skill required for holding on to blocks of information and switching across them. Once the processing is over, the individual can cease to be aware of the data and the execution plans, or drop them out, and become aware of the final results so that they can be stored, documented and used for communication or as a piece of information for use in further processing.

(4) Visuospatial buffer memory refers to the cortical areas, which are used for perception and storage as well as those areas where the inputs blocks of information are held for processing. The secondary association areas and other relevant verbal areas are the domains for holding the blocks of information, which require processing. The data held so may be sensory-motor imageries or recognized patterns, ideas, symbols or entities in different sensory modes. When one or more pieces of information are selected for further mental processing, they are held as well as attended to or processed, and this is considered to happen in the buffer memory. It is a buffer memory as the information is held only temporarily there. These stages of attending to execution plans, and selecting and attending to relevant blocks of information could go on in steps in a continuous manner in each individual.

Central Executive in Encoding

Encoding is the unique brain process used for creating meaning from the sequential and other causative relationship that may exist across units and array of signals received in the brain. Even recognition is a basic form of mode specific encoding, as it helps to assign a meaning to the sensory inputs recognized. Encoding leads to learning new information or developing memory traces with new internal models. Encoding is essentially a verbal process using words and their assemblies for creating semantic interpretations and meanings of sensory events and motor expressions. When the inputs are in verbal mode, the process is called encoding, while transcoding is the verbal process of assigning meaning to nonverbal inputs. Creating relationship between two sensory events or motor expressions is the most significant characteristic of the encoding process. Encoding is a working memory processing, as assembly of words are done for creating specific meaning from the combination of words. The syntactic assembly of words may be considered a working memory execution of a plan for creating a desired meaning from the assemblage. Several different meanings may be imbibed or made out from different set of words in a sentence, connecting the different meanings to create yet another meaning from the total assemblage. Online creation and recreation (comprehension) of the different blocks of meanings require holding on to the different blocks, recreating their meaning and the relationships across blocks of information for recreating the total effective meaning. Creating meaning is indeed not an automatic physical process, but involves contextual, experiential, and conceptual interpretations. Hence, all these factors are to be considered while assembling words for encoding. The table 6 below shows the mean and the percentage scores of immediate reproduction of left and right lesion patients when two passages with 19 and 21 blocks of information were read out to each. The left frontal and nonfrontal lesion patients have maximum difficulty to reproduce the blocks of information compared to the right lesion and the community control participants. These patients did not have any receptive or expressive speech disturbances.

Table 6: Showing the mean and SD of immediate recall scores of brain lesion patients and normal community controls

Group	PASSAGE 1		PASSAGE 2	
	RCS	% of Tot	RCS	% of Tot
LPF (n = 30)	5.9 (5.3)	30%	6.1 (5.7)	29%
RPF (n = 30)	11.4 (4.9)	57%	12 (5.2)	57%
LNPF (n = 11)	9.5 (4.9)	48%	10.1 (5.3)	51%
RNPF (n = 11)	11.1 (3.4)	56%	12.4 (4.2)	59%
NC (n = 30)	11.6 (3.6)	58%	13.2 (3.8)	63%
P	<0.01		<0.01	

RCS—Recall Scores

The inadequacy seen in the left-brain lesion patients in the test is not because of speech receptive or expressive difficulty. They comprehended less as they could not hold on to the words heard for processing them or recreating their meaning and hence could not reproduce those blocks of information. Since experiencing is a subjective reality verification method for every individual brain, and what most people can readily apply in life, interpretations based on experiences have a significantly higher personal value to each individual. Encoding may take place with conscious deliberations or automatically. When the encoding is done with awareness, it is said to be an exercise in working memory. On the other hand, if one is emotional and under stress, one may only partly be aware of the meanings created, and one may not succeed in isolating the unrelated events for encoding, with the result that unrelated events or observations may also be bound in the relationship created. Emotional arousal associated with experiences, and deductive interpretations are important aspects that affect the meaning encoded.

Another important aspect is the process related to transcoding when one verbalizes nonverbal experiences, which result in the creation of a verbal meaning, which one can easily interconnect with other stored experiences and documents, as well as use for communication. Retrieval of a verbalized document may often be easier and faster than remembering an autobiographic episode with recreation of imageries, using its source memory, and then transcoding the nonverbal details retrieved, all over again (Mukundan 2007a). Encoding is discussed elsewhere in the book to explain its characteristic features and outcomes. Encoding is essentially an online mental process, and the process is considered to use the Central Executive of the working memory. One has to initiate it as well as hold on to the different bits of information for creating a wholesome meaning from the words or the units of information received as well as retrieved, for recreation and creation of meaning respectively. One can recreate a meaning, which one believes is the idea or concept, which another person wanted to convey. Encoding may take place in all sensory modalities and one may understand or assign meanings to the signals. Thus visual recognition of what is verbally expressed as a square is different from the visual recognition of a rectangle. One understands and may respond to a square and rectangle differently, without conceptualizing and transcoding the differences between them. Verbalization as square and rectangle is part of transcoding of the visual perception. One transcodes all sensory and motor components of experiences, and use the transcoded details for personal documentation of the experience as well as for communication. Perception or understanding the organization of the inputs during encoding facilitates their learning and the units of information being written into memory (Bor et al. 2004, 2003). Organization of information at all stages helps their orderliness during storage and hence retrieval is made easier. An important aspect of stimulus perception is to encode the organizational structures in the incoming array of signals while converting them into units of information, and create relationship across sequence of units of information. Understanding the organizational structure of the array of signals helps to create an effective and stable meaning. This happens most effectively while taking in verbal signals for recreating meaning (comprehending) of spoken or written speech and while speaking out and writing down meaningful ideas.

Frontal Lobes and Working Memory

Holding or attending to units of information and execution plans, and switching across units of information for their processing, and initiating and monitoring the processing are the important functions that we ascribe to the Central Executive of the working memory. Processing may take place at functional, concrete, and/or abstract levels. It may require skills and abilities like arithmetical skills, visuospatial analysis and synthesis/construction skills, route finding skills, language skills, etc., which need to be called in from other centers in the brain, using which the action plan is executed on the blocks of information mentally held on. There were several earlier studies, which demonstrated the nature and degree of frontal lobe involvement in working memory operations. D'Esposito et al. (1995) demonstrated that working memory was required when dual tasks were to be carried, while each alone did not require a working memory involvement as demonstrated in earlier PET studies. The two tasks used were a semantic-judgment task and a spatial rotation task. Normal subjects were instructed to perform these tasks concurrently while they were monitored on the PET. The results showed that concurrent testing was associated with bilateral dorsolateral prefrontal (areas BA 9 and 46) activation. Activation was also seen in some subjects in the anterior cingulate and in the left premotor cortex. Prefrontal activation was absent when the tasks were individually carried out, indicating that the dorsolateral prefrontal cortex participation is specific to concurrently attending to the two tasks and not needed specifically for processing the data. By additional testing, they were able to demonstrate that the prefrontal activation was not a function of increased workload but indicates the involvement of the CES. Increase in mental effort produced an increase in posterior activation. The findings of the studies were in conformity with the earlier suggestions of a frontal lobe (Owen et al. 1996, 1998, 2005; Petrides et al. 1993; Morris et al. 1998) and a mid-dorsolateral prefrontal activation during CES function. Their study has shown the possibility that the same neural structures are at least partially used in CES operation as well as buffer memory engagement.

There have been several functional neuroimaging and clinical studies, which have shown involvement of the Prefrontal cortex, especially the Dorsolateral Prefrontal cortex during the Central Executive operations. Though Baddeley and Hitch (1974) did not propose that working memory as a function of the frontal lobes, findings of several later studies could propose and support the dorsolateral prefrontal involvement. Studies by Petrides and Milner (1982), Owen et al. (1996, 1998, 2005), Ruchkin et al. (1992, 1995), Petrides et al. (1993), Jonides et al. (1993, 1998), Andreasen et al. (1995), Cohen et al. (1997) were the early ones that revealed a Frontal cortical involvement during working memory operations. Prefrontal participation especially that of the dorsolateral areas, in working memory operations has been demonstrated in several later neuroimaging studies (Baker et al. 1996; Braver et al. 2000, 1997; Cohen et al.

1997; Courtney et al. 1996, 1997, 1998; D'Esposito et al. 1995; Jonides et al. 1993, 1997, 1998; McCarthy et al. 1996; Owen et al. 1996, 1998, 2005; Paulesu et al. 1993; Petrides et al. 1993; Rypma et al. 1999a, 1999b; Smith et al. 1996, 1998; Smith, Jonides, 1999a, 1999b; Iidaka et al. 2000; Miller, Cohen 2001; McElree 2001; Curtis, D'Esposito 2003; Babiloni, et al. 2004; Kondo et al. 2004; Osaka et al. 2004; Pernille et al. 2004; Rajah, D'Esposito, 2005; Schonwiesner et al. 2005; Collette et al. 2005; Sauseng et al. 2005; Narayanan et al. 2005; Bledowski et al. 2009). The non-frontal parts of the brain especially the lateral and posterior aspects (temporal lobes, parietal lobes, and occipital lobes) may also be used for temporary storage. A dynamic model of the working memory indicates interaction of the prefrontal cortex with rest of the brain, which was supported by the findings from most of the above studies.

Working memory came to be regarded as an essential functional mode of the brain for holding information and their mental processing in various contexts. Mental execution involves conceptual handling of ideas and symbols in verbal, visual, or other sensory modes of problem-solving. It may also have motor accompaniments, in which motor acts are performed according to a predefined cue or plan of action held in the working memory. Common areas of the brain are activated in verbal and visual working memory, though it uses modality specific buffer areas for holding the information. Studies by Jonides et al. (1993), Cohen et al. (1997), Andreasen et al. (1995) have shown that during verbal working memory tasks, activation is seen in the dorsolateral, inferior frontal, supplementary motor, premotor, and parietal cortices. Squire et al. (1992, 1998) and Buckner et al. (1999) found right lateral prefrontal activation (area 10) during long-term cued recall of written words. Jonides et al. (1993) observed that right cerebral hemisphere (right prefrontal, parietal, occipital, and premotor cortices) is associated with visual/verbal short as well as long-term working memory. Petrides et al. (1993) observed bilateral activation of lateral frontal areas in visual and verbal memory tasks. Tulving et al. (1994, 1994a, b) found extensive right prefrontal activation (areas 10, 46, 44 and anterior 6) when normal subjects were presented with sentences, which were to be compared with the sentences presented 24 hours earlier. Nyberg et al. (1996a, b) also found confirming results in their study. Based on the neuroimaging study findings on memory, they proposed a "hemispheric encoding/retrieval asymmetry" model (HERA). According to the process specific HERA model, the left prefrontal cortex is selectively involved in encoding new information into an episodic memory, whereas the right prefrontal cortex is involved in the retrieval of episodic memory. Shallice et al. (1994) obtained evidence for left prefrontal cortex and retrosplenial activation during acquisition and right prefrontal and precuneous activation in the retrieval of information. Kapur et al. (1994a, b, 1995) demonstrated that the left inferior prefrontal cortical (areas 45, 46, 47, and 10) areas were involved in semantic memory encoding in comparison with orthographic discrimination. Fletcher et al. (1995) observed during encoding of auditory episodic memory, activation of left prefrontal cortex and retrospinal area of the cingulate gyrus, and during retrieval activation in the precuneous bilaterally and prefrontal cortex on the right side. Cabeza et al. (1997) also obtained evidence for a left frontal and retrospinal area activation during verbal acquisition or auditory encoding and right prefrontal activation during retrieval. Study by Wickelgren (1997) showed that the degree of prefrontal activation is a function of the amount of memory stored or held at any time in the working memory. The amount of information that can be held in the working memory varies according to the processing needs as well as the quantity of information that needs processing. The hypothesis that the left Prefrontal cortex is more involved in the encoding of verbal information, whereas the right Prefrontal cortex is associated with its retrieval was reformulated (Habib et al. 2003) to indicate that encoding and retrieval do have such left and right prefrontal lateralization, but there is no material specificity. Both verbal and nonverbal information arc encoded better on the left and they are retrieved more effectively by the right prefrontal cortices respectively. What is retrieved is a function of the quantum of information encoded and hence poor encoding would always result in poor retrieval. However findings of several studies (Miller et al. 2002; Lee et al. 2000;

Epstein et al. 2002; McDermott et al. 1999; Kelley et al. 1998; Wagner, et al. 1998; Owen et al. 1996) supported lateralization between left and right prefrontal cortices, based on material specificity of the information rather than processing specificity. However, in our own study of left and right frontal lesion cases, encoding was significantly impaired in left frontal lesion patients in both verbal and visual learning tasks (Tables 11-14) as seen in their recall scores. Babiloni et al. (2004) tested the HERA model of asymmetry using EEG activity and found that encoding resulted in significant lateralization changes seen only in the gamma activity in the left posterior parietal leads, whereas greater right parietal activity was seen during retrieval.

The degree of involvement of different brain areas would depend on the nature and complexity of task demands or the skills and abilities required for processing. Bledowski et al. (2009) postulated that interaction between mnemonic retrieval and attentional requirements decide the nature of engagement of frontal cortical areas and posterior areas. They found selective modulation of the task demand and attentional requirements resulted in range of activation from the caudal superior frontal sulcus and parietal cortex to rostral superior frontal sulcus and posterior cingulate/precuneus areas. Osaka et al. (2004) found the effects of increasing visual task demands during working memory applications decided the engagement of anterior cingulate cortex, left inferior frontal gyrus, visual association cortex, and superior parietal lobule. Tanoue et al. (2012) differentiated between externalization and internalization of attention and the respective demands on the frontoparietal networks during selection of attention direction, with greater frontal cortical demands during internalized attention. Complexity and nature of workload engaged in working memory operations may be considered to decide the nature of cortical engagements and the network selected van den Bosch et al. (2012). Workload may be visual or verbal and they may require skills ranging from mere detection, semantic interpretations, arithmetical skills, visuospatial analysis and synthesis, and reasoning at abstract and non-abstract levels.

Working Memory Deficits

10

Working memory impairment causes severe disability in mental-cognitive processing. Such impairment is a common outcome of several brain disorders, especially when functioning of the frontal cortex is affected by the lesion. It is true that modern inventions make man less dependent on mental processing. Internal processing has its own limitations, as the quantum of information that can be held at a time is limited, whereas we deal with huge arrays of information requiring complex and extensive processing, which can only be carried out by external tools. However, working memory operations have its uniqueness, as we still need and use this mental capability to identify new relationships and create new meaningful ideas. Only through creative thinking, such online processing to bring out unique results can be made. The Frontal cortex has to share its resources for holding blocks of information, action plans and monitor their execution, and switch across blocks of information. Greater the amount of information held, lesser may be ability to process them to create new relationships. On the one hand, modern inventions have made it possible to have greater opportunities to use mental resources for creation of new ideas instead of using the mental capability for attempting to find routine solutions. It is now possible to hold and analyze enormous amount of data externally. Brain is not to be used any more as the great storehouse of information. The brain holds a huge FAT table, which provides man with instant details of what, when, and where the huge blocks of varied blocks of information are stored, using which one can retrieve huge chunks of data instantly from the external source. This indeed gives him greater time and opportunity to be more creative and for finding greater emotional resources and their applications in life. There is no need for experiential verification of most of the ideas created, as they can be experimentally verified. Mental processing ability, especially the ability to hold on to large chunks of information is seldom emphasized as a desired ability. There are normal individuals socio-economically doing well in life, but who need aids for even multiplication of single digit numbers or for multiplying two digits with a single digit. This is no more considered a handicap, provided one knows how to find solutions quickly.

One of the working memory tests for clinical neuropsychological assessment was developed in the mid-1970s (Mukundan et al. 1979a, 1987, 1991; Mukundan 1996), as part of the NIMHANS Neuropsychological Battery. The examiner presents a patient an arithmetical problem in auditory mode, viz., "add 5 and 6 and subtract the sum from the sum of 7 and 9", and the patient is expected to mentally solve the problem spontaneously and speak out the answer. It is important to ascertain, before presenting the arithmetical problems that the patient do have the necessary arithmetical skills and does not have any dyscalculia. The test was originally called "Delayed Response Ability" test. The test contains 14 items. Mentally solving such problems will require, to start with, a person to hold on to all the numbers and the three execution plans. Once he has done "5 + 6 = 11", he can drop the numbers 5 and 6 and hold on to only 11, and the remaining numbers and the execution plans. While holding on to 11, he must do the second part, i.e. "7 + 9 = 16". Then after, he must hold on to 16 and the next action plan, and drop out the numbers 7 and 9. Once this stage is completed, he has the numbers 16 and 11 and the next plan of action of subtracting 11 from 16. Once he has the answer, he can drop the remaining numbers also and hold on to just 5, which he will speak out to the examiner. Interestingly seldom normal individuals remember the original problem, if they are asked to repeat it, though they have solved it correctly. The typical difficulty seen on this test is the inability to hold on to the second parts while processing the first. The patient may then ask for the repetition of the second part, as he does not remember it. The test findings showed that Prefrontal lesion patients, with focal or diffused lesions have severe difficulty in the test. All average intelligent normal individuals can successfully do 80% to 100% of the problems. Lesion patients invariably ask for repetition of the problems more than once and may often give up solving them, saying they cannot hold on to all numbers and instructions at a time. He may often solve the second part (7 + 9) of the problem, which was heard last and wonder what the first part was. Interestingly, working memory application is not required for one to solve just "7 + 9" or a similar single level mental operation, except one should listen to the inputs fully. Even asking a patient to repeat digits forward and backward is a simple effective test of working memory. Patients with moderate severity of frontal lobe lesions and deficits were found unable to repeat more than 2 digits, whereas several of the normal controls would repeat 4-7 digits forward and 4-6 digits backward.

The two essential roles of the Central Executive, therefore, are: (1) holding and switching across blocks of information and (2) to switch between or among mental execution plans as well as engage the necessary skills to mentally act on the units of information held and switch to the next action plan. Other than the switching across plans of actions and blocks of information, the central executive helps to hold on what is relevant. For example, we do not have to hold on to the first part of the mental arithmetic discussed above once they are already used, as they have become irrelevant for the remaining part of the task. For example once number 7 is subtracted from 11 and the answer 4 is obtained, there is no need to hold on to 7 and 11. The extensiveness of the use of working memory or the amount of information that one could hold in awareness depends on practice. Use of working memory involves a conscious process, though most of the processing could become automatic by practice. Mesulam (1998) proposed a model based on "supervisory control" or conscious control required for working memory tasks, which depends on nonfamiliarity/novelty of the task attended. Familiarity makes it possible to have automatic control and the attentional control could be reduced to minimum levels, mainly for detecting any change in the predefined and expected outcome. The less the task is familiar, greater will be the need for conscious control. Task complexity is another factor that plays an important role in deciding the need for the right degree of conscious control. Estimate of complexity may also be influenced by practice, which could determine the demand for conscious control. A carpet maker would be able to spend hours knitting a carpet automatically, without giving much thought to the intricacies of the design that he is weaving as he has already made several such pieces, even though he would detect even minor defect in the ongoing activity. Lesser the magnitude of conscious control deployed at a given time, greater will be availability of such control for sharing other concurrent activities. Multitasking is said to divide attention across the different tasks. We need working memory operations for all critical thinking and related cognitive processing, which are consciously accomplished. Working memory represents the problem-solving domain of human mind. Working memory helps to allocate attention into segments for executing almost mutually exclusive tasks one after the other. In other terms, one maintains awareness of several blocks of information and executes them in sequential manner as per a plan of action. The Tables below give the finding on the Working Memory Test (Delayed Response Ability test) results in Left and Right Frontal lesion patients, Bifrontal lesions with Left and Right dominant lesion patients, and Left and Right Non-frontal lesion patients and Normal Controls.

Table 7: Working Memory in Brain Lesion Patients Mean Delayed Response Ability Test Scores in Left and Right Frontal and Bifrontal Lesion Patients. Total number of items = 12

DR	LFL	RFL	BFL LD	BFL RD	LNFL	RNFL	N	
n	32	32	10	10	11	11	35	F
Mean	6.6	6.8	6.5	7.0	9.7	11.7	12.0	7.24**
SD	4.7	4.7	5.9	5.9	4.00	3.3	3.3	
	<0.01	<0.01	<0.01	<0.05	<0.05	NS		

Table 8: Working Memory in Intra-Frontal Lesion
Mean Delayed Response Test Scores in Intra-Frontal Lesion Patients
Comparison with Community Controls (N)

DR	Dorsolateral PFCL n = 18			Anterior Medial PFCL n = 14			Posterior Medial PFCL n = 17			N
n	18	Lt (9)	Rt (9)	14	Lt (7)	Rt (7)	17	Lt (8)	Rt (9)	35
X	8.11	8.11	8.11	7.43	5.86	9.00	6.12	4.87	7.22	12.0
SD	4.43	4.73	4.40	4.97	5.20	4.86	4.92	4.36	5.38	3.3
P	<0.01	<0.02	<0.01	<0.05	<0.01	<0.05	<0.01	<0.01	<0.05	

PFCL - Prefrontal Cortical Lesion cases; N - Normal Controls

Interpretation of Findings of Working Memory Tests

Results in the Tables 7 and 8, show that both left and right frontal lesion patients have done poorly on the working memory test. The right non-frontal lesion group's performance is as good as that of the normal controls, whereas the left non-frontal lesion group performance is significantly different from that of the normal controls or that of the right non-frontal group. The performances of both bifrontal lesion groups are again significantly impaired, and there is no significant difference between the right and left frontal lesion groups. Within frontal lesion groups, the posterior medial PFC lesion group's and then the dorsolateral PFC lesion group's performance were the most significantly impaired. Overall, the left and right Prefrontal Cortical lesion groups do not have significant difference in their impairment. This is a simple clinical test of working memory, which can be effectively used for detecting impairment in the function. However, effective working memory operations are required on more number of neuropsychological tests, and the patients who have difficulty on the above test would indeed show difficulty on the other tests.

Working memory deficits adversely affect occupational efficiency and daily life habits. Careful interviewing of the patients and their informants could throw light on the deficits, if present, in the patients. Working memory deficits will also be accompanied by other cognitive and personality deficits indicating frontal lobe involvement. The personality and emotional changes in the patient will have definite history in terms of the changes that others living and working with the patient started noticing.

The effects of impairment will also affect performance in the clinical interview as well as all other neuropsychological tests. If the same tests are given in writing, interestingly the patient will be able to perform the tests correctly on the paper. The digit forward and backward test and the serial subtraction tests are commonly used as routine tests in mental state examination of psychiatry and neurology patients. The Delayed Response (WM) ability is a test designed to assess the efficiency of the Central Executive, especially ability to hold on to three small action plans and sequentially switch across them. In moderate and severe lesion cases, the patients almost fail in all the items of the test. Instead of the numerical test, even if the patient is presented with simple problems related to shopping, the difficulty to hold on to the relevant information is very apparent. This problem could be "if you purchased 5 glasses and 4 plates from a shop, and another 8 glasses and 5 plates from another shop, how many glasses and plates have you bought?" It is important to demonstrate the typical impairment a patient has by repeat testing, without making the patient feel agonized about his difficulty. They manage to carry out several of the single digit arithmetic operations like addition and multiplication with relatively less or no problem at all. Maximum impairment is indeed present in bifrontal lesion patients and then the left frontal lesions cases. Impairment is severe even in left nonfrontal lesions, partly due to the presence of minimal difficulty in the direction of dyscalculia that may not be clinically present in some of them. The left posterior lesion patients have difficulty to manage numbers mentally, even if it does not appear as definite dyscalculia. The test cannot obviously be given when the patient has dyscalculia. Greater impairment in the arousal of attention seen in the right frontal lesion patients than in left frontal cases could be responsible for the impairment in the test in the right lesion cases. Inadequate attentional arousal could leave a patient unable to receive all the sensory inputs as they occur and this make it difficult for meaningfully processing them as required.

Information used for processing may be held in awareness online, only as long it is required. However, it does not mean that working memory is used only transiently. Long-term applications of working memory may be found in the retention of daily schedules and retaining other intentions in a person. Every morning, some of us make a mental notes (many may prefer to have a written schedule) of the activities of the day. We are aware of what we should do at the different points in time in the day and keep executing them as per the mental schedule. We keep a written schedule only when it is too complex to hold them on mentally or we know that we may forget it because of reasons best known to the person. What is important is the fact that one does not have to recall what one has to do at different points in time. However, there are individuals, who have had poor working memory self-training, who has not cultivated the ability adequately for such needs of everyday life. It is posited that rote-learning skills contribute to the ability to hold on to blocks of information. The attentional allocation to be used for holding on to these schedules may be very limited, so that we can still attend to the remaining tasks and execute them. Simultaneously attending to more than one task, or dividing attention and focusing on to different tasks are a common need of everyday life for many, unless a certain performance is that important that one attends to the needs of that performance alone. However, this decision is made by each person based on the personal significance of the schedules of the day. Once an activity is carried out as per the schedule, there is no need to keep that appointment or engagement in mind any more. The entire process is like writing the different appointments of the day on a piece of paper and sticking it up somewhere in the mind. All that is required is to look up at this mental note to know what to attend next. Impairment in working memory, therefore, affects daily working habits easily, as the individual will find it difficult to cope with the need hold the mental note as well as to look in the mental notebook, even if present, and read the next scheduled program. Working memory difficulties are often seen as a preclinical feature in dementia, even before clinical manifestation of impairment and other symptoms take place. Impairment in working memory ability could also be the result of excessive emotional arousal. Under stress and in anger, depression, elation, etc. working memory efficiency may be easily eroded. The person under such conditions will find cognitive processing, decision-making, or multitasking, etc. tiring and may not realize the inadequacy of efforts put in. One may have the insight of the gradual loss in the ability in the beginning, which may disappear, as other clinical symptoms start aggravating. Uniform and controlled emotional tone is therefore an important requirement for efficiently attending to, holding, and switching across blocks of information and execution plans in preset sequence.

We divide our attention for simultaneously attending to and processing of multiple tasks, as in the case of listening to music, while watching the TV, sipping tea or juice, and talking to another person sitting next or on the phone, as well as simultaneously play monopoly game or knit a sweater. This ability may be attributed as that of the central executive. This is possible only if the multiple tasks are familiar ones, which could be executed almost automatically. If there is a demand for greater attention to any specific task, the division of attention may fail momentarily. The individual is geared to take in or invest greater attention to the one demanding it. Multitasking need not be across different sensory modalities alone. It could be across issues requiring different types of internal processing and decision-making in the same sensory mode. For example, problem-solving using thoughts of different problems and strategies for solving those problems require such allotment of attention across tasks. Multitasking uses parallel processing of different sensory inputs or multiple inputs in the same sensory mode. Association areas in the different sensory modalities have the capacity for receiving multiple inputs from different synaptic connections (Clemo et al. 2008, 2007; Lee, Winer 2008; Mereditch 2004; Mereditch et al. 1986; Saleem et al. 2000; Seltzer, Pandya 1980) and conduct parallel processing of multiple sensory inputs. This makes it possible for the brain to integrate the multisensory perceptual inputs and create wholesome view of a stimulus or stimuli. We assume that the

Central Executive switches across these centers and processes them independently. It could easily switch across different tasks and process diverse information using variety of principles and mandates, which may not have commonness. Brodmann's areas 39 and 40 along with 5 and 7 have the capacity to mix and process multiple sensory inputs as well as limbic input to produce unique multimodal experience. However, multitasking or processing multiple tasks by partially attending to each task may be efficiently carried out only when the blocks of information processed are familiar to the individual and do not require highly focused processing. Otherwise multitasking will obviously reduce the efficiency of processing as it becomes necessary first to make an internal model of the hitherto unknown sensory inputs.

Retraining in Working Memory

Patients who suffered from Traumatic Brain Injury, surgically treated frontal lobe patients, patients with focal epileptic discharges from the frontal cortex, patients who suffer from fronto-temporal dementias and other disorders in the early stages, and ADHD children are helped with working memory retraining programs. Restoration of impaired working memory could be total or near total in patients with minor to moderate levels of severity of lesion, whereas patients who had severe frontal lobe injury/lesions, the benefit may be lesser or minimal. The working memory retraining allows the patient to relearn the three functional roles of the Central Executive, viz., (1) holding on to blocks of information and plan(s) of action, (2) sequential execution of the plan(s) of action, (3) set shifting or switching, and (4) initiating or engaging the necessary skills for execution of the plans of action (Mukundan 2012; Mukundan, Hemalata 2011c; Christina et al. 2009). Lesions in the nonfrontal areas may result in the loss of cognitive skills viz., language, arithmetic skills, visuospatial perceptual and constructional skills, as well as reduce buffer memory capabilities for holding verbal and visual information for internal processing.

Responses and Actions: Motor Programming

11

We differentiate between motor outputs made as a response initiated by an external stimulus, and action initiated from within because of a need state. These have been called the Stimulus-Response System and the Complex Motor Programming System. A response is released as a conditioned response by the detection of a conditioned stimulus. The stimulus-response strength helps the release of the response. The psychomotor controls needed for actions, originate in the premotor area and the necessary motor components are executed from the primary motor cortex. Action is initiated from within for the gratification of an internal state, which we commonly call the need or the drive state. The most basic needs are survival needs related to hunger, thirst and sex. Human brain has learnt to create several other needs, which are considered their aspirations and desires, which are unconnected with basic biological survival. Achievements of these aspirations and desires individually and as a team have become the essence of life. Most of the human beings consider these achievements superior to the satisfaction they receive quenching the routine biological needs. If a wishful thought or desire propels a person to action, it is indeed not a mere wish or desire; it has become a need, which has the potentiality to initiate the necessary action. Two structures of vital importance in this respect are the Lateral Supraarcuate and Arcuate Premotor Areas and the Medial Supplementary Motor Area (MSMA) in the premotor cortex, which regulate the sequence and the intensity aspects of the complex program that are expressed as motor acts.

Psychomotor performance refers to motor activity associated with mental processes. Motor effects can be produced as conditioned responses to conditioned stimuli or as an automatic response of the brain as in 'flight or fight' to fear evoking stimuli without their perception or awareness. The third types are actions generated from within the brain, which are part of complex motor programming and executed with action plans so that sequence of actions are initiated and expressed accordingly, for navigating oneself for achieving specific goals. A biological need state automatically initiates brain activation triggering motor responses, which lead to saturation of the need. The need states are essentially biological survival conditions in animals, though they assume psychobiological dimensions in human beings. The responses to biological drive states like hunger, thirst, fear are genetically determined and learnt in the animals and the responses are automatically expressed. The biological need refers to a derived condition whereas the drive is the prerequisite for the initiation of actions. Raised drive level triggers brain responses, which will lead to the expression of familiar responses that would culminate in the saturation of the need state. It is not different even in human beings, even though the offspring may receive greater attention and care, and hence quickly learn the responses required to saturate the need states. Additionally, the human offspring learn to develop various other forms of need states facilitated by their psychosocial interactions and superior intellectual capabilities. However, activation of a centre in the motor cortex must take place for the initiation of a corresponding motor response and this requires sending signals to the motor cortex from the brain areas, which provides the drive to act in the living system. This initiation is the most important function about which we know only a little from the neuroscience point of view, except the clinical profiles seen when there are lesions in some of the cortical areas. The initiation of action must take place automatically by the drive to act, when need state reach certain level of discomfort, survival threat, or intensity. We have already discussed how lesion in the Anterior Cingulate Cortex deprives the individual of emotions and activity, and how the patient becomes apathetic, loses initiative to eat, talk, move around, and does not even experience pain. Human beings have learnt to have multiple needs related to various aspirations and desires in life and they even consider achieving these aspirations as more important than taking care of their routine survival needs. Many would sacrifice taking care of biological needs for the sake of achieving other drives in life. These needs related to personal aspirations and desires, drive people to varied actions and to their destiny. A need arises because of deprivation or aspirations created in the brain and the brain responds to a need state by self-arousal, activating the motor system, which initiates appropriate behavior. The final saturation of such needs and drives may occur in steps. For example, one may leave work and walk down some distance to drink a glass of water or a cup of coffee. However, several of the actions taken for satisfying many of the personal aspirations and ambitions may be akin to the satisfaction that they seek with regard to sexual needs rather than hunger. One may remain patient and go through several steps seeking final closeness and intimacy. Once the motor output is powered, actions follow in strategic steps so that the individual finally achieves the goal. This is seen in animals also at a smaller level, as the persuasion may be only for satisfaction of sexual drives.

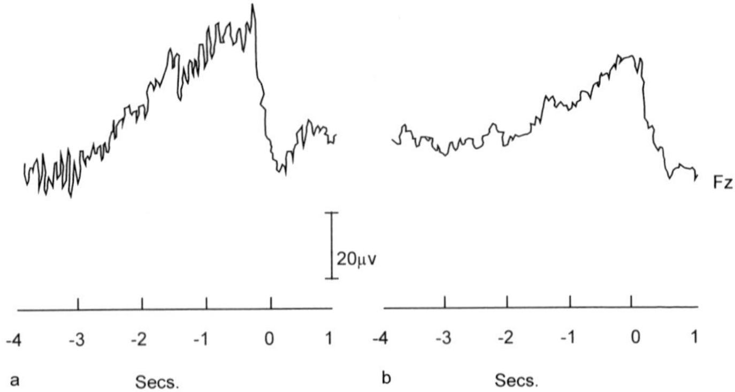

Fig. 10

Bereitschaftspotential in a button press paradigm in (a) normal volunteer and (b) in alcohol dependent subject. Onset of movement (Movement Potential) is between -1 and 0 sec. BP onset is at about -3 sec in the normal volunteer (a) (Mukundan et al. 1986c).

Intention

Intention is the awareness of a state of wanting to carry out an action. Verbal expression of awareness of intention emerges after the cognitive appraisal of the drive aroused by the need for an act or response. The act or the response can satiate the drive and hence it is experienced as a need. Intention is therefore a self-report and the resultant verbal awareness of the presence of the increased drive present, which is experienced as the need to act or respond in a certain manner. When the drive level increases, it may reach a point when the neural activation of the act or the response is automatically initiated. Mere wish to act does not result in the initiation of the act, if it is not accompanied by drive of adequate strength. One becomes aware of the response or the action initiated only when the action occurs. One my express the presence of drive as intention, though it may never be executed. One can control execution of action only by controlling the associated drive. Learning to control drive is an important component of the neurodevelopment of the brain. Awareness is therefore, of the intention to act or the drive of wanting to initiate an action, occurring well before the drive state initiates the specific motor response. Awareness allows one to interfere with the specific motor response already triggered. If it occurs well before the initiation of the action, the intended action can be aborted. This can easily be ascertained by asking individuals, especially young people to observe themselves closely during those moments of carrying out an action. This effect is demonstrated by several Bereitschaftspotential studies (Libet 1978, 1985, 1999, 2001; Mukundan et al. 1986; Khanna et al. 1989; Madhavi, Mukundan 1999), which clearly demonstrate that the neural process, which results in the execution of the response initiates well before one becomes aware of the action. The option to withdraw the motor output is an immense functional capability of the human brain, as each person may have multiples of needs, even though they are not related directly or indirectly to any of the biological survival needs. The needs may give rise to actions, which may reinforce and facilitate one another or cause conflicting effects. However, response inhibition can be achieved only by controlling or inhibiting the drive to act and not the act itself. The action or the response is automatically executed when the drive reaches or crosses certain level of potentiation. This option for response inhibition or withdrawal of the drive may be considered the essence of free will. A need state can automatically initiate or release motor responses, and hence we may accept that actions and responses have an unconscious origin and we become aware of the intentions to act, only when the specific actions and responses are triggered from the primary motor cortex. However, each brain must cultivate and acquire the ability to become aware of and then cut off, inhibit or withdraw the drive to act, which would otherwise automatically trigger the response, if allowed to increase in strength. Response inhibition is studied only when it is disturbed and for understanding the various types of motor disinhibition symptoms that occur in various brain disorders. The entire process of socialization of a developing brain in a growing child may be considered as efforts to cultivate such ability in each brain for nurturing as well as training to hold, withdraw, and release drive in various social contexts. This training shapes and controls their socialized behavior as well as initiatives for achievements in life. This would mean that an infant brain does not have the capability for such controls, as it has to be acquired through training. Response inhibition is considered the controlling ability of the prefrontal areas (Anterior Cingulate Cortex and the Orbitoprefrontal Cortex) over the rest of the brain. There is need to study and practice response inhibition as a unique positive functional capability of the brain, and develop and strengthen it in each human being. Biological drives of hunger, thirst and sex are normal drives, important for the preservation of the body. However, one must learn to keep these drives under control and release them for initiating socialized actions for their gratification.

We invariably encode all our psychological needs, which further help design execution plans and goals for fulfilling the needs. One becomes aware of the entire encoded need state, wanting to act, goals and action plans, and call all the planned actions as intended actions. Intention is primarily an awareness of the act or response one is about or wants to make and encoding the intentions makes it available as an idea. The needs of private and public organizations of people are such encoded and articulated intentions to act or engage in execution of planned actions. They are shared by large number of people, who work in each organization. It may be the need of the whole society, and they unite and resort to strong actions for achieving the goals. Intentions of executing various strategies may be different at different levels of an organization and they may remain isolated and not shared by all concerned. However, a cluster of meaning gets associated with every intention because every action may have purpose and specific goal. There may be more than one purpose served by a goal-directed act, and not all may be aware of all the purpose. The goal allows one to define where the act must take one to or what should be the outcome of the act. Purpose serves as a justification for the goal directed actions and gives the person justification for willing to act. However, we often use the word intention only when we are aware of the goals and the acts, as we consider that the intended action needs justification, as it is a wilful one and the justification for the acts must come from the goal that one achieves, and the purpose served by the outcome of the actions. As purpose and the goal justify the action initiated from within, and as these are encoded or verbally or symbolically expressed, purpose and goal are considered the basis for intention to act. We consider that the action intentionally carried out is a wilful expression. One may act out without such explicit awareness, when it may be called an unconscious wish or impulsive act. Therefore, presence of intention is indicative of justification for the action. Therefore, intention to act only means the awareness of the presence of the drive to act. Action itself is initiated only when the drive reaches the necessary level to trigger the action. The neural process of action initiates well before one becomes aware of the execution of action.

The Supplementary Motor Area (SMA) has a high topographically organized connectivity with the motor cortex, while the connections from the Supraarcuate and Arcuate Areas are less intense. The SMA of each hemisphere projects to both ipsilateral and contralateral primary motor cortex, and to the corticospinal tract (Macpherson et al. 1982; Murray, Coulter 1981). It receives inputs from primary and secondary somatosensory areas, parietal association cortex, and auditory association cortex (Bowker, Coulter 1981; Petrides, Pandya 1983; Godschalk et al. 1984; Galaburda, Pandya 1982). The subcortical dependence of the Stimulus-response system is on the cerebellum whereas the Complex Motor Programming is dependent on the Basal Ganglia. Various sensory areas send their input to the SMA, which in turn, are used for motor controls. The connection of SMA with the corticospinal tract indicates its direct participation in the control of musculature. Goldberg (1985) summarized the role of the SMA as (1) predictive in control and anticipatory in action mode, (2) simultaneous in bimanual control, (3) has propositional semantic dependence with regard to speech, and is associated with spontaneous speech output, and (4) is intention dependent in skilled motor actions. It has subcortical connection to the basal ganglia. Basal Ganglia refer to a set of nuclei viz., caudate nucleus and putamen, globus pallidus, substantia nigra, nucleus accumbens, and subthalamic nucleus (James 2008) situated at the base of the forebrain with connectivity with cerebral cortex, thalamus, and other brain areas. These structures help inhibitive control of motor activities, procedural leaning eye movements, cognitive and emotional (reward learning) functions and the release of inhibition facilitates activation of the respective motor activity (Alexander et al. 1986, 1990; Cummings 1995; Andrea et al. 2010; Weyhenmeyer, Gallman 2007; Chakravarthy et al. 2010). On the other hand, the lateral premotor area is responsive in its performance and utilizes feedback of actual effects for control, and is interactive in action mode. It is serial in manual control and has nonpropositional auditory dependence, and is associated with repetitive speech output and is input dependent in skilled motor performance. Its subcortical connection is to cerebellum. The stimulus hooked responses have high dependence on the corpus callosum for the transfer of signals to the opposite to the hemisphere, where such dependence is selective and hence low in the case of Complex Motor Programming.

Movements are the expressions of the body, which are needed for maintenance of balance and posture, which facilitate body equilibrium and reception of sensory signals for establishing physical contacts with the external world. Movements of the body, limbs, eyes, speech, and gestures are some of the typical motor expressions. There are three categories of movements, viz., the involuntary reflex responses, rhythmic movements, and voluntary movements, which we indulge in. Reflexes are conditioned responses as seen in closing the eyelids when a puff of air is blown into the eye or withdrawing fingers if they tough a hot substance. Rhythmic movements are used in walking, running, and chewing food, etc. They may be initiated and maintained voluntarily, but the movements themselves are rhythmically carried out without conscious deliberation. Voluntary movements are initiated by intentions and examples are dancing, driving, walking from place to place, combing, writing, drinking coffee, using tools, playing all games with or without tools, etc. They are learnt over time, with purpose and great amount of practice. They need learning for controls in conscious and deliberate manner. Once the concerned motor skill is learnt, some of these movements may be executed in an automatic way. During learning to drive, movements of the hands and legs are carried out intentionally and consciously in order to steady the wheels, change the gears, and the speed. Intense concentration and conscious control are needed in the early stages of learning to drive, which gradually becomes automatic and one learns to carry out with much less conscious deliberation, when we call them implicit actions, as one may not have to carry out the skilled activities consciously, unless there is an unexpected need. Voluntary movements are essentially propositional. The propositional movements are endogenously initiated and are mainly guided by anticipated effects as the movements take one forward in time, whereas the nonpropositional ones are initiated as response to stimulation and they may be guided mainly by the stimulus inputs to the brain. The propositional movements are called feed-forward type while the nonpropositional uses feedback information. Movements in dancing, singing, and playing musical instruments involve propositional movements, while movements in driving and riding have mainly nonpropositional motor components. When there is stimulus input to which the action is initiated and directed, it is called nonpropositional. When one carries out sequence of movements without any compulsion to act, they are propositional. Human behavior consists of both propositional and nonpropositional movement components. All movements are controlled by the motor system of the brain and the spinal cord. They are regulated by the inputs from the sensory system in a direct or indirect manner. Regulation refers to initiation, maintenance, termination, guidance, and appropriate applications of force and dexterity. Such action regulation can be achieved only by using a feedback of anticipated and the actual effects. The premotor area has very significant role to play in the executions of voluntary movements.

Movements are controlled either by phasic or tonic controls. Movements involved in reaching out to a glass or a book on a table and pressing a switch on a wall are examples of the phasic stage of the movement. A phasic movement may employ ballistic or ramp (graded) type of movement. Extension of the hand to reach out a glass is a ballistic movement, while holding the glass or pressing a key will require graded movement. Tonic control is applied for achieving stability of the body as in balancing body posture while sitting or walking.

Motor Programming

Ability for voluntary regulation of ongoing motor behavior using the anticipated effects and the actual outcome of behavior is the chief aspect of complex motor programming. The concept of control using anticipated effects was first postulated by Sperry (1950, 1952; meta-analysis—Mukundan 2007a). Anticipation is the perception or awareness of the outcome of the intended act, even before the act is executed. Anticipation of the outcome is an extremely important aspect of motor regulation as motor acts are carried out to arrive at a specific goal. This takes place in time as the ultimate outcome can occur only after the lapse of seconds, minutes, hours, days, months, or years, during which actions have to be continuously executed. Sensory information facilitates an action plan and having the anticipated effect of the action allows altering the plan of action even before its execution. Monitoring the actual effects of actions during the course of actions allow changing either the course, the choice of action, or even the goal to achieve. Anticipation at every stage of a complex sequence of actions can regulate the actions. Anticipation is a process of predicting an outcome; the brain carries out the prediction based on stored information and online sensory inputs. The brain may indulge in moment-to-moment prediction of what it expects, and compares anticipated effects with actual effects for deciding the discrepancies between the two effects. This process helps in redefining the strategy of movements, if required, and to learn the principles to be used for increasing the accuracy of prediction, which can lower the quantum of errors, if any present, between anticipation and actual outcome. Any motor activity requires continuous afferent inputs into the concerned muscles, lasting as long as the motor output is present, which means that even though body, limbs, and mouth are executing movements, the expressions are continuously acted out in the brain. The inputs are controlled, changed, and terminated depending on the needs of the drive state, harmony and smoothness of the muscular movements required and executed. This involves the participation of several motor areas and their sequential controls. Some of the important features of the motor programming systems are discussed in the following section. Motor programming explains how actions are composed, synchronized sequentially for achieving predefined effects.

Association between Intent and Action in Speech and Limb Movements

Expressive speech deficits could be demonstrated easily in a patient with lesions or functional impairment of the SMA during a clinical interview. For example, the patient may have no difficulty for providing answers to direct questions such as "What is your name, age, etc.?" He will respond promptly to the simple questions and instructions that may be used in a typical clinical examination. However, difficulty arises, when the patient is asked to describe an event, or the nature of his work. He would find it difficult to describe the nature of the work in an organized manner and in detail and instead use minimum number of words to describe a complex activity. The following is the description given by a patient who works on a metal cutting lathe machine: "Fix metal..., run lathe..., cut metal..., several pieces..." Luria (1966b) described the neuropsychological deficits associated with SMA lesion in a patient "Ch", and the major deficit was what he called "Deautomatization" of speech and limb movements. The patient responded quickly and directly to questions, which did not require elaboration, but had difficulty in elaborating ideas beyond simple answers. When questioned about the difficulty in fluent and spontaneous speech, the patient remarked, "thoughts do not enter my head" (Luria 1966b). This effect has been further reported by several other clinical researchers too (Alexander, Schmitt 1980; Rubens 1975; Brown 1977). The main feature of the syndrome is the absence of spontaneity in conversational speech, when the patient has to initiate and maintain speech from within. As the speech structure itself is not impaired, the deficit is often referred to as "partial mutism" (Damasio, Van Hosoesen 1980; Jonas 1981). Jonas (1981) reviewed literature on clinical features of speech deficits in SMA lesions and summarized that SMA lesion patients during recovery showed that "nonpropositional 'automatic' speech may be initiated easily, even involuntarily, while initiation of propositional speech is still difficult or impossible". Jonas hypothesized that intact SMA facilitates and controls the initiation of propositional speech, while it may suppress the "emission of nonpropositional 'automatic' speech". McCarthy and Warrington (1984) proposed a dual system for speech output. They suggested that (a) spontaneous propositional and endogenously originated speech involving semantic analysis will take a route involving the SMA and (b) nonpropositional speech will take a route from "auditory/phonological transcoding" centers to articulatory output, which will involve the Arcuate Premotor Area. The latter involves a direct "route between the auditory images of words and the motor images of words" (Bogen 1979).

Impairment seen in movements because of brain lesions are of great importance for understanding the immense functional features of the motor system in the brain, as they are true deficits in the functions, and understanding of which can throw light on the existence of unique features of the functions in the human brain. Luria (1966a, 1966b) further reported the difficulty observed in his patient for spontaneous and smooth limb movements. The patient could not execute "smooth movements composed of chain of successive links" and had difficulty in using coordinated bimanual control. Bimanual or simultaneous use of both the hands and legs require regulation through the SMA. These are continuous skilled movements involving fluent and sequential execution of the components of movements. Stimulus-Response system from the Arcuate Premotor Area controls alternate movements of the two hands or the legs as they are input driven and segmental rather than continuous as in the former type of motor execution. Luria cites the example of a typist who has difficulty to type smoothly, but is able to type out each letter separately. Yet another interesting finding was that the patient was fully aware of his difficulty and the discrepancy between intentions and actions. The patient felt that his hands did not belong to him and he could not make them do what he wanted. The components of a sequential activity were carried out in isolation and they were devoid of the "kinetic melody" which bound the components together for rapid and smooth performance. Goldberg et al. (1981) reported that in two patients with SMA lesion, they observed during execution of skilled movements, conflict arose between the actual organized goal directed movements of the contralateral hand and the internal verbal intent. The extra-volitional nature of the movement was called the "alien hand sign" (Goldberg et al. 1981). This phenomenon has been further reported and studied by several other clinicians and researchers (McNabb et al. 1988; Goldberg, Bloom 1990; Doody, Jankovic 1992; Chan, Ross 1997; Martí-Fàbregas et al. 2000; Scepkowski, Cronin-Golomb 2003). It has been widely suggested that the role of SMA in initiation of voluntary action is similar to its role in the initiation of spontaneous propositional speech. Luria (1966b) commenting on the common features of the motor disturbances produced by lesions in the premotor area, stated that "the program of the actions to be performed in all cases of a lesion of the premotor areas of the brain remains intact, but the performance of the movements is defective and these disturbances are based upon defects of the organization of complex movements in time with considerable difficulty in the inhibition of some movements and the smooth changeover to others".

The SMA controls skilled movements, allows both learning as well as expression. Learning of sequence of movements and their simultaneous expression as in dance and music require participation of the SMA. The SMA is also needed for the unfolding of the learnt components of movements in their original and/or improvised sequences. Such internal control is needed for not only the movements in the above situations but for new learning complex information, speech, and all goal directed behavior, in general. Therefore, the entire process is called Complex Motor Programming. On the other hand, environmentally controlled behavior is nonpropositional and dependent on stimulus inputs. For example, while driving a vehicle, a red road signal is expected to elicit a prompt response of jamming the break. Socialization and social conditioning in all its varied form represents environmental control of the individual achieved through stimulus-response conditioning. Such social controls facilitate and reinforce the development of behavioral patterns needed for the perseveration of the human society. Governmental controls, organization controls, control from family, community, and the society are examples of external origin and exercise of controls on man. The internal control is navigational in nature while the external control involves piloting. Piloting needs continuous stimulus contact, whereas navigation is based on a plan of action, which allows the person to arrive at goals after navigation, for which the navigational controls need to be exercised from within.

Bimanual Control

Bimanual control refers to utilization of both the hands in a synchronous or asynchronous manner. Each hand is controlled by two independent motor systems. Movements of each hand involve (a) the SMA of each hemisphere with its ipsilateral and contralateral projections to the motor cortex, and (b) the lateral Arcuate Premotor area in each hemisphere with its ipsilateral and contralateral connections to the motor cortex. Each hemisphere has therefore, two control systems directly responsible for the movement of limbs on the contralateral side. Voluntary control of each hand will normally involve the activation of contralateral SMA and therefore two independent motor programming systems with each involving the corresponding SMA and the lateral Arcuate Premotor motor area are to be considered. As the SMA is connected to the motor cortex in a homologous manner, if two hands are to be independently controlled in a synchronized manner, the SMA in one hemisphere has to activate contralateral limb and suppress the ipsilateral limb. The motor programs in each hemisphere can oppose each other creating a conflict situation unless one center takes a dominant role. Such dominance is achieved by one of the SMAs by control of the contralateral limb through its projections to the ipsilateral motor area and suppression of the potential influence of the other SMA by interaction through the corpus callosum. Bimanual control may involve simultaneous and coordinated movements of the two hands. The coordination is with regard to the temporal and spatial components of movements of the two hands. The spatial characteristics of the hand movements may be independently controlled, whereas temporal coordination or interlimb coupling of movements may depend on proprioceptive feedback from the two limbs (Verschueren et al. 1999). Eliassen et al. (2000) proposed that anterior and posterior fibers of the corpus callosum are involved in distinct contributions to synchronization of bimanual hand movements. This is achieved by temporal precision of bimanual coordination, specifically the initiation of the hand finger movements in the two hands. One hand may lead and the other one may play supportive role in several of the bimanual controls. However, this may not be affected by hand dominance of the individual (Elizabeth et al. 2002). Research in this area has brought out a new line of investigation in which bimanual control is achieved by cognitive components rather than by the integration of the sensory inputs and motor outputs. Neural interferences are considered to affect largely the integration of sensory inputs and motor outputs, which debilitate the efforts of coordinated and harmonious bimanual movements (Kelso et al. 1979; Marteniuk et al. 1984; Sherwood, 1994; Spijkers, Heuer 1995; Cattaert et al. 1999). Several studies (Schöner, Kelso 1988; Turvery 1990; Kelso 1995; Bressler, Kelso 2001; Beek et al. 2002; Swinnen, Wenderoth 2004) have examined the higher levels of bimanual applications, and have proposed that various conceptual features, which are part of cognitive processing, have greater influence on bimanual coordination than sensory and motor components. These controls come from emotions and other complex mental states, which one wants to display using bimanual movements of limbs. Such controls indicate the immense control and effects mind can cause on the brain and the motor outputs of the brain. These controls need to be learnt through intense practice. However, when there is a brain lesion, coordination at more basic sensory and motor levels may be affected causing impairment in bimanual controls, which need to be elicited in a clinical examination of a patient.

The coordination must be executed in a harmonious and smooth manner, which is described as "kinetic melody". Communication and interaction between the two SMAs through corpus callosum is important for such bilateral and synchronized movements of non-homologous muscles, which ensure coordinated and complimentary movements of both the hands. An alternative bimanual control using visual guidance is proposed by Jones et al. (1978) and Pandya and Kuypers (1969). This alternate circuit through the intrahemispheric corticocortical connections involving the lateral premotor area is considered slower as the two channels may function out of space, despite the visual guidance. The SMA plays critical role in the production of skilled movement sequences as in playing a music instrument. Though the movements may be complex, they will hardly require visual gating. The sensorymotor schemata of the movements are "precompiled" (Angel 1976) and executed in a feed-forward mode using anticipatory cues. The feed-forward and predictive unfolding of movements (Rolls et al. 1979) relies on its own sensorymotor schemata for online monitoring and error correction. Luria (1966b) has labeled these schemas "abbreviated kinetic schemas" based on which the movements are executed. Critical points in movements are linked to select sensory inputs (Angel 1976) and the basal ganglia plays an important role in detecting the task relevant sensory events (Baddeley, Hitch 1974).

Stimulation of premotor area, in contrast to stimulation of the motor cortex, does not give rise to movement of small muscles. Complex and gross movements can be generated by stimulation of premotor area, e.g., stimulation of area 6 and 8 causes deviation of head and eyes to the opposite side and complex movement of limbs (Goldberg 1981). Stimulation of certain parts produces depression of ongoing movements and alterations in muscle tone, which indicates a higher level (frontal) control of lower level movements (Goldberg 1981). Total removal of premotor cortex does not give rise to paralysis, but produces spasticity, rigidity of movements, and disorders of grasp reflex and vasomotor functions along with disturbances of skilled movements. Simple clinical procedures, which can be used for eliciting difficulty in bimanual controls is discussed in the next section.

The neural connectivity for cognitive and emotional control of movements that exists in the brain is an important medium for feedback controls of emotions and cognitive states through movements. The psychological effects of movements deployed in dance and playing instruments have been understood and well utilized (Hanna 1995; Cassileth 1998; Cohen, Walco 1999; Dance/movement therapy fact sheet. American Dance Therapy Association Web site-http://www.adta.org/,; Castaneda 2003; Sandel et al. 2005). Dance therapy has proved its usefulness in the control of disturbing emotional states or stress reduction and accentuating emotional stability in individuals, and it has become an extensively used method, as a self-enhancing and rehabilitative measure.

Psychomotor Impairment in Prefrontal Lesions

Luria (1966a, b) described several psychomotor tests, which can easily elicit impairment indicating prefrontal lobe involvement in patients. Some of these are for eliciting psychomotor perseveration and disturbance in kinetic melody, which can be demonstrated using simple clinical procedures with a patient. The examiner must take care to know that the patient has understood the instructions and the best course is to demonstrate each procedure to the patient and make him repeat it the same with examiner. Limb movement, especially gesture controls is known to relate closely to oral motor development associated with language development in children (Alcock 2006; Bishop, 2002; Hill, 2001; Bates et al. 1979), and when limb movements of the type discussed here are impaired, there is possibility of impairment of oral praxis and disturbance in expressive language functions in patients. For purpose of testing a patient, motor functions are subdivided into—(a) motor functions of the hands, (b) oral praxis, (c) speech regulation of motor acts, and (d) rhythmic movements in perception/motoric reproduction of pitch relationships and of complex rhythmic structures.

Perseveration

Perseveration is the repetition of a response, when the individual is expected to switch across different responses. Perseveration can be clinically seen in the use of words, phrases, gestures, in writing, drawing, and expression of other motor responses. Perseveration disables a patient to change response mental set and execute different motor responses. In speech, this can make a patient repeat the same word or the phrase. In a simple drawing or writing task, the patient will keep drawing repeatedly the same word, or figure, as the patient is unable to switch to the next words or motor responses. The repeat expression of the response is not either cued or instructed. Psychomotor perseveration can be easily demonstrated and elicited in (a) motor alternation tests and (b) continuous drawing tests. One method of testing motor alternation involves instructing the patient to first stretch out his right hand or preferred hand (Luria 1966a) and show a fist and then put the hand down, and stretch out again and show a ring with the thumb and the index finger. The patient must alternatively keep performing this act several times until the examiner is satisfied that the patient can carry out the task smoothly and rhythmically, and the alternate steps are correctly maintained. To start with, the examiner may demonstrate the movement of hand and even train a patient to carry out the limb movement. Impairment is seen as inability to continuously alternate when patient will throw a fist or a ring alone. An equally easy procedure is to instruct the patient to hold the fist and open and stretch the index finger, and fold it back and then open and stretch out the ring finger. He is instructed to fold it back and repeat the whole movements with the index and ring finger alternatively. A patient with impairment in this function will not be able to alternatively fold and open the two fingers. However, it is important to test and assure that the patient has no rigidity of the hands and fingers before instructing to carry on the motor tasks. Patients with dementia may invariably fail to understand the subtle instructions and hence may fail to carry out the tasks, even though they may not otherwise have the difficulty.

Sequential Motor Activity: The test measures the ability of a patient carry out different motor responses in sequence. The patient is first asked to draw small circle, triangle, and a cross on a sheet of paper one by one. Once the examiner is satisfied that the subject can draw these with ease, the patient is instructed to draw the figures as the examiner calls out their names. The examiner then calls out the names at random order from a prepared list. Keep the pace convenient for the subject to draw the figure fully. Impairment will be inability of the patient to change the figures as and when they are changed by the examiner. The patient will be seen drawing the same figure repeatedly. This is recorded as perseveration.

Perseveration of the above type is seen generally when there is extensive lesion of the frontal lobes especially in the Orbitofrontal areas. Perseveration of this severity can impair all performances in DAL. Even in less extensive lesions, perseveration may be seen in other performance tests such as the visuospatial tests viz., Bender Gestalt test and other drawing tests during assessments.

Kinetic Melody Disturbances

Kinetic melody refers to the ability to make rhythmic movements. Tapping with fingers is an easy and efficient method to elicit impairment in kinetic melody. To test kinetic melody, it is necessary for the examiner to first instruct/ demonstrate the patient how to tap rhythmically on the table with the fingers of the two hands. The patient must tap twice with the right hand, and tap once with the left hand fingers and maintain the rhythm for about a minute. Very seldom, a patient may be seen, who does not understand the instructions for finger tapping. If the patient can spontaneously tap after the examiner has demonstrated, there will be no further need to test the patient. Sometimes it may be necessary to increase the complexity of tapping especially if the patient is a musician who has a special musical ability. The number of tapping can be then changed, for example, tap thrice with right hand and twice with the left or changing the rhythm and timings, which the examiner must demonstrate first. As impairment is a significant indicator of a frontal lobe involvement, a hasty decision about it is unwarranted. It is also extremely important to know that tapping ability can also be impaired in cerebellar lesions. In this case, the tapping may become rigid and devoid of smoothness and at times the patient may be unable to move the hand at all for tapping. Therefore, it is essential to know if the patient also has a cerebellar involvement before arriving at a conclusion about frontal lobe involvement. Perseveration could be also the

Table 9: Number and Percentage of Patients in FL and NFL groups with Impairment in Sequential Motor, Fist and Ring, Fist and Outstretched Fingers, and Tapping Tests.

MOTOR TEST	LF	RF	BF-LD	BF-RD	LNF	RNF	X^2
n	32	32	10	10	11	11	
Sequential Motor Test	12	2	8	8	1	0	28.73*
n - (%)	38%	6%	80%	80%	9%	0	*
Fist & Ring Test	15	8	8	8	1	0	17.96
n - (%)	47%	25%	80%	80%	9%	0	**
Tapping Test	23	24	8	8	0	1	4.73*
n - (%)	72%	75%	80%	80%	0	9%	

LF - Left frontal, RF - Right frontal, BF-LD: Bifrontal-Left dominant lesion, BF-RD: Bifrontal-Right dominant lesion, LNF - Left non-Frontal lesion, RNF - Right non-Frontal lesion. n = Number of Patients; * $P < 0.05$ ** $P < 0.01$

factor that impairs ability to maintain the rhythm rather than losing perception of the rhythm and the ability for its reproduction. Luria described impairment in kinetic melody because of premotor area lesions. The results of some of these tests in patients with focal cortical lesions are given and discussed in tables 9 and 10.

Table 10: Number and Percentage of IFL and NF Lesion patients with Impairment in Sequential Motor, Fist and Ring, Fist and Outstretched Fingers and Tapping Tests

Lesion GROUPS	No. of Patients	Sequential Motor Test	Fist and Ring Test	Tapping Test
Dorsolateral	18	0	5	10
		0	36%	71%
	Lt (9)	0	4	4
		0	80%	40%
	Rt (9)	0	1	6
		0	20%	60%
Anterior Medial Frontal	14	2	3	11
		7%	21%	78%
	Lt (7)	2	2	4
		7%	67%	36%
	Rt (7)	0	1	7
			33%	64%
Posterior Medial Frontal	17	7	8	13
		41.17%	47%	76%
	Lt (8)	7	7	7
		100.00%	88%	54%
	Rt (9)	0	1	6
		0	13%	46%

Finger Tapping test is the one, which is found to be most significantly affected in frontal lobe lesions in right handed patients. Non-frontal lesion hardly has any effect on the test. This is followed by Fist and Ring test and Sequential Motor test respectively. However, within the frontal lesions, there is no clear indication of lateralization of the deficit, except in the case of Posterior Medial lesion patients. In these patients, the left Posterior Medial lesion appears to have very significant impairment compared to the right lesion cases, except in Finger Tapping test.

Encoding

12

Encoding is a complex cognitive process in the brain. In the neurocognitive context, it is referred to as the process of assigning meaning to sensory signals received in the brain and generated from the brain. On the one hand, encoding would therefore refer to the neural process of coding the sensory signals received, which would mean interpretation of the signals, when the signals are converted to information in the brain. On the other hand, the brain creates auditory and visual signals and even body movements assigning meaning, which is also an important part of encoding. The process of assigning meaning to signals received in the brain and the reverse process are based on the knowledge database available in the brain. The knowledge base is acquired in the brain experientially and conceptually (Mukundan 2007a). Encoding would therefore include relating the incoming signals with the assigned meanings to the existing knowledge and experiential base. Encoding is the first processing step carried out by information already stored in the memory on the sensory signals received in the brain. Recognition is therefore the first encoding step that happens in the brain. Recognition can be a complex process as the signals may be interpreted using a huge data bank and the recognized entity may have meaning in a large spectrum of relationships. Thus, one who sees a dog running first and then a boy running in the same direction after a few seconds may recognize the event as 'boy chasing the dog'. However, recognition and encoding cannot be equated to the same neurocognitive process. For example, one may see a creature somewhere nearby, and he has the following options of recognition: (1) it is a human being,

(2) it is a male or female human being, (3) it is a child, adult, or old person. On the other hand, one may recognize the creature as his daughter or wife and not just as another human being. There is an ocean of difference between the recognition as another human being and as one's daughter. When we listen to a speech, we recognize the words spoken. However, what we listen to are not the phonetic images of the lexical configurations. We listen to the meaning conveyed through the words and respond to them. Detection of meaning and assigning meaning are the true encoding process, both involving wide spectrum semantic interpretations.

Meaning is a reference to an entity, its physical and functional properties conveyed symbolically or semantically using symbols and words. Names are used for identification of each entity, their physical appearances, and properties. Words are used to refer to their movements and interactions. Meaning may be generated at concrete, functional, and abstract levels. The Global Language Monitor states there are more than one million words in English language, though the number was a little more than half of this about 100 years back. These are words and meanings created by human brains over hundreds or thousands of years. A word is an auditory expression made orally, using sounds by an infant. Starting with babbling, the child learns phonological strategies, and utters more appropriate word sounds. Interestingly the child learns to comprehend mainly through operant conditioning, the contextual meaning of sounds and words before learning to utter words. Later the child learns to make an orthographic representation of the same word. Use of words for representing internal and external conditions, like pain and heat respectively are learnt later in the development. Once words are learnt, the child starts using the words for referring to the objects and persons in speech as well as mentally. After using auditory or verbal equivalents for names, words are learnt to express a state of the object, which could be the self or an external object or entity. These expressions could be "baby hungry", "baby paining", "baby hot", etc. Development of self-identity and learning language helps the child to become more expressive and use the language differentiating self from the rest and say, "I am hungry", "dog is hungry", "dog is running", etc. Further developments in language skills bring about amazing capability to use language for communication and thinking. Need to babble and utter words, is quite intense in normal developments. The child displays feelings of achievements. Language development and brain development progresses simultaneously and language for communication and thinking may become the most important tool in many children. Simultaneous developments of psychomotor and visuospatial skills through drawing and constructive performances contribute to the development of other cognitive processing abilities in children. Mastering competency in the use of language can turn out to be an immense experience requiring extensive practice and need of knowledge of the several complex language algorithms.

One has to learn the words and their meanings and learn how to compose the words to convey meaning. These are the words and symbols used to refer to atomic particles and their properties, physical materials and their properties, plants and their growth, animals and their behaviors, human beings, their behaviors and emotional and intellectual pursuits, and biological basis of life. Encoding is the neurocognitive process of recreating and creating meanings for communication and as part of creating (thinking) new ideas and relationships for explaining various phenomena in the world. When one sees a figure and calls it square, the brain of the individual has identified certain relationships in the signals received, which qualify it to be called as square. The process of creating complex meanings and relationships could be a long and continuous process. Organized verbalization is made as per the choices and the language resourcefulness of the individual, and according to the needs of a situation perceived by the individual. Emotions play an important role affecting articulation and semantic interpretations and may be present in varying degrees as per the choice of the speaker. One who listens or reads the sentence has to decode the meaning or recreate the meaning, which one anticipates was the meaning created by the speaker. Both intellectual and emotional empathy play important roles in recreating the meaning, which the listener anticipates or claims that the speaker wanted to convey. This is done by recreating a meaning using the same words so that one believes that he has comprehended the meaning created by the one who spoke or wrote the sentence. Words are joined for creating or recreating meaning using information already stored in memory. If stored information does not help to recreate or create a new meaning, it would mean creating new relationships, which may start with the use of available information in the knowledge bank and progress towards defining new relationships hitherto not known. Relationships verbalized may be imaginary and conceptual, or with reality verified features of the world. Hence, such encoding of imaginary happenings or events need not necessarily have reality verified solutions. When encoded relationship reflects reality, it is by choice. We can encode or conceptualize situations, conditions, features, and objects, which are purely imaginary and not rooted in the known real world. Encoding therefore facilitates creation of new possibilities, concepts, and hypotheses. It may be possible to create new realities using those hypothesized relationships, provided we succeed in creating the materials and the unique functional relationships, which form the hypothetical model. Encoding helps in creating new organizations at conceptual and reality levels. Organizational structure of the meaning or the ideas verbally created depends on the sequential arrangement of words and constructs created using those relationships.

Gershberg and Shimamura (1995) reported in one of their early studies, impairment in the organizational strategies during free recall of related and unrelated items in patients with frontal lobe lesions. Their study showed that both encoding and retrieval processes are impaired by frontal lobe damage and they suggested that CES has a role in the formation of organizational structures in the meanings created. Neuroimaging studies have shown significant left prefrontal activation in association with encoding tasks (Tulving et al. 1994a, b; Fletcher et al. 1998a, b, 1997, 1995) and they observed that the left dorsolateral prefrontal area was engaged in the mediation of formation of organizational structure involved in the abstraction of relevant semantic attributes of information. Fletcher et al. (1998a) observed that the left dorsolateral prefrontal area was engaged in the mediation of formation of organizational structure involved in the abstraction of relevant semantic attributes of information, and they commented that, "This abstraction enables an assessment of the commonalities and differences which is the basis for segregating and grouping material to optimize encoding." Encoding involved in perception of familiar entities may be simple and based on retrieval of already known and relevant information. However, encoding new relationships may be complex and difficult both for creation as well as for understanding. There is generally greater demand for deducing relationships or meanings in the events occurred and occurring. Creating statements related to plans of actions, which cannot be easily detected and monitored are always difficult. Creating such relationship using semantic interpretations is indeed encoding at the most complex level of thinking, as in subjects like mathematics, biological sciences, and physical sciences. Thinking is the encoding process in which meaning is created using internally spoken words. Creative encoding does not have to be only at verbal or semantic levels. It could be part of creative visual arts such as painting and sculpturing. Nonverbal sensory experiences, responses, actions and emotions are generally verbally transcoded, which help their communication as well as self-analysis. Such transcoding may not generally take place online while the individual is acquiring the experience. One transcodes the experience after the autobiographic episode is over or at a later stage while remembering the same episode. Encoding is therefore, the most significant cognitive process in the brain which makes perceptions meaningful, and which allows creation and communication of ideas and concepts. Encoding helps to create the major repertoire of the human mind in which one is always engaged in meaningful dialogue and interaction with the self, others, and the word.

Language Systems of the Brain

Language represents the ability of the brain primarily for communication with other brains. Though children learn language as an auditory molded verbal skill, they learn visually represented language fast in the early stages of development itself. Language is the ability to attach meaning to words and symbols and use them for expressing meaning as statements and ideas. As language is used by everyone, a common code is evolved to communicate the meanings, ideas, and concepts using common words and their organizations. However, language is a changing tool encapsulating the needs of the time and the people and their ideas, and hence it goes through continuous changes. Though primary use of language is for communication, it has become the tool for self-expression. It is used as tool to imagine by which one can create ideas and hypotheses, which can be reality verified or one can leave them as fictional thoughts. An imagined idea need not be part of reality and there is no compulsion for its reality verification. One can imagine for the sake of imagination; and through imagination, one can create a world of choices, which need not be governed by laws of nature. It has helped to propose alternate possibilities and hypotheses explaining realities, which can be tested for reality verification. The proven hypothesis denotes the law of the universe and the knowledge of universal laws has enabled humanity to control and change nature.

Language processing has been traditionally related to the Wernicke's and the Broca's area in the left cerebral cortex. The Wernicke's area and the Broca's area have been called the listening center and the talking center respectively of the brain. The two speech centers have been traditionally considered interconnected by arcuate fasciculus. There is also the Geschwind's territory in the parietal cortex, which indirectly interconnects the Wernicke's and Broca's areas during the developmental stages of the brain. The anterior segment of this connection interconnects Broca's area with the inferior parietal lobe and the posterior segment interconnects the inferior parietal lobe with the Wernicke's area (Catani et al. 2005; Catani, ffytche 2005; Anderson et al. 1999). The extensive anterior posterior interconnection in each cerebral hemisphere by superior longitudinal fasciculus, which interconnects the posterior temporoparietal junction with the ipsilateral frontal cortex, serves to exchange signals across, and the signals are available to the contralateral hemisphere through the corpus callosum (Makris et al. 2005).

Three speech systems that have localized representations in the brain are the phonetic system for recognition of speech sounds, the Broca's system responsible for producing the motor images of words, and the Lexical system responsible for storing the words for use at the speech receiving and expressive junctions in the brain. These three functional systems are based in localized brain areas, whereas semantic interpretation may need inputs from extensive frontal and temporal areas in the two hemispheres. The Wernicke's area is the speech reception center whereas the Broca's area is the speech expression center. The Lexical system was proposed by Damasio et al. (1996, 2004), who proposed the lexical systems at the storage of memory of different categories of lexical representation of words. The lexical system is proposed as an independent nonspecific system, which accesses the right words based on the orthographic or phonetic image of the word, but on its own does not use any modality specific information, expect providing the name or the word. The lexical system reconstructs the phonemic structure of the word from the concept used. Concepts are of actions, names of persons and animals, and the name of objects. The concepts of actions are represented in the left frontal areas, and the concepts of names of persons and animals in the left temporal area. Names of objects are represented in the left parietal areas. Lesion studies show that lesions in one of these specific areas produce area specific impairment to reconstruction of words (Damasio 2001, 2000; Jobard et al. 2003).

Language Processing in the Two Cerebral Hemispheres

Semantic interpretation is the core processing function of language used for recreating meaning for understanding and creating meaning for communication and expression of ideas. Several clinical and neuroimaging studies in the past two and half decades, have established the involvement of extensive left and right frontal and temporal cortical areas in language processing, though the left frontal and temporal involvements are considered stronger (Cooke et al. 2006, 2003; Cutting et al. 2005; Humphries et al. 2005; Dietz et al. 2005; Crinion, Price 2005; Hoeks et al. 2004; Martin, He 2004; Constable et al. 2004; Capek et al. 2004; Friederici et al. 2003; Heim et al. 2003; Jobard et al. 2003; Ruchsow et al. 2003; Booth et al. 2002; Baumgaertner et al. 2002; Friederici 2002; Homae et al. 2002; Roder et al. 2002; Keller et al. 2001; Saykin et al. 1999; Wildgruber et al. 1999; Chee et al. 1999; Dalla Barba et al. 1998; Wise et al. 1991; Demonet et al. 1992; Petersen et al. 1988). From the processing point, syntactic and semantic processing are the main functional roles played by the cortical areas. Of these, the semantic processing is of vital importance as this consists of encoding for creating and recreating meanings from simple to complex levels. Semantic processing involves sequential use of words appropriately connected with each other, according to syntactic rules, so that intended meaning can be created or recreated. Comprehension of written and spoken speech involves semantic interpretation for recreating the meaning, which one considers as the intended meaning conveyed by the person who has spoken or written the document. Semantic processing may also be significantly influenced by emotional state of the individual. Speech comprehension or semantic understanding takes place spontaneously, or through sequential processing. Contextual understanding may play important role in creating and recreating (for comprehension) the meaning. As in the case of visual perception, only minimal information (Biederman 1987) may be generally used by one to recreate the meaning while hearing/reading a familiar conversation or topic. Sequential and deductive processing are two important reasoning methods used for creating meaning. Non-articulated speech expressions constitute the thinking process, the enigma of human brain-mind. In an earlier study, Petersen et al. (1988) demonstrated that auditory and visually presented words engage multiple and parallel routes in the brain during the different stages of phonological processing and semantic encoding. Auditory sentence comprehension is associated with the primary auditory reception, in which the left Wernicke's area is activated (Crinion, Price 2005; Rodd et al. 2005; Kuchinke et al. 2005; Jobard et al. 2003; Heim et al.

2003; Chee et al. 1999; Stowe et al. 2004). Crinion and Price (2005) could also find activation of the right lateral superior temporal region during sentence comprehension. They elicited evidence for the right temporal lobe participation in narrative speech. Study by Cutting et al. (2005) also revealed right hemisphere participation in sentence comprehension, though the involvement of the left temporal area was stronger than that of any right side involvement. Visual inputs of verbal materials access the same audio processing centers for comprehension (Hall et al. 2005). They found that auditory speech was seen to activate bilateral superior and middle temporal gyri. They could find activation of the left middle temporal gyrus, the inferior parietal lobe during lexical processing in spoken speech. During auditory speech generation, bilateral activation of the superior and middle temporal gyri was elicited. Dietz et al. (2005) could elicit bilateral activation in the motor, auditory, and extrastriate cortex in the read aloud condition in comparison with read silent mode condition. Capek et al. (2004) found that audio-visual presentation activated the right anterior and middle lateral sulcus. Bilateral activation of the angular supramarginal gyri was seen during stimulation by non-words (Homae et al. 2002), whereas phrases produced activation of only the left inferior and middle frontal gyri.

Language is more than what speech represents, though the language function has developed in the brain as a sequel to speaking. Speech is an expression of language, as brain can conceptualize a mental world and the multiple interactions in that world through language. Speech is essentially used for communication, whereas the orthographic representation of speech has values far beyond mere communication. Music is evolved from the same speaking abilities, though music grows into an independent domain for experiencing and expressing emotions of love, happiness, sadness and many more, including some sublime states, normally identified as spirituality. That one can speak without articulating, i.e. think, is another immensely rich functional capability. Additional functional endowment arises from the fact that one can think as well as concurrently follow it up by listening to the thoughts created within, knowing its source of origin as the same brain. This functional capability becomes the launch pad for the development of verbal awareness (Mukundan 1999, 1998) in the individual.

Prosodic Effects in Language Processing

There have been several neuroimaging studies, already discussed above, which have demonstrated that some of the language functions are processed by the right frontal and temporal areas of the brain. The emotions and the context in which speech is spoken and heard have a premium effects on the meaning created and recreated. Emotionally modulation of speech is part of speech intonation, which is called the prosodic effects of speech. Decoding the meaning based on the emotional content of speech is equally important aspect of communication. This appreciation of the emotional contextual meaning of the words is interpreted by the right brain (Ladd 1996; Buchanan et al. 2000; Friederici 2002, 2001; Mitchell et al. 2003; Taylor, Regard 2003; Stevens 2004; Poeppel et al. 2004; Humphries et al. 2005). Buchanan et al. (2000) posited evidence to confirm that prosody is lateralized to right frontal and temporal areas. Friederici (2001) reported that inferior frontal and temporal areas bilaterally supported auditory language processing. He further observed that the neural effects of syntactic-prosodic interaction preceded the effects of syntactic-semantic interactive processing in auditory speech. The right hemisphere involvement is required only for the detection of the emotional effects in speech but also for mixing the emotional effects into speech. Activation of the right middle and superior temporal gyri in prosodic tasks was reported by Mitchell et al. (2003). The right hemisphere involvement in language processing was demonstrated by Taylor and Regard (2003) using split visual field reading studies, which has important indications for language rehabilitation of aphasia patients. What the listener finally comprehends is the combined left and right hemisphere processing effects. Recognition of emotional contents in speech provides the true meaning used by the speaker. Stevens (2004) differentiated the neural mechanisms of voice recognition from word recognition, which he proposed is lateralized to the right cerebral hemisphere. Using separate voice and word recognition tasks, which included memory for tone as non-speech comparison, word related activation was seen mainly in the left frontal and bilateral parietal areas. Voice recognition related neural changes were seen in the left temporal, right frontal and right medial parietal areas. The author concluded that partially right lateralized Frontoparietal network engaged in the rapid recognition of the tonal quality and identification of the voice and it is different from the verbal working memory seen to be associated with the left temporal and parietal neural structures. It has been also found that predictive perception of spoken or written words as often described as spontaneous understanding is also controlled by the right areas of the brain. Poeppel et al. (2004) observed that left hemisphere engages in lexical decisions whereas the right hemispheres carries out recognition of frequency modulated tonal quality of the words. A semantic interpretation can only follow these two types of recognitions, though recognition of prosodic aspects may be needed only in selected conditions. Humphries et al. (2005) reported that detection of prosodic effects was associated with activation in bilateral superior temporal gyrus in the dorsal regions of the anterior temporal lobe. Detailed meta-analysis of research findings in this area is available in Mukundan (2007).

Studies have shown that right frontal and temporal lesions take away the ability of a person to appreciate humor and wit. Deductive reasoning is yet another important aspect of understanding, which requires participation of the right hemisphere areas. Logic specific speech network as in the case of left hemisphere speech areas has been postulated in the right frontal, temporal and basal ganglia structures. The engagement of the right hemisphere is therefore very important for all deductive reasoning, which may form backbone of all creative efforts in science and technology. The left hemisphere specializes in the semantic interpretation or transcoding of the results of the right hemisphere contributions not only in speech but in all diagrammatic and visual representations of various phenomena investigated.

Thinking Brain

13

Mind from Language

Thinking is encoding using words and we call the mental products 'thoughts'. Thoughts are one of the several of the following viz., transcoding details of experiences, or new plans dealing with problem-solving, decision-making, new adventures, or mere unfocused thoughts. There are people who find it difficult to think, whereas there are those who are always filled with thoughts. Thinking easily becomes a habit, if learnt to practice it in the early years of growth. Irrelevant and untimely thoughts can interfere with other cognitive processing and performance. Thinking is also called inner speech (Morin 1993, 1995; McGuire et al. 1996; Siegrist 1996). The neural processes that take place in silent reading and thinking have common features, as they both require semantic interpretation by the fronto-temporal areas. The medium used are mostly words, even though thinking or internalized encoding may take place using symbols and visual imageries. When words are not articulated, i.e. expressed using the voice cord, they are still expressed mentally or within the Broca's area in brain and hence it is called internal speech. As there is no articulation, another person has no objective indication that one is thinking, though thoughts can be listened to and monitored by the speech receiving centers in the same brain. Hence, though thinking remains a private process, which we call a mental process, it is self-monitored. In other words, thinking can be considered a method of developing a mind. In thinking, there is a clear effort to use words and symbol for expressing an idea. The idea is mostly meaningful to the brain it creates it, though one may often wonder about the meaning of the thoughts created within, especially they are created by mere indulgence. As part of thinking, one often creates images of visual designs and then transcode the visual designs, though such transcoding may sometime take long periods as one may find it difficult to encode the visual relationships using words and symbols. One may use the picture of a square or circle as symbolic expressions for the benefit of the self or for communication to others. Use of language for understanding the realities around develops into an infinite domain of the mind, as mind is developed using the resourcefulness of the brain and from the ideas created. Language is used as the instrument for the development of knowledge in each brain. Language serves as the medium for communication across brains and documentation for each brain. Language is the medium used to understand the various relationships that constitute reality or the real world. Language helps to conceptualize all natural phenomena, their compositions, and interactions. The two dimensions of existence of reality of the universe known to the brain are that of time and space. Both are important for knowing the happenings in the universe and the rules of physical existence and changes in the two dimensions of existence. Information created about any change in reality must be organized in terms of their temporal and spatial relationships. When information created by mind is organized in terms of temporal sequences, it is considered to reflect the real relationships in reality. Learning language for communication is different from learning to think. Thinking is an internal process and it is used for creating strategies and solving problems. Thinking may be in a positive or negative direction in some. Negative thoughts have highly disturbing effects on emotions and behavior. Over encoding, under encoding and defective encoding become the personality basis for negative attitudes and development of negative stress reactions in many individuals. On the other hand, spiritual thoughts may serve as positive thoughts in many facilitating hope and personal strength to handle difficult life situations. Words and meanings used as part of cognitive behavior therapy, psychotherapy, and counseling have immense effects on the thought formulations and contents, and emotional states of clients or patients. As these need extensive discussion from the point of view of stress controls and emotional management of people, they are not attempted here. As thinking can be self-monitored, one can become aware of the thoughts created and it gives the immense opportunity to change the thoughts and encode desired or most effective meanings, before they are expressed or executed. Thinking takes place intentionally, or unintentionally as it becomes habitual. In unintentional thinking, thoughts are generally related to the self and topics of interest to the self. It is considered immensely worthwhile for children to learn to think, as it is in the early years, one must acquire the habit of thinking.

Reductionism, Rational Thinking and System Approach

Physical sciences and mathematics can be understood only by knowing the sequence of changes that occur over time and by learning to relate those changes and deriving the principles contributing to the changes. Once the principle or the rule that determines changes across time is understood or derived though thinking, then explanation of the observed phenomenon becomes possible. This would mean that one must go forward or backward, but strictly sequentially breaking down events or phenomena until one is able to derive the principles that contribute to such natural sequences, and they are formulated and expressed. Knowing the sequence of changes that occurs in reality is different from knowing or deciding the sequence of signals into the brain, as it could always be influenced by personal biases and subjective interpretations. The latter cannot be said to align fully with the sequences that exist in reality. Experiences of the brain are affected by several interpretive biases in the brain; the sequences cannot be accepted as true, unless the sequence is experimentally proven. However, these are domains, which constitute the framework for scientific disciplines.

Language ability allows the human brain build a mental world of its own. The human brains learn to restructure the external world according to the values mentally defined. There is no way they can alter the rules of realities and needs of survival, but they can accomplish the same using imagination, which make the journey adventurous and creative. Instead of drinking water from a lake, men builds castles, where they sit in highly decorated air-conditioned courts and drink specially purified water from silver glasses, even though there is no natural lake for hundreds of miles around. They can travel far beyond their feet can take them. Though they cannot fly, they have built vehicles, which can fly and take them across the planets. The biology of the natural and created needs is the same, but the needs associated with desires and ambitions are accomplished in the style created by them. Purpose, as a creation of the human mind, needs to be defined first. This can be done only using language. Once a purpose is defined, then it becomes necessary to identify achievable goals and plan the strategy to arrive at them, for serving the purpose. This is the context for considering the entire purpose driven and goal directed journey of life. This can be understood, defined and carried out only within a different model of existence, which we call the 'system' model. Working within the system model, we learn to understand as well as develop the principles that must be followed for such achievements of life. The concept of the system model used here may be considered different from the ontological and epistemological views of the General System Theory models proposed by Ludwig von Bertalanffy (1962, 1974) and several others. The major effect of the manifestation of purpose directed behavior is the need for self-regulation. As behavior in the System model cannot be always explained by stimulus-response conditioning principles, it is necessary to evaluate the navigational pursuits and reward effects of the spectrum of behavior on the brain. Judgments and decision-making based on personal values are important features of system thinking, as system represents groups of individuals with specific purposes and navigating in different directions for achieving their goals. Judgments and decisions are to be made for facilitating such navigation using goal directed behavior.

Purpose is defined as a justification for the continuous efforts, one is expected to engage in covering long periods of life, for achieving specific goals. Such purposeful acts bring out specific results and achievements, facilitating sustenance of the purpose within individuals. We have learnt to create institutions for serving such purposes for the entire society. We speak about the purposes of learning and education, marriage and family, working and serving an institution, etc. Man needs to define all purposes incorporating the assets and liabilities of human behavior, which would help to determine and serve each of those purposes. We learn to manifest large spectra of behaviors for serving the non-biological needs, generated by our desires and creative thinking. Though the system approach may have a large spectrum of psychosocial components, it is also interlinked to the psychobiological states of the body and the brain. It is indeed the human brain, which consciously and unconsciously desires, speculates, and struggles to achieve the goals, and finally attain the satisfaction and pleasure of those achievements. They need to work with the natural forces in these endeavors, which would mean knowing the realities of the nature, and developing expertise to alter as well as create new realities, which foster the systems they build. Each of these endeavors may be unique requiring immense amount of thinking for planning and designing models of strategies for developing vehicles to take them to the targets. These thinking efforts may need to be highly creative as well as productive, and hence may involve different thinking strategies and algorithms. Reductive thinking is obviously the most powerful method, which takes one near every particle of reality and changes in the various domains. Water becomes steam when it absorbs enough heat, and if water loses heat, it becomes ice. Water cannot become ice absorbing more heat; such reversal can never happen and the idea is against law of nature. The amount of heat required to change the state of water may vary in different conditions. This form of analytical thinking forms the base for understanding the reality of the nature. For creating new phenomenon or a reality, we must learn to imagine creatively and then make them a reality. Whatever physically created would only follow the physical laws, but the products created serve manmade purposes, which are unique to the human mind, though not part of the rest of the nature. Therefore, purposive behaviors need to be analyzed using non-reductionist point of view. This is where system thinking which incorporates parallel or holistic thinking is required, and human behavior has to be understood from a system point of view. Efforts to change behavior and cultivate new behavior need a system support. The values of life are created through thinking. They are creatively encoded for specific purposes with specific goals and navigational plans for achieving them.

Estimation of Time by the Brain

The brain has no biological clock using which one can read or become aware of the events that took place at a particular point in time or by which it can go to a particular point in time and retrieve the information stored at that point in time. Each brain indeed may have a huge data bank of knowledge, which constitutes its knowledge of the world, and from where it has to retrieve the required blocks of information. We call such retrieved information as experiences or autobiographical episodes or conceptual information. The brain is a time locked machine, which can go to its past only event or episode wise (Mukundan 2007a). Retrieval of conceptual information have immense knowledge value for dealing with various exigencies of life. Remembering experiences acquired in the past allows one to bridge the present with the past. We infer the time of occurrence of the specific events from their remembrances. Brain computes time as the difference between episodes or experiences. Subjective time estimation may be severely impaired in several neurological and psychiatric disorders (Sadock, Sadock 2008). Inability to remember past events take away memory of those times and subjectively the present is detached from the past. This is generally discussed as a memory disorder. However, the loss of subjective time estimation has a highly debilitating effect on the individual's perception and understanding of the organization of the sequence of life events and capacity to make reality contacts and verify the contacts.

It is very important to note that external reality and the dynamic changes and movements of the parts of this reality occur even if they are not perceived by the brain. The brain learns to acquire information of these changes using the capabilities it has, and the tools it has created. It is a truth that the world we know is the world sensed through the tools we use. Time is an inferred knowledge, unless one keeps track of it using external measures. There is no direct perception of time though we commonly speak about knowledge of time elapsed. The concept of time arises only when there are two events and it is the difference between the occurrences of the two events. Time and space are accepted as relative references, since the theory of relativity was propounded by Einstein. Time is the difference between two events. Time is estimated or inferred when body movements and external movements are perceived. The difference in the occurrences between two heartbeats is understood as the dimension of time. There are several bodily rhythms related to respiration, food intake, and wakefulness, which one experiences, and the difference between two consecutive rhythmic events is understood and estimated as the time elapsed. Time and space are mutually dependent relative notions, which join matter or reality. Experientially, each brain has its own estimation of time and therefore, one cannot objectively communicate subjective sense of time. We remember the sequence of events, what came first, second, and so on. As the brain cannot go back in time, it goes backwards event wise during retrieval. The events may be complex ones like an experience of immense joy or sorrow, or of any other personal significance, or a simple one like remembering or listening to piece of conversation, or reading a passage. Time estimation of past events can be made simple and accurate, if the events are documented with appropriate records of timing of their occurrence, which is called the source memory. Once an event is to be remembered and its time of occurrence thereby established, then one can make a subjective estimation of the timing of other antecedent and precedent events. The temporal and spatial (place) coordinates of past events known to one are part of the source memory, which serves as the gates to the past events. There is nothing like perception of a past time. The present may be perceived moving faster or slower according to the movements of sensory-motor effects, one perceives, and it may be a function of the patience/impatience, one has for achieving the goal. If the brain fails to detect a change in an experience, like sensory-motor effects, it fails to know the passage of time. The mental state of timelessness or time staggering occurs, when one fails to notice movement. Social movements are more important than mere physical movements for knowing the elapse of time and its estimation (Mukundan 2007a). It has been reported that long social isolation (Wadhavan, Mukundan 1985) resulted in the loss of passage of time in the participants who were subjected to such isolation, though they could move around, read, write, and carry on with physical exercises. The participants could not make mental estimation of the time they spent in each activity and the interval between two, and if it were day or night. The mental state accompanying mental and physical activities have a direct influence on the mental perception of time. Time appears to stall in monotony and boredom whereas it speeds up in challenging intellectual and physical activity. The only way to correctly measure time elapsed is to detect it as multiples of a fixed interval of occurrence of a physical activity, which moves or occurs at constant speed or rate.

A simple example of time locked brain can be demonstrated by the following example. If the participants in a workshop, are asked to comment on the correctness of the following statements, almost all will readily say that the first is wrong and the second is indeed right. The problem is "if x = 10, then x = 30", and "if x = 5, then x = 5". The question that easily arises with regard to the first statement is "'how could x be equal to 5 when it equal to 30?' or how x be equal to 10 and 30". Interestingly, any computer will accept this statement as correct and accept it, because it will take that if x = 10, then x assumes the value of 30, as these are conditions occurring at two different points in time. If x = 10 at a given point in time, it can take the value of 30, the next moment. X can continue to have the value 5 at different points in time, and hence the second statement too is acceptable. We perceive several things occurring around us at the same time, as we are often looking at the same objects and entities, and hence fail to see any appreciable change occurring in them at different temporal points. We presume that many objects and entities do not easily change their physical states and hence continue to appear the same, even though time is continuously changing in relation to all events. State of reality and accompanying conditions keep changing even though the brain may fail to detect the progression of reality and the related elapse of time.

Despite the fact that the brain is time locked, it learns to recreate the past as well as anticipate the future. The brain recreates the sensory and motor imageries of experiences or episodes earlier participated, which allows the brain to relive or re-experience the past. Tulving (2002), who pioneered and developed the episodic memory formulations called episodic memory a "marvel of nature". Remembrance of the past bridges the time gaps between the past and the present, and makes one experience the present as continuation of the past.

Serial and Parallel Processing

Computer analogies of sequential and combinational circuits connecting inputs and outputs are too complex and difficult to use as examples of information processing methods commonly used by the brain for various experiential interactions with the reality. These manmade processing algorithms do indeed function in various contexts, indicating their accuracy, acceptability, and possible presence of the same methodology as part of the physical laws in the universe and in the brain. However, the focus here is on the algorithms, which each human brain consciously cultivates and applies in everyday life. These applications are experiential, and form important part of establishing personal contacts and verification of reality. The merit and superiority of a manmade computer is essentially the amount of data and the complex mathematical steps it can process, for which, the brain is a poor example. Neural signal processing within the brain and encoding of the neural signals forms different methods as the latter is dependent on the recognition of the neural signals and the information each brain draws from the signals received or created in the brain. There is no doubt that the neural signals received from the sun and the moon in the human brain or in many animal brains is the same today and thousands years back. However, what the sun and moon mean to these brains today and in the past are not comparable, as the amount of information encoded from these signals are massively different. What the brain recognizes is determined by the knowledge base available in each brain, and the knowledge base each brain uses has been continuously changing or expanding. There is no evidence to consider that the brain is genetically endowed with any certain specific processing (thinking algorithm) method, which would expresses itself, as several other functions are developed and expressed. Thinking or more specifically encoding ability has to be cultivated and taken to higher levels through constant exercises. The brain does have the immense natural capacity to learn and develop rational processing capabilities, unless clouded by other emotional needs, both of which no other manmade system presently has. The brain can make critical decisions based on the sensory-motor effects encoded in the brain, and they can be assembled to create novel ideas or notions. The brain can engage in complex sequential and parallel processing almost simultaneously as it encounters realities. It learns to interpret the incoming signals using huge knowledge bank acquired and stored in the memory. The brain finds inadequacies and errors in its own explanations and creates new logical relationships, which can offer better or more accurate explanations. The relationship interpreted may belong to the present, the past, or the future between sequence of events and across multiple events occurring in succession and simultaneously. Available knowledge base is used for explaining the relationships detected, or they are predicted or hypothesized, requiring further verifications. Explanations using linear relationships are adequate for understanding most of the phenomena of the physical world, whereas they may altogether fail when it comes to explanations of human behavior. Large spectrum of human behavior has their origin from within the brain, as they are not initiated by external stimuli and conditions. Such behavior need to be understood from a system point of view, as such human behavior cannot be explained in terms of a biological survival model of "flight-fight" reactions. Human emotions of love, affection, compassion and forgiveness, and readiness to offer the self (self-sacrifice) instead of resistance change the whole algorithm of human behavior from what is seen applicable in the rest of world. The realities of the world within which it finds happiness and sorrow, are mostly its own creation.

The dichotomy of serial and parallel processing has its origin in the differences in auditory and visual signal inputs into the brain. Auditory inputs are always serial, one after the other and the only relationship the brain can encode is between two signals, in the order they arrived. On the other hand, visual signals pour into the brain simultaneously from large spatial contexts, and one has to always compare one signal with the adjacent ones and the total effect is to be drawn from the arrays arrived in the brain. The temporal sequence is the main characteristic of the auditory inputs whereas spatial parallel effects are the features of visual inputs. A Gestalt perception is the normal outcome of the visual inputs, whereas we strive to understand two auditory stimuli or words from their temporal relationship. The need to explain all events in the world from a serial point is understood because of their temporal sequencing and the opportunity to break down large spectrum of stimuli into temporal array where we can sequentially follow up the changes. The human brain is habituated to creating information for explaining the multitudes of physical changes that occur in the world. Thinking is the method used for creation of such logical information. Thinking reflects the use of various processing dynamics described under serial and parallel processing, known also as inductive and deductive thinking. While listening to another person or to a voice delivery system and while reading, the verbal comprehension that takes place within the brain involves holding on to the words heard or seen for short periods so as to assemble them and create meanings from the assembly of words. The meaning created is the information created and comprehended. A meaning can be extracted only by considering the contextual and other accompanying details that occur in the same timeframe in the individual. Either the whole sentence must be held in the span of attention or one must hold on to some of the words, which one considers significant, so that an anticipated meaning can be recreated. While listening or reading, it is a recreation of the meaning as a meaning has been already intended by the one who generated the sentence. The listener has to recreate the same meaning from the inputs received. However, as in the case of all perceptions, one can anticipate or predict what one has yet to hear and recreate the meaning even before one has heard or read the whole sentence or the text. This is often called the intellectual aspect of empathy (Richard, Grinder 1975a, b; Goldberg, Goldberg 2002). When the meaning cannot be anticipated, it becomes necessary to carefully examine the word assembly and recreate only the relevant part or unit of information, which may have been created by the words assembled by the one who made it. If there are other meanings, one may recreate them too, but not accept them as the intended meaning. However, this needs a very critical attitude to the processing, which may not be present in many, because of which they may infer meanings that were not conveyed. The meanings extracted can directly influence self-evaluations, interpersonal relations, and personal well-being of individuals. As human mind thinks in terms of strategies for fulfilling self-generated wishes and ideas, which aim at creating new comforts and realities, it is necessary to think within a system model. Rational thinking must also consider a new dimension as it has to incorporate navigation for achieving the self-defined goals. One has to start with intentions and acquire skills and knowledge all through the journey to the goals. Rational thinking falls short as the process cannot incorporate self-defined purposes and goal directed behavior. Reaching goal is definite only if a path exists and one knows the path, and one may have to learn to create a path according to one's wishes and plans. 'Game theory' (John von Neumann) is an excellent example for system thinking, which takes into account all self-made strategies and goals (Aumann 2008; Dutta 1999). This makes it imperative for one to anticipate effects of planned actions, as well as the effects of realities that may emerge from the endeavors of other minds working with the same frame of interests. Such thinking would demand the participation of both the left and right cerebral hemispheres. Luria (1966a, 1970, 1999) had earlier described this as bilateral speech as it required frontal lobe involvement bilaterally.

Independent comparison of serial and parallel processing is possible, though the brain may use them concurrently, and several neural structures may be commonly involved in both the processing. Even though semantic interpretations forms the foundation of language, the signals interpreted incorporate large amount of visual inputs. Therefore, serial and parallel processing methods are constantly needed for understanding large part of the world that we live in. Serial processing is the choice method when we deal with the large spectrum of physical phenomena, whereas we resort to methods that are more comprehensive when we deal with the behavior of other individuals and their organizations. Both sequential and parallel processing may be used in several neurocognitive tasks such as speech production, speech perception, thinking, planning, and problem-solving, etc., which are the methods of processing used by the brain as a computing organ while dealing with the world outside. Choice of processing depends on individual preferences and the abilities acquired and deployed by the brain. The processing methods used can be brought under conscious control and self-analysis and hence they can be applied or withdrawn intentionally. However, biological propensity in the brain is to learn behavior as well as response patterns through conditioned responses and operant conditioning, as they are important for survival and growth. The left hemisphere superiority in sequential processing and the right hemisphere superiority in parallel processing have been already discussed in the earlier sections. Michael Wertheimer's (2000, 1989) immense contribution of the Gestalt theory is a unique and important principle that speaks about brain's propensity to perceive the visual world in totality than in parts.

Retrieved information from the knowledge base serves as the basis for encoding. Words are identified using their auditory images during reception of speech and the meanings of the words and their contextual references are used to generate meaning of the spoken speech. Encoding therefore helps in recreating familiar meanings or new meanings. However, when new meanings are to be created, it would require careful sequential processing and understanding of the context facilitating creation of new meaning. This is always a slower process as any error in understanding the sequential relationship can result in gross errors in comprehension. Therefore, when new meanings are to be created, predictive encoding may not always be the best choice. Encoded meanings may be directly written to linked memory base or remain isolated when such links cannot be established. Encoded information may be impersonal or personal as it may form part of autobiographic episodes or may have only conceptual value. Errors in encoding viz., overencoding, underencoding and defective encoding, etc. lead to severe cognitive dissonance and produce resultant emotional and behavioral problems. These have to be understood and managed by learning the strategies developed in each brain, and the capacities and limitations that exist with regard to information creation in each brain. This has been the subject of studies leading to development of therapeutic efforts for cognitive restructuring in individuals (Beck 1975, Beck et al. 2003, 1979; Ellis 2004, 1994, 1977; Ellis, Grieger 1977). Cognitive restructuring therapies have established as one of the most effective psychological treatment for various disorders viz., depression, anxiety, phobia, borderline personality disorders, and ADHD, etc. (Frojan-Parga et al. 2009; Pull 2007, Kanter et al. 2005; Taylor et al. 1997; Linehan 1993).

Efficiency in encoding is determined by the speed of comprehension and the extensiveness and accuracy of the meaning that one may generate while listening and reading, as well as while thinking, writing, and speaking. Encoding is therefore, a cognitive ability that one must carefully learn and develop. Encoding may be carried out at concrete, functional, and abstract levels using words or symbols. One may understand meaning of an event or expression even without expressing it verbally. However, the efficient use of encoding helps to analyze critically the various components of the event or the phenomenon. This can be documented and used for communication with others. The major effort of encoding is to find and express a rule or a principle that would explain the occurrence of a phenomenon. This can be done after careful examination of several events or cases and if they all show the same sequential relationship, i.e. a condition is preceded by another condition or state every time, the first condition is considered to precede and indicate or determine the following event. The three inner angles of several triangles of different shapes can be measured and when they are always found to sum up to 180 degrees, then it is considered to define the principle that determines a triangle. Similarly, we know that the sum of inner angles of a square is 360 degrees. This is considered a general principle or a fact and that said conclusion could never be altered in any place and time. On the other hand, an inference or conclusion can also be made based on an accepted general principle, which may not have been verified and accepted as fact. The former uses inductive type of reasoning whereas the latter uses deductive reasoning. If the general principle drawn from the induction method is used for explaining a specific event or observation, its accuracy may be as accepted, as the general principle has been already verified in several independent repeat observations. However, this cannot be said about general principles that we draw from experiences, especially when the experience has not been verified by repeat occurrences in other individuals and different occasions.

Diagrammatic Representation of Language Processing

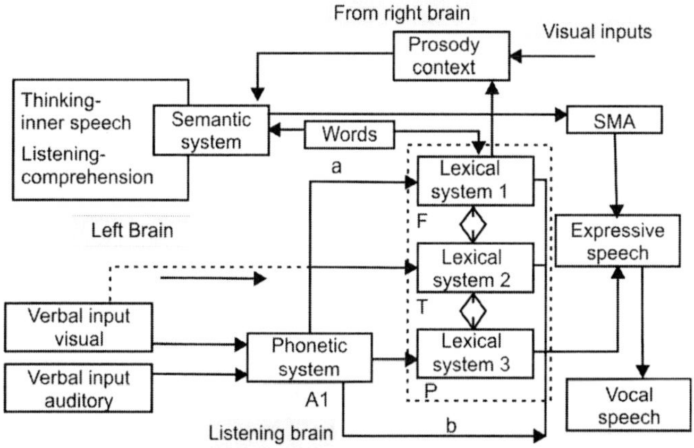

Mukundan (2009)

Verbal Monitoring

Awareness is proposed as the knowledge, the brain comes to possess of the sensory-motor processes taking place within. Since it is the knowledge of a processes taking place within the brain, it occurs only online, i.e. when the processing is on. It is the brain coming to know of what the brain-mind is processing, an outcome of self-monitoring. The brain does not automatically develop awareness of an ongoing process. It has to monitor the process for becoming aware it. The state of knowing taking place while monitoring may be called awareness. Awareness in this sense and context is to be differentiated from perception-recognition. Becoming aware of is to be differentiated from the knowledge base possessed by the brain in the memory. Awareness is an online development of knowing that the brain is engaged in sensory-motor activities. Awareness can occur only when the brain is monitoring itself while processing.

One monitors the sensations produced by various muscular activities like breathing in and breathing out, chewing, swallowing, movement of the limbs, etc. The perception of sensations produced by these movements takes place in wakeful condition and the sensory experiences are a way of knowing the bodily activities and the body making contacts with the external world. The sensory experience serves as a modality specific awareness of the movements. One can move the hand or imagine that one is moving. However, the neural activation pattern associated with the movement of the hand can be produced by actual movement or by imagination of the movement. Normally one can differentiate between the two. There cannot be awareness of hand moving, without moving the hand unless one is imagining the movement. However, imagined experience of movement is indeed different from real experience of movement as reality contacts are not established in imagination. It is not the neural activation pattern of motor activity that differentiates the two, but the fact that one allows contact with reality, which could offer continuous and varying degrees of constraints and opposing effects, whereas the other is an imaginary contact with reality. Imagined sensations do not take one to achieving the goals and help redefine realities. The brain has to come to know from the sensations that it is in the process of moving the hand, once the process is initiated. Preference to experiencing the reality to imagining the reality develops as a personality trait in individuals. Explorative risk taking encounters with reality are part of adventures of individuals, which take them to discoveries and creation of new realities. Awareness is the same as online recognition of movements and it ceases when the movements are stalled. The brain learns to infer the stalled state, when sensations are not recognized. There cannot be awareness of a processing when the processing itself has not taken place. One may remember processing taking place earlier and even could recreate the imagery of making efforts to process. One remembers an earlier attempt to process and may remember even having awareness of the processing, though may not remember the contents of the processing. This indicates that the occurrence of awareness of a processing is stored, though the contents of the processing cannot be reproduced from that awareness.

Verbal awareness has the same etiology, except the contents recognized and monitored may be own thoughts generated as inner speech or articulated and written speech. Since the source of thoughts is within or in the same brain, which is engaged in recognizing them, verbal awareness is a special ability, as it is a form of self-awareness. As the human brain develops the ability for verbalization as the chief method of communication, and verbalization is used for creation of ideas and they are stored as orthographical documents, verbal awareness of these and their remembrance form large spectrum of continuous mental activity in most individuals.

Transcoding

Transcoding is verbal encoding of all nonverbal experiences. Transcoding may take place online or while remembering the experiences. Recognition without transcoding forms the primary level of perception.

Level 1—Perception: Recognition without naming—clock, painting, photos, flowers, light, switch, books, paper, pen, computer. Recognition may take place in other sensory modes viz., olfactory and somatosensory too, while eating, moving around, etc. Most of people make attempt to name them only when they need to communicate with others. They would recreate the imageries if there were need to remember them.

Level 2—Verbalization (Encoding): Recognition with naming—clock, painting, photos, flowers, light, switch, books, paper, pen, computer. Verbalization needs additional mental efforts. When recognition is of objects and entities in familiar surroundings, one often recognizes them without verbalizing them. One may transcode them later during their remembrance, if there is a need. One often passes through familiar routes and places, without making efforts to name the familiar objects and persons encountered.

Level 3—Verbalization (Transcoding): Nonverbal experiences are transcoded. Online transcoding requires greater mental efforts, as one has to select the words and encode them to create a meaning. There are some individuals who habitually transcode, whereas most do not online transcode. They go through routine sensory experiences without making any effort to verbalize their experiences. Interestingly, during remembrance, one recreates the imageries or recalls the transcoded details, if it were attempted in the earlier occasion, without recreating the imageries. The latter is indeed faster, though the accuracy of the transcoded details may pose problems if the original experience were provocative or emotionally disturbing. This is the platform for all cognitive therapies. Accuracy of transcoded details are also questioned and debated in eyewitness evidences.

Had the sensory-motor experience been already transcoded online, one can straightaway recall the transcoded details instead to recreating the imageries and then start transcoding the imageries, which may use much lesser brain resources. Recreation of imageries is a sure and reliable method for remembering several types of information, which have clear visuospatial correlates, in everyday life. This may be easier, than the retrieval of verbal details, as the former can be done even without accessing the source memory, whereas verbal recall can be isolated and accuracy depends on the efficiency of the original transcoding, carried out while the brain was also processing the sensory-motor components of the experience. Later transcoding induces people to find justification for the actions witnessed, and the possibility of erroneous judgments is high in those who do not critically review their transcoding. There cannot be a verbal awareness of any experience without transcoding the sensory-motor components of the experience. However, even a hearing and speech handicapped person may learn to express the act of looking at an object by gestures, and would use it for self-monitoring.

Development of verbal skills provides the unique capability for verbally transcoding the visual, somatosensory, olfactory sensations and all motor effects in subtle manner and polished manner. Additionally, it has made possible to develop complex monitoring and regulation plans in the form of syntactic rules (Caplan 2006) for verbal expressions. The visual effects can be verbally planned, and the executed visual effects, monitored by the visual system can again be verbally transcoded and analysed. This supportive and interactive help can be used by all other sensory systems along with verbal transcoding and using the accompanying verbal analysing and synthesizing abilities. Verbalization of most of nonverbal sensory effects and motor effects takes place almost automatically in most individuals. It explains the dominant position of transcoding and the immense scopes of verbalization in exercising sensory-motor controls. Without verbal or thinking support, animals do indeed learn to overcome physical impediments for sensory search of the external world. Thus, a monkey or a rabbit would climb over a tree or a blockage to have a better vision of the area blocked by a natural growth or wall. If transcoding does not take place online during an experience, people normally carry out the transcoding during the remembrance of the episode. This may be carried out for communication, documentation, or as part of personal indulgence during a remembrance session. Transcoding helps to relate the various components of experience, the presence and the behavior of self and others, emotional effects, and thoughts that controlled and propelled the actions and the specific context of the episode in the life of the person. These various aspects can be related to one another only through transcoding. However, the advantage of transcoding is the resultant awareness, which help one to understand, judge, and explain own behavior. Awareness helps to rearrange the transcoding for critically justifying own understanding and behavior. On the other hand, if it is a planning of an action, most of it occurs at a conceptual level, except using the imageries of familiar entities and person and connecting them with all other variables.

Speech Receiving Centres Monitoring Speech Expression

Auditory verbal medium is the most powerful platform for the brain to engage in communication with the other members of the human society. Wernicke's area was identified long back as the centre for speech reception, and the Broca's area as the centre for speech production. Speech processing requires involvement of several other areas. The talking brain and the listening brain are interconnected through the arcuate fasciculus and the pathway through the left inferior parietal cortex (Geschwind's territory, Catani et al. 2005) so that the processed signals in the two centres are easily exchanged with each other. Both speech reception and expression require lexical, syntactic, semantic processing. Of these, the semantic interpretation has the widest scope and hence the involvement of brain resources for such processing is found maximum. Contextual and emotional effects in semantic interpretations play very important roles. The same functional systems in the brain contribute to these diverse processing needs at the receiving and the expressive ends. Thinking and speaking are common in many respects except absence of articulation during thinking. The most significant aspect of speaking is the communication of own thoughts, whereas thoughts remain as inner speech and they may not be controlled by the effects of speech produced in the listeners. When thinking is in process without adequately defined objective, thoughts may occur in parts and unconnected, though one can work on these aspects later. The interconnecting pathways allow the listening brain to monitor the thoughts created and this was postulated to produce verbal awareness of the thoughts as they are being created (Mukundan 1996, 1999).

Since the same syntactic and semantic systems are used for interpretation of meaning of speech and thoughts, self-created, as well as received from other sources, the knowledge source serves as a common repertoire and their expressions lead to verbal awareness of the thoughts and speech expressed. Listening to the thoughts created or recreated facilitates their verbal awareness, which helps in monitoring their meanings and making judgments of their appropriateness in terms of syntactic accuracy and anticipated effects. Habitual talking enables each one to express words almost automatically while speaking in familiar situations. In several situations, one may have to think and talk i.e. create and recreate meanings using words until one knows (becomes aware of) that one has made the best meaning possible and then speak them out. However, for listening to the thoughts created within the self, one need to attend to them and listen to them as one would listen to speech heard from outside. This may need one to withdraw attending to other stimuli from outside world so that attention can be directed inward to the thoughts being created.

Words used for thinking and speaking may not be always discretely selected, especially in information situations; several words and their expressions may be used more as habit. As thinking is a private affair, these effects may be significant. Automatic expression of words or speaking is a common phenomenon in all individuals in selected situations. These expressions are made most commonly as responses to others. One may not often have opportunity to select the words and speak, because of pressure of time, exigencies and associated anxieties, and one will then listen to the words only after they are articulated, provided one makes effort to understand what they really said. If one has the chance or habit of selecting words before they are articulated, the listening brain has the chance to monitor them and help the brain anticipate their effects and select the most appropriate words to create the best effects. This process may take time, which one may not have during a normal conversation or discussions, unless one is a trained and habitual thinker. However, one can practice and develop the habit of creating quick internal rehearsal with selected words and assemble them, which one considers most appropriate and effective in a given situation, and then speak them out. Thinking and writing are therefore important methods for creating new ideas and concepts as it allows one to reformulate the words used and their assemblage any number of times, until one is satisfied about the content or the meaning created. This is indeed the best method for becoming aware of them and for their recreation to achieve the best and critically most accurate effects. Since one may think or transcode one's own state of mind and emotions, comforts and discomforts, needs, desires and ambitions, goals and plans, and the actions which one intend to execute and responses already executed, one has the opportunity to become verbally aware of large domains of the self-related conditions and activities. One may even think about earlier efforts to think and remember, even if one may not recall their exact contents, as already mentioned. Since we keep frequently transcoding our sensory-motor experiences, the same transcoded verbal details are monitored by the listening centres and produce a state of continuous verbal awareness of those transcoded experiences. Vivid remembrances and their verbal awareness together could become intensely traumatic. Creation of verbal awareness facilitates self-monitoring as one has the opportunity to develop verbal awareness of various nonverbal processes and closely monitor the sensory-motor effects. Listening to own thoughts and speech therefore, creates verbal awareness of the self and its activities, which remain private and personal until and unless they are expressed to others. This helps to change action plans before they are executed and even during execution. Awareness of the thoughts provides important matrix for their critical examination and making decisions. One start practicing thinking intentionally in the early stages of development, but soon it could become a habit in most, when one keeps verbalizing everything one sees, hears, feels and does as a habit without any efforts. However, this does not mean that verbal awareness would follow automatically, as there are many who fail to report verbatim what they were thinking, as found in large personal surveys of thoughts of individuals in connection with cued remembrance of experiences (personal communication, Mukundan 2010, 2011a). That would need special efforts and time to monitor what one thinks and says which probably not all develop. Those who readily speak out may not bother to monitor what they have said, whereas those who speak out less, but speaks within (thinks) have a greater chance to monitor their own thoughts. This would develop faster when children are encouraged to practice critical thinking, which can be ensured in the early stages if they are asked to speak out their thoughts or ideas about specific observations. One can think critically only when one monitors what one thinks and says, i.e. when one learns to become aware of what one thinks and says. Only a few would pause and monitor own thoughts, many would not do it. The ability needs to be cultivated as part of educational programs. However, verbalization of imaginary and anticipated experiences and the verbal awareness that follows may make it appear real and inflict trauma to the individual, if one does not know how to resolve the conflicts and stress created by it.

Learning to Think

Learning to recognize speech sounds and articulate them referring to external objects, persons, and drive states of hunger, thirst, etc., are the earliest milestones of language development. The child learns to use words explicitly and implicitly and the implicit use of words develops into thinking. Streams of thoughts keep occurring in some children, whereas some have to be facilitated to think. Each child develops a unique language style and thinking pattern. Thinking becomes a habit in many and they wonder how varied thoughts keep occurring without efforts. Many children, especially girls are known to become verbose from very early years of development, articulating words and small sentences, which they have learnt from parents, for self-controls and as warning to anyone else whom they observe may need them. For example, a two and half years old girl speaks out “be careful when you walk there” not only to herself, but anybody else she sees walking in a certain place. Speech generation becomes a conditioned habit for many, depending on the habits of parents and teachers, and the encouragement they provide the children with, which facilitates both encoding and transcoding skills as reflexive self-controlling processes. What a growing child learns to start with is to verbally transcode experiences and needs, rather than encoding. Use of language may start and end with mainly transcoding in many. Encoding is a complex process used when language skills are used during verbal communication and for creating meaningful concepts and ideas. Using language for relating other persons, objects, other entities and events take place at concrete and functional levels. Using language at abstract level needs intensive training and practice, which is imparted mainly in classrooms. It is indeed important that one must learn to engage in disciplined thinking in later years, as one learns to discipline oneself in terms of responses and expressions at the behavioral level. This does not easily happen as thought creation is not monitored by others, and it does not often become a matter of concern for individual's social discipline and preservation of social norms. It is equally important that growing children be trained in not only learning to observe social norms, but also learning to think and reflect on the need for the same. Training children in developing various conditioned responses may be easy, but making them think about the need for the same behavior could indeed be difficult. There is also need to think intentionally for creating meaningful ideas, carry out problem-solving exercises, which can explain reality relationships. These exercises are extremely more important than learning solutions, as it helps to train them in creative thinking for problem-solving, in the early stages of development. Intense emotions, anxiety, and tension could have a detrimental effect on creative and positive thinking. Once practising encoding and transcoding become habitual, it becomes easier to channelize and organize these effects. There are also those, who visualize more and transcode and encode less, and may be nonverbally creative. It is often claimed that there is a visual and/or nonverbal presentation of new ideas and relationships, which may remain submerged for long periods, before one is able to verbalize—encode them for the person to becomes aware of them. The visual inputs bring signals directly from the visual reality and one may recognize important relationships in the visual inputs, though one may not be able to verbalize them. Verbalizing those relationships needs very creative and persistent efforts. This is when some individuals feel and express that they have something to say, though they are unable to explain, as they themselves are not aware of them. One struggles mentally to give expression to the 'unknown idea' (?), until one succeeds in expressing it as an idea. Once the thought is created, one can become instantly aware of it, and can work more on the idea. Artists may express the 'unknown idea' through colors and lines or through sculptures.

Once the habit of thinking is developed, one needs to be careful to see that thoughts are about relevant matters. If thinking has become a habit, then positive efforts have to be made to regulate the contents of the stream of thoughts, and that one does not indulge in thinking about irrelevant, violent, and antisocial matters. Thoughts also trigger emotions and imageries and they may have their own effects on the individual and his behavior. Irrational and provoking thoughts may have distracting effects reducing the accuracy of other voluntarily initiated thoughts. Indulgence in unlimited and uncontrolled thinking and creation of fantasies could take one away from making reality contacts and reality verifications. Thoughts can become disturbing when they arouse negative emotions, which may again interfere with efficient critical thinking processes, and even sleep. An easy method, many follow when thoughts prevent them falling asleep is to "count sheep", or repeat words, or chant phrases. When one intentionally engages in such activities, other thoughts and their disturbing effects recede and the person falls asleep.

Semantic Interpretations

Semantic interpretation is the method of assigning meaning to each word and creating meaning from the syntactic assembly of words. Semantic interpretations may be therefore, for simple communication across people, or for creating definitions and scientific explanations, for imaginative poetic narrations, etc. and the relationships or the meanings may be assigned at concrete, functional, and abstract levels. Other than linguistic semantics, we speak about the semantics in programming language, formal logics used in scientific explanations, and the use of signs and sign processes in non-linguistic sign systems of expressions. The semantics used in poetry is significantly different from the semantics used in normal communications. Only a few may have the poetic imagination and creative thinking required to encode the semantics of poetry, whereas there may be more who have the capacity to appreciate it. Semantics of sciences or logical thinking can be practised only after learning the fundamentals of each speciality. The non-linguistic sign systems comprise of the entire range of signs, movements used in various dance forms, and the communications expressed through movements in animals including insects (Beynon-Davies 2010). Understanding the semantics of movements in dance is again complex as only a few learn them and practice. Each child learns the semantics of normal communication from infancy and hence it is the strongest in most. Meanings may also be drawn from facial expressions, body language, and emotional effects used in spoken speech. However, during critical thinking, the extraneous effects and biases are to be excluded or not considered, so the meaning is created by words and symbols according to the best possible relationships that could be sequentially established, simultaneously considering the effects of different factors that may influence the relationships. The role of the Frontal cortex for creating meanings or semantic interpretations of all forms is obviously clear, and this may be considered the most unique advantage human brain has developed over all other known brains.

The knowledge base already available in the brain and that the brain can access from external sources are always used for interpretations. It becomes extremely important that those who want to share the meaning created by another must understand the meaning from the same platforms in which it was originally created. Semantic interpretation during creation and understanding a meaning could equally be scientific or may need same experiential resources. Creation of meaning may depend on mere identification of a known meaning or creation of a new meaning in parts or full. Creation of new meaning takes place when new relationships are elicited. The process may go on until one has a rationally satisfactory statement or explanation of the new phenomenon. These new relationships may be an attempt to explain a physical, physiological, psychological, or social phenomenon newly recognized or experienced by an individual or an effort to apply better explanations to an already known phenomenon. The new explanations may be based on already known processes, knowledge of reality, or they may open new vistas of understanding and possibilities, which need to be verified. Human history is full of instances of varied explanations of life and the universe created from the varied knowledge banks available to them from time to time. Understanding is only part of the game for human beings, their true achievement is in learning to control and create reality from the knowledge base they have created. The neural involvements used for large spectrum semantic interpretations in the brain may have wide area-wise representation, though speech reception and expression have specific localization. Extensive frontal, temporal, parietal, occipital, and subcortical engagements have been established during applications of different aspects of language. The role of the frontal and temporal lobes in complex semantic interpretations have been established in several studies (Cooke et al. 2006, 2003; Cutting et al. 2005; Humphries et al. 2005; Dietz et al. 2005; Crinion, Price 2005; Hoeks et al. 2004; Martin, He 2004; Constable et al. 2004; Capek et al. 2004; Friederici et al. 2003; Heim et al. 2003; Jobard et al. 2003; Ruchsow et al. 2003; Booth et al. 2002; Baumgaertner et al. 2002; Friederici 2002; Homae et al. 2002; Roder et al. 2002; Keller et al. 2001; Saykin et al. 1999; Wildgruber et al. 1999; Chee et al. 1999; Dalla Barba et al. 1998; Wise et al. 1991; Demonet et al. 1992; Petersen et al. 1988). These bilateral frontal and temporal involvements in language processing have been discussed earlier, other than the specific roles of parietal and occipital lobes in language reception. One may use the entire potentiality of the brain in such creative efforts. Large sections of the brain, especially the frontal cortex is found to be involved in the recognition of novel effects and their interpretations. Study in hypnotic trance (Mukundan et al. 1999, 2013) has shown how recognition can be significantly altered or totally blocked by hypnotic suggestions and how the suggestions affect the electrophysiological functions of the brain. The changes seen are the effects of influencing the interpretive role of the frontal cortex, even though the processes associated with sensory registration remained intact (Gruzelier 2006; Mukundan et al. 1999, 2013) in the participants. The Frontal cortex is the primary resource center of imagination and all creative efforts are the products of that imagination. The human brain can also transport several of the ideas from the imaginative levels to reality.

Imagined ideas are expressed at verbal level, or using shades of colors and lines as in artistic works, or using body movements. There may always be unique methods of expression of imagination. Auditory and orthographic verbal expressions are made using words and symbols and the meanings are made at various levels of understanding. Language allows us to use words for representing persons, other living species, hundreds of thousands of objects, conditions, changes that occur at physical and functional levels and multitudes of relationships that exist across space and time. Language is used to represent and express the customs, attitudes, value systems, and beliefs of the people, which distinguish and separate the psychosocial, cultural, and religious practices and abnormalities of the people dwelling on the earth. Rapaport (1998, 1999) proposed while dealing with the mind-brain relationship that the mind is an abstraction implemented in the brain. He equated the whole process of semantic interpretation to a process of implementation of a program in a computer, which processes and implements a specific idea using various rules of data management and computation, at abstract or concrete levels (Rapaport 2005).

Monitoring Nonverbal Expressions

There is no evidence to consider that a verbal type of awareness may occur in nonverbal modes. For example, can a visual awareness of visual recognition be present? Can we differentiate a phase of visual awareness different from visual recognition or visual imagery? Visual recognition takes place only when a known entity is externally identified. The term perception is used to refer to the entire sensory processes that start with the sensory monitoring of the external world, when sensory signals are transferred from the receptors to primary sensory cortex, creation of the external sensory model, and the process of its identification from the memory traces, if a matching internal model is present. If recognition fails, perception leads to creation of a new internal model, which forms the basis of learning in the brain. Perception is also used to refer to the way one looks at behavior and ideas of others.

Monitoring the External and Psychic Worlds

Attention is considered the state of processing in which the number of independent sensations processed by one may reduce to a minimum of one, when one considers attention most focused. As the number of items attended increases, attention is said divided, as the system has more related or unrelated pieces of information for independent processing. Attention shifts from the focused one to another, either because of the stimulus characteristics of the intruding stimulus or intentionally, as per a system demand. The complexity of the information processed may be considered an independent challenge to the system, as mere reduction in the attended items alone does not contribute to enhancement of information processing demands. Attending to own breathing or any other singular process alone does not enhance information-processing capability of the system. It may indeed train the system in selective attention. True challenge to information processing is in the ability to simultaneously attend to variety of blocks of related or unrelated information and the capability to detect unique relationships across the blocks and even process them independently. This indeed needs utilization of greater brain resources, which is not achieved by mere reduction in the number of stimuli attended. Attending to the inputs from the external world as well as attending to own thoughts and remembrances are the two domains between which the direction of attention shifts in an individual. Both are equally important for every human system, though task demands and their preponderances change across systems and situation to situation. A soldier or volunteer, who is given the responsibility to watch a territory or activity, should not withdraw or shift attention to within, unless it is very important (?). On the other hand, one who is engaged in a mental problem-solving task is not expected to attend to any external stimulus, unless there is a survival (?) threat. The ability to switch attending between the two is learnt during the neurodevelopmental stages. However, the challenges one may face during the developmental years may emphasize on one pattern rather than utilizing the two domains and switching across them. A child may obtain little opportunity to reflect back and introspect if he is forced to attend to external stimulus inputs all the time. On the other hand, another child may be prevented from facing the varying environmental inputs and forced to look into the self and fantasize, because of social and other pressures from the environment. A biological etiology cannot be ruled out, though this has not been singularly isolated and identified. However, discarding legitimate demands of attending to and processing of the external and the internal worlds could only result in biased understanding of the two worlds. If it happens in a growing child, it could become a pattern, which we would call a personality profile. The dimensions of extraversion and introversion may be the outcome of developing such dominant selective attending and processing profiles and its consequent effects in the individual. Carl Jung (1921, 1995) who was the proponent of extraversion and introversion, considered an extraversion characterized by "concentration of interest on the external object" whereas introversion is characterized by focus on "psychic activity". Eysenck (1967) who worked extensively on these factors as the basic personality dimensions considered sensitivity of the mesolimbic dopamine that extraverts have low cortical arousal and hence they seek greater social engagements. Sensitive mesolimbic dopamine activity resulting in higher rewarding effects was proposed by Depue and Collins (1999) in extroverts. A study by Johnson et al. (1999) demonstrated greater blood flow in the anterior cingulate gyrus, temporal lobes, and posterior thalamus of extroverted individuals, whereas introverts have greater blood flow in the frontal cortex and anterior thalamus, postulated to be linked with internal processing of executive functions viz., problem-solving and planning. As they prefer solitude and focus on psychic matters, they indeed may have poorer social engagements. Increased social interaction seen in the extroverts is considered a positive factor (Lucas et al. 2008). Nevertheless, these are in extreme cases, where socialization has built extreme attentional biases in some individuals. Normal socialization ought to make the individual competent to attend to both external and internal domains of the world equally smartly and efficiently, failure of which results in the differential attentional preferences.

Continuously attending and making judgments of own sensory-motor expressions make them personally more effective than carrying out the living process automatically without any or adequate self-monitoring. Such continuous attending or self-monitoring can become habitual, if one practices monitoring of the sensations of motor effects in a continuous manner, the associated experience becomes a lot more effective and satisfying. However, this does not mean that any separate awareness of the activities is generated. We learn to carry out several routine activities in automatic manner without specially attending to them. Thus, we may eat our routine breakfast, lunch, etc., walk around, and handle things in the workplace and at home with minimal attention, as they have become habitual acts. If one is mentally engaged in some other positive activity, this may be acceptable. However, if one is not mentally engaged in any other activity, and the routines are carried out automatically, then one may easily lose control over own attentional capabilities, and living can become an automatic process. Several recent studies and their reviews (Jain et al. 2007; Arch, Craske 2006; Brown, Ryan 2003; Jha et al. 2010; Garland et al. 2009; Wallace, Alan 2006; Piet, Hougaard, 2011; Manicavasgar et al. 2011; David, Kabat-Zinn 2008; Grossman et al. 2004; Bedford 2012) have shown that the practice of meditation, especially the practice of "mindfulness" type of meditation enhances the ability to focus attention and reduces stress responses. This in turn improves working memory performance and enables people to perform at their optimal efficiency, and brings in the satisfaction and happiness of doing their best. Attending to the bodily sensations as practised in 'mindfulness' makes a person becomes continuously aware of or recognize those sensations. Recent study by Hölzel et al. (2011) showed that practice of 'mindfulness' increased the grey matter density in the posterior cingulate cortex, the temporoparietal junction and specifically in the left hippocampus. The positive effects of practice of attention have been reported in superior performance, stress reduction, and positive thinking. Several recent studies have reported positive effects of 'mindfulness' practice coupled with cognitive behavior therapy in patients for the treatment of depression (Segal et al. 2002; Ma, Teasdale 2004; Piet, Hougaard 2011), insomnia (Heidenreich et al. 2006; Yook et al. 2008); cardiac rehabilitation (Griffiths et al. 2009), cancer rehabilitation (Foley et al. 2010) and psychiatric disorders (Chiesa, Serretti 2011). Continuously focusing attention to an online sensory-motor activity brings in only the continuous sensory awareness or recognition of the activity, which one learns to accept and acknowledge.

Nonverbal expressions may occur automatically as a biological response of the brain or one can learn highly sophisticated methods of nonverbal expressions. Facial expressions, body and limb movements, painting, sculpturing, and dancing are some of the methods used for visual expressions by human beings. These visual expressions can be mixed with emotions and they reach unique levels of meaning, which we may altogether fail to express verbally. Expressions and communication through visual medium is important especially when verbalization of an idea cannot be adequately accomplished or when one wants to support the verbal expression with a visual parallel effects. What are communicated in the verbal mode are not sound bursts and orthographic design, but specific meanings using words and meaning created by the assembly of words. We know that children and adults with problems in listening and speaking learn to communicate through gestures, writing, typing or printing. Several of the relationships verbally encoded in speech can be visually expressed and communicated. They learn to visually imagine those gestures when they want to carry out what we call thinking. They may be able to read instead of listening and write instead of speaking. A sign language is immensely useful for persons with auditory handicaps. The whole purpose of a sign language is for communication and for use of the visual signs indicating equivalents to names and verbs. One can assemble the signs and gestures to make a meaningful equivalent of names and actions and through them express an idea or concept. Using sign language and visual and somatosensory sensations for a meaningful and strategic control of behavior may not involve explanations at varying spatial and temporal coordinates. Most important is the fact that emotions in these individuals are intact and normal. Coordinating events at visual and somatosensory levels may be difficult, but possible, though it may require very creative efforts. If these handicapped people develop such capability, they may not only overcome the debility caused by the handicap, but may also develop extraordinary capability to handle their intact sensory-motor assets. They learn to interpret and create meanings using their own skills and get close to what others may reach through verbal expressions. They acquire not only knowledge from recognitions, but also learn to understand the personal significances of even small things whatever they recognize within themselves and outside. There is no independent knowledge system exclusively accessed by the handicapped, which is not shared by others. We cannot say the same about emotions that one may experience and express when verbal skills are absent. The visual expressions can be monitored and regulated only by the same visual system deploying appropriate motor coordination.

Logical Fallacies of the Mind

The property of a living physical structure to interact with its physical surroundings directly and indirectly has opened a new unique phenomenon in the universe. This is accomplished by the near 3 KG organic substance inside the head, which we call the brain in human beings. As the brain learns to explain and interpret semantically the experiences of the external realities, it learns to create new ideas and concepts, which form the foundation of the mind; the mind expands to unlimited horizons as human beings learn to live with reality using the meanings created in the mind. The physical world becomes integrated with the meanings in the mind, which guide their behavior. That the brain can create infinite number of semantic relationships results in the creation of statements imbibing both feasible logical relationships and logical fallacies, depending on the accuracy of critical thinking employed by each. The former may be reality verified, whereas the latter become fallacies, as they have irrational and unverifiable relationships and fail in verifications. However, the brain has the capability to create ideas in an infinite manner and thereby expand the mind; the creative capability of the brain-mind is not normally bound or controlled by the realities of the universe, unless the brain fails in the endeavor. There could be a relative causative effect in every creation, which we learn to scientifically explain and verify for formulating the relationships. However, reality verification of the explanations need to be carried out independently or the explanations may be attempted only after reality verifications. Scientific verification of the proposed relationships helps to systematically recreate them in sequential manner and create new physical realities, which becomes the power of human mind. The new physical realities created change the logistics, adventures, and expeditions of life, and the lifestyle. Experiential verification of reality indeed is the choice for making reality contacts and verifications in daily life, though taking this approach beyond the needs of practical living may result in erroneous explanations and judgments, and such explanations may become mere logical fallacies.

The semantic formulations and their expressions are used for creating symbolic relationships, used for communication of complex ideas to one another, when logical explanations fail. Thus, science fiction stories and movies, and many religious stories are full of paradoxical and ultraparadoxical entities and relationships. The processes and the contents of the mind attain infinite and independent dimensions. The mind enjoys making them stand apart from realities or as distortions of realities, as they contain ideas and meanings, which cannot be physically presented. The meaningful ideas or concepts created by the brain and the art of their creation constitute the human mind. If these ideas are taken away, what remains are only basic emotions, which may not differentiate the human beings from most of animals. Meanings are created by each brain and they share them and thereby developing a medium for sharing their mind, social practices, culture, and civilization. There are several thousands of meanings not shared by all brains and hence they do not share the same mind, even though they all have the same brain structure and neural processing. As the mind is not automatically evolved, but created from the brain, it makes the mind an independent creation and entity (?). The creation of the mind may be made through logical relationships, which are verified, or symbolic creative efforts, which may become logical fallacies. Such logical fallacies are often considered important domains of religious faiths. The most intense and explicit result of accepting, experiencing as a method of reality verification is the very development of immense faith in the experience. Faith in the experience one has had and the associated explanations may become the strongest reality verifying method for all, and many may believe that faith in experiencing is the only alternate choice for reality verification, as critical thinking and experimentation cannot be used at such levels and for such concepts, which they consider supernatural and extra-terrestrial. Faith may be the most powerful self-induced suggestive state of mind, which may affect all interpretations of a person influencing his recognitions and all other related experiences. Faith may provide immense mental strength to the one who entertains it, as the emotions attached with it can drive one almost endlessly towards the goal one has set for the self, without needing critical appraisal of any happening on the way. Some of the aspects of this experiential and individualistic pursuit may obviously be outside the domain of scientific understanding of mind and behavior. Intense sharing a faith or idea by a group of people may result in a process of group thinking (groupthink), when many individuals think and work together in a common and shared manner and they may fail to know the fallacies in their logics. This is an important construct of social behavior and needs consideration in System Theory approach to the study of behavior. Such thinking in harmony by a group, ignoring or sacrificing individual critical evaluation, could result in the formation of cult groups and their behavior. Group thinking may be considered an ideal method to achieve higher levels of dedicated work output in an organization, whereas such thinking may bring together people with logical fallacies in religious cults (Turner, Pratkanis 1998; Wexler, Fraser 1995).

Verbal Awareness

14

The presence of separate centres for auditory sensations and expressions has produced a unique functional system in the brain. This could be considered an extension of the characteristics of the physical attributes of auditory stimulation. The spatial and temporal characteristics of visual stimuli make them unique, but the brain cannot directly produce a visual stimulus. The visual world emerges in the brain because of the reflective effects of electromagnetic energy within certain frequency ranges, to which the retinal receptors respond. Even if the visual world does not exist if a functional visual receptive system (the eyes) is not present, the physical characteristics of the world indeed exist. Sensitiveness to light energy and the ability of the brain to monitor the physical characteristics of matter in various forms resulted in a visual world and the development of intriguing capabilities for visual analysis and synthesis in the brain. However sound, which is a by-product of vibrations is a unique form of mechanical energy, which may not directly contribute to any essential physical interactions in the universe. Unlike light, sound can be generated only in a medium and it needs a medium for propagation. Biological systems indeed use vibrations, for the detection of presence of obstacles, threat, and other living systems in the surroundings as well as for communication. These systems have developed necessary biological mechanisms for producing and receiving vibrations. Insects, water and land based animals detect vibrations and it is an important accessory for survival and communication within those species. Vibrations are produced and received by organs placed close to or outside the brain. The brain is used for the interpretation of the vibrations. It superimposes specific meanings or signals for communication on the vibrations, which their own organs produce. It necessitates that the biological signals produced by the receptors must be sent into the brain for their processing and evaluation, and the corresponding signals from the brain must be passed back to the vibration generating organs for creating similar meaningful messages. The capability of the brain to receive and produce sound has developed into extraordinary functional system in the human brain, which is beyond comparison with all other non-auditory modes of stimulus reception and processing. For example, we can hardly produce 'music' and take it to such heights of performance and appreciation using other sensory signals. Audio generation of music is easily accompanied by extensive motor skills, which results in the generation of musical notes using body movements and instruments. Change in small ranges of frequencies and intensities produced by the vocal cords create magical effects in the brain of the person who generates them as well as in the listener. Using the same principle, each brain develops millions of auditory or phonemic images, each with specific auditory structure and meaning. Our knowledge of speech centres in the brain is rather recent. Paul Broca in 1861 was the first to speak about a speech centre in the brain and then came the knowledge of speech reception centre from Carl Wernicke's (1874) works, that there are separate brain centres in one hemisphere, which came to be called the dominant hemisphere for the reception and expression of speech. A recent study (Dronkers et al. 2007) using neuroimaging technique has shown that expressive speech impairment is caused by lesions in the medial insular cortex. Control of articulation is important not only for speech but also for music. The clinical lesion studies show that lesions in the Broca's area almost specifically impair speech production ability, though it is not because of deficits in the vocal cords, and this deficit does not cause impairment of speech comprehension.

There is no evidence of an independent self-reflective state as awareness, though it is often used as an independent dimension of mind in philosophy. Verbal awareness in essence, is a self-reflection of the thoughts created or recreated.

Differentiating the world outside from own body and attributing it with the mind created through semantic interpretations is an important method of developing a self-concept and differentiating it from the rest of the external world. This referencing method helps to identify various sensations, responses and actions, emotions and thoughts as of the self. Self has been a difficult proposition in neuroscience as it has no structural basis, and it is not a functional state either. Brain does not appear to have any special processing associated with awareness, even though speculations have been made about such activation. Awareness is the brain knowing its own processes, and in that sense, it may be said to be a state of knowing. Thus, recognition is awareness, and hence contents of awareness are modality specific as the original inputs are modality specific and available only in the brain. The advantage of verbal awareness is that it happens when the motor outputs created as speech and thoughts are received back by the same brain and it comes to know online what it has been thinking or speaking. One can indeed draw or paint and visualize it, as it is in progress and after it is created. This visual awareness or recognition does indeed help to understand visual creation of one's own and that of others. One encodes meaningful relationships through the verbal medium and the faculty helps each brain to create ideas about everything that can be sensed and interacted across the universe, and concepts and ideas are created at functional, concrete, and abstract levels. Thinking is a continuous brain process in many, and the thoughts and their meanings help to create a mental world in each individual. Sensory and motor experiences linked with the thoughts created and the associated emotions become an intense representation of the self-creation.

From Sound Image to Meaning

A close analysis of generation of speech from sound helps to understand the nature of receptive and expressive speech functions. A growing child learns during the early years of development:

(1) Development of abilities to recognize specific speech sounds and express the same for referring to the self and

various external objects, and as instructions for specific response from self and others.

(2) That the speech sound or the word represented by it has a specific meaning, as each word refers to a specific object or movement (Skipper et al. 2007, Fadiga et al. 2007, Craighero et al. 2007). Meaning of the word is the ability one develops to remember a specific object, entity, condition, or the need to make a specific gesture, rcsponse, or action, whenever the word is heard or repeated by the self.

(3) Language develops when we start using sounds as:

  (a) Words (names) are used along with what they represent.

  (b) Words (verbs) are used when a specific action, response, or gesture is carried out.

  (c) The child is trained to execute or make the same response to the words (verbs) used.

  (d) Words are used to indicate the differences in size, weight, height, etc.

  (e) Words are used to indicate quality of objects, tasty food, sweet milk, etc.

  (f) Words are used to relate one object with another. This may be for comparing their physical structures and qualities, like one object is greater or smaller in size, weight, height, etc. compared to another object.

  (g) A word may refer to an object—the word makes one remember the object. A visual or somatosensory imagery or concept is produced when the word is heard.

  (h) A word may refer to an action—the word makes one remember the action. The motor imagery or a concept of action is created by the word.

Soon use of language becomes a method of programming the brain as Rapaport (1998, 1999, 2005) suggested. The brain soon learns to understand the meanings used by others using words and learn to create them by itself. The meaning is used as either a name or state of movement, with vast spectra of variations in each category. The meaning is understood only by the brain and hundreds of thousands of brains share the same meaning and learn to use words carrying those meanings. A meaning is indeed different from the word, and the associations are purely manmade though the quality of sounds used may have reflection on the meaning imbibed. We know that words are identified from the phonemic structure or orthographic design and the meaning is retrieved. Words are stored separately and appear to have greater localization in storage, whereas meanings have wide representation in the brain. On the one hand the brain learns to extract the meaning from the words heard, and on the other hand, it learns to express the meaning using words. Meaning can be established only after the selection of appropriate words, and only when one knows the physical and other relationships one wants to express, i.e. A is taller than B. When relationship is physical, it is at concrete or functional levels. Such relationships have functional values and one can gather the meaning experientially. When relationship cannot be physically represented, then it is said to be at a conceptual or abstract level. If there is a visual understanding of the relationship, one tries to express it using words. If the relationships can be easily visualized, then the verbal expression may be easy. However, if the relationship is not directly detected at a physical level, then verbalizations becomes complex and difficult for specification. Verbalization becomes even more complex when one wants to deal with concepts and conceptual issues and relationships. The speech reception involves extracting meaning from the words drawn from the speech sounds, while speech expression involves using the words for creating meaning and then internally and externally articulating them. Inner speech or thinking creates motor imageries of the words, though they are not articulated. Speech sound reception and expression are carried out by thc ears and the vocal cords respectively. Both speech reception and expression access words and their meanings from common repertoires stored in the brain dictionary. Meanings generated by assembly of words have to be created or recreated every time. This could be a complex and time consuming process, unless the brain can anticipate and predict a meaning, as it happens in normal conversations. Words selected and the meaning created may be expressed externally, orally or orthographically or they may remain internal, when we call it thinking or inner speech.

The expressive aspects are affected in the classical Broca's aphasia, which disables their oral and orthographic expressions. Similarly, in receptive aphasia, the process of accessing words and their meanings from the word images produced in the brain fails. This would mean that in expressive aphasia, the patients have difficulty in some type of inner speech, before it is sent down for articulation. They have no difficulty to make use of their voice cord and produce sounds, but cannot produce speech sounds. They understand words and their meanings, but have difficulty to carry out the reverse process of using words. Those frontal areas, which provide the semantic and syntactic interpretations, can still carry them out as long as the words are received in the brain, but their resources are not employed by the area or the centre for creating the stream of thoughts, which need to be expressed. A more recent neuroimaging study by Dronkers et al. (2007) revealed that the area affected in expressive aphasia is the medial insular cortex. What the expressive speech centers in the brain accomplishes is to select and produce words for creating the meaning supplied by the rest of the fronto-temporal areas and initiate the motor controls needed for the movement of vocal cords to produce articulation of the words. In nonpropositional speech, words are accessed spontaneously and automatically (McCarthy, Warrington 1984; Goldberg 1985), whereas in propositional type of speech, sequential selection of words are required for creating a desired or planned meaning. The latter indeed requires greater neural inputs accomplished by other areas like the SMA and the dorsolateral frontal cortex (McCarthy, Warrington 1984; Goldberg 1985; Nakai et al. 1999; Chee et al. 1999; Gyung et al. 2005; Alario et al. 2006). However, this means that words selected by the Broca's area are passed on for expression by the movements of the vocal cords. In writing, the mode of expression of language is through the hands and fingers, though the planning and generation of words and meanings follow the same rules as that in the inner speech. Distinctive receptive and expressive speech impairments clinically seen indicate that the functional impairment of the above two centers because of lesions or failure of functional capabilities. The two centers are interconnected, which help them to interact with each other. The involvement of left frontal and temporal areas in semantic interpretation indicate the extensive representation of speech in the brain. However, semantic interpretation may be considered to have larger contextual and emotional references, supported by the right frontal and temporal areas, indicating extensive left and right frontal and temporal involvement for creating meaning by words as part of language function.

Awareness of Remembrance

During remembrance, when one makes attempt to retrieve an autobiographic episode, the remembrance is further strengthened by the recreation of imageries and the retrieval of source memory. Such recreation of imageries and source memory are not needed when simple conceptual information is retrieved. Recreation of imageries is also a process of retrieval, as the imageries are stored as perceived and experienced by the person and hence may be recreated in full or part, with or without the same clarity. When one wants to remember a person, an object, or a place and if the name is not retrieved readily, we recreate the sensory imagery and then search out the names. One may retrieve the name of a person, object, or entity readily, when it is not necessary to recreate the imagery, making the recognition faster. This can happen only when the names are familiar and confirmative. If the name is recalled first and there is uncertainty about the content, then the brain may need to retrieve or recreate the associated imagery so that it confirms the name with the imagery. Failing to retrieve the name of a person, object, or a place after successfully recognizing the same is also a common experience. Recreation of imagery may often take place almost automatically and the retrieval of the linked name follows. The visual and verbal memory traces are stored in different locations in the brain and the two needs to be retrieved together, or one after the other. The two processes are initiated together by neural binding effects. Experience shows that visual imageries are stronger than verbal names in most individuals. Recognition and responses from the brain can take place most often automatically, even without having a verbal awareness of the same. The brain has to cultivate the capacity for self-monitoring, which leads to the creation of verbal awareness.

An equally important, but not well understood aspect is the temporal characteristics of remembered information and imageries. When a visual profile is remembered, or when the imagery is recreated, it appears, as reported by several individuals in their interviews (personal communication), that they can keep visualizing the imagery continuously, and most of them thought that clarity of the visual imagery was best when they first recognized the imagery. One can re-examine the visual imagery searching for the presence of different components! On the other hand, during retrieval of name, the auditory image appears transiently, though they can retrieve them (recreate the auditory imagery) any number of times. They cannot hold on to the auditory image of the retrieved name, as they can hold on to a recreated visual imagery. One transcodes the imagery as it is recreated, as well as attempts to retrieve its verbal description, if available. One becomes aware of the transcoded details as well as the retrieved information, and realises the discrepancy if it is present. One would remember the effort to remember a name or a piece of information during earlier occasions, even if one does not remember the content of the remembered item. Thus, one may remember several times, the earlier efforts made to recall a name, even though one failed to remember the name itself. One may even remember the details of how the name was finally retrieved from another source in the earlier attempt, and still not remember the name.

Awareness in Working Memory

Auditory signals enter the brain in sequential manner, unlike visual signals, and they generally have short temporal presence and then disappear cease to exist. Auditory units carrying verbal information indeed are very short; lasting for one or a few seconds and hence the online encoding must take place almost simultaneously. However, this makes it necessity that one must hold on to the different auditory blocks to encode them or extract information for further processing, in a sequential manner. Working memory operations are a product of this necessity. One learns to become aware of the verbal mental process, which facilitate their monitoring and corrections. Articulated or mental repetitions of the problems allow one to get back to any segment of the blocks of information and process them in any desired sequence. Presence of verbal awareness of a brain-mind process can be communicated by only one who is aware of the process. Recognition takes place often without verbal transcoding, and it serves as the awareness or knowledge of the source. Verbal transcoding most often used for giving a name for the recognized entity and one can instantly become aware that one has recognized the entity known by the particular name used. This may be followed by the transcoded details of the actions or movements recognized. Attention is directed to the external source during recognition, whereas it is directed to the blocks of information and plans of action, if any, held internally during working memory operations. Continuously attending to the internal blocks of information is a necessity for their proper processing. This stage of attending to internal information has been often described as the process of mentally 'holding' on to blocks of information (Mukundan et al. 1979a) and the executive plans. Information itself may be internally recreated or received from outside. Most of the working memory operations may require sequential processing and hence holding on to blocks of information that are being processed and still to be processed becomes necessity. The brain must first create the imagery for attending to internal information. These imageries may be mostly auditory or even orthographic and one may additionally have to attend to visual and other signals as part of processing. The processing demands are either externally received or self-assigned. Verbal working memory processing allows working directly with the meanings of the blocks of information. Interviewing individuals engaged in working memory tests has often revealed (personal communication) that they repeat the blocks of information, whenever required in the working memory operations, and they call this the ability to 'hold' on to the blocks of information. Holding on to the blocks of auditory information in this manner is carried out by mental repetition of the blocks of information. The blocks of information that need processing may have no other personal significance to the individual. Equally important is the fact that the processing or the execution of the action plan, when present, is done continuously without break. However there are indeed limits for the length of the array or blocks of information that can be mentally held on (Chen, Cowan 2005; Cowan 2001; McElree 2001; Mukundan 1996). Ability of the brain to recreate the same information repeatedly in quick sequence is used for such online processing. As discussed before, we acquire this ability for quick repetition through rote learning practice from early childhood. It is proposed the rote learning practice is important for developing the ability for working memory operations. One learns to repeat the same pieces of information in quick succession without being affected by their meaning, as long as the process is not interfered with any other intruding process or other blocks of information. Learning verbal materials by rote learning may therefore strengthen working memory ability. Working memory operations are important not merely for mental arithmetical problem-solving, but for all creative thinking when one searches for new relationships across variables. One needs to hold on to daily schedules, and other important assignments, which contribute to personal organization required for various achievements in life. Plans of actions received from outside and self-defined need to be held on for their timely execution. The plans and the blocks of information one may need to execute change according to contexts and responsibilities one share with family, friends, peer groups, and organizations. Working memory utilization for self-organization is important in every stage of life for disciplined performance and growth of each individual. The amount of information one can hold on and the complexity levels of processing determines the quality of performance and achievements of individuals. The execution carried out may not always be at the mental level, they may be associated with the initiation of actions and response in various contexts of life. One may use other skills, both mentally and externally expressed for applications/solutions of working memory problems. Many persons hold on to along list of appointments or work schedules for each day and for different periods in life. Normally, one does not have to remember the schedules intentionally, as one becomes aware of each action plan in the right time for one to execute it. Once executed, one does not have to hold on to the plan or other related information. Impairment in execution occurs if one cannot develop the awareness of the details of the mental task, if one fails to repeat the inputs and misses the correct details of the problems. It appears that most people carry a mental notepad with various daily schedules and appointments scribbled, and one keeps watching these notes for keeping up with the appointments and for carryout the different assignments in a sequential manner. Mentally holding on to such blocks of information may not most often require any further mental processing. One needs to hold on to such assignments only as long as one needs to attend to them. Mental execution is the second working memory phase, which could be a complex one as it may involve sequential processing of segments. This would make holding more difficult, as one may have to hold on to the subsequent blocks of information while processing an earlier block, as well as hold on to the results already obtained and proceed with processing in sequential manner.

Working memory is a necessary 'mental information management' ability required for all mental problem-solving and hence contributes to the intelligence of the individual, though specific abilities and skills required for processing must be acquired separately. The processing may require other skills like arithmetical skills, physical and biological engineering skills, visuospatial skills, language based and mathematical reasoning abilities. Verbal awareness developed while mentally repeating the problems and other semantic interpretations of a problem contribute to the monitoring of the accuracy of the working memory executions. Impairment in execution occurs if one cannot develop the awareness of the details of the mental task, if one fails to repeat the inputs and misses the correct details of the problems.

Awareness in Meditation

One can have a combined awareness of the results of the sensory-motor effects, their transcoded/encoded details and other neurocognitive processes such as remembrance of experiences, and their combined processing may contribute to higher levels of processing results. The difficulty in investigating awareness is because it cannot be isolated from perceptions, cognitive processes, and monitoring of motor effects. One must avoid the presence of all other activities in the brain, so that one can attend to the sensations produced by a single sensory process. Traditionally this has been called the practice of "mindfulness", which has become an extremely useful concept and method to enhance awareness of specific mental and physical activities originating from the brain. Practice of "mindfulness" trains one to continuously attend to a process and develop the awareness of the process. Thus, one learns to continuously recognize the small bodily processes like chewing a gum, movements of the chest and the body associated with breathing, walking down, making sequential movements of a dance, or the more intense mental activities related to thinking and problem-solving. Singularly-monitoring these activities provides opportunity to experience the specific sensations and the related movements, for applying greater controls on the total processing. Generating a mental state of happiness and tranquillity allows one to become aware of the happy and tranquil state of the brain-mind. A mental vacuum may bring about an awareness of emptiness, which may become disturbing. What is disturbing is not the absence of processing or vacuum, but the knowing that brain is not engaged in any activity. It is important that one must first train the brain to engage in neurocognitive processes and learn to emote positively, so that one can become aware of the processing states and changes, the details of processing, and learn to enhance the performance levels.

Meditation and awareness has been always postulated as closely linked; meditation facilitating normal and altered states of awareness. All practices of meditation are considered to enhance focused attention and remove creation of irrelevant thoughts and preoccupations from the emotional states of the mind. All forms of meditation teach a person to focus attention on a single thought or a movement process in the body, so that all other thoughts slowly subside, filling the mind with the awareness of the single thought or recognizing a single body process like breathing in and out. The practice of repeated mental (internal speech) chanting of special phrases or producing certain sounds during 'meditation' serves as good examples to illustrate the formation of related verbal awareness. One of the main aims of all systems of meditation is removal of the occurrences of irrelevant thoughts and focusing attention on a specific theme expressed as a phrase or cluster of sound. As one gets habituated to random recreation of words in everyday life, it becomes almost impossible to suppress voluntarily thinking, which may be irrelevant to the person in a given context. The option of not speaking out enhances thinking in most individuals, as thinking is private. However, many find it difficult to avoid thinking about unconnected matters while intentionally processing specific mental tasks. Interestingly such irrelevant thinking recedes or may even subside when one executes bodily movements. Thinking may be propelled and guided by emotional needs and absence of habit for focused thinking. It may continuously occur when one has to engage mentally and physically in specific problem-solving tasks and psychomotor acts. Compulsive or persistent thinking becomes a habit in many persons, especially when one has cognitive challenges requiring highly critical thinking for problem-solving. One may be aware of irrelevant thinking taking place, but may seldom be aware of the contents, unless makes special effort to monitor the thoughts. Thinking on its own is not intentional but incidental (Kapur et al. 1994a, b) and habitual, and it is made intentional by need states. Biases can be generated because of intentions and expectations, though these factors will speed up the process of encoding and the thoughts may be subjected to greater errors. However, during intentional thinking, awareness of the thoughts created is in the focus, which helps critical examination of the thoughts and their corrections. Awareness of these thoughts may become persistent and stressful for many, rendering it difficult to move out of thinking of those stressful themes for engaging in focused actions. Persistent awareness of these thoughts may trigger unpleasant affective states, all of which could affect ability to solve problems and meet other challenges in life. Knowing the source of the thoughts, that the thoughts are generated from within, is a strength and comfort to the individual and facilitates further evaluations of the thoughts already created. Not knowing the source of the thoughts from within, make the individual think that they are placed from outside (Hubl et al. 2003; Dierks et al. 1999; Cleghorn et al. 1992). Occurrence of series of words and ideas in uncontrolled manner is indeed different from creating or recreating meaningful ideas using words. The latter is indeed like learning to accomplish complex movements for a dance performance, with or without accompanying a music recital. Being able to run around or jump around do not automatically make one a dancer, who needs to learn complex steps and movements practicing them over years before achieving professional standards. Similarly creative thinking needs disciplined practice. One of the aims of meditation in the early stages is to learn to abstain actively from unwanted thinking during meditation and not to indulge in any challenging problem-solving. This is slowly achieved by mentally engaging or continuously attending to a simple and specific mental task. In some Indian systems of meditation, the meditating person chants or repeats mentally a small verbal passage or sound. In the initial stages of meditation practice, irrelevant words keep pouring in as one attempts to engage in the task. One has to repeatedly verbalize a specific phrase at a certain phase and keep mentally observing or become aware of the same being carried out. Automatic generation of other intruding and irrelevant thoughts retards slowly and ceases, and the awareness of the words repeated becomes clearer, sharper, and dominant, as it is the only theme of awareness. One can easily monitor and become aware of those thoughts. It is claimed that in intense and heightened states of meditation, one may also lose self-identity momentarily or the presence of own body and the mental process of monitoring the focused words. During such stage, one may cease monitoring or attending to normal bodily sensations, and one may even cease to monitor the efforts put in to carry on with the focused thinking, and the awareness of the thought created alone will persist. The awareness of the theme becomes powerful and merges with self-identity and one becomes what one is thinking. This is a state often referred as 'self-realization' in the Hindu methods of meditation.

In another form of meditation like the 'Vipasana', the subject must merely observe the process of breathing, and one initially recognizes or become aware of several body sensations viz., flow of air or breath in and out, the movements of the chest, the stomach, and the head. As breathing become regular and slow, the focus slowly shifts to monitoring the gradual origin of body sensations of taking in the breath and how it passes away. The meditation facilitates experiencing very specific sensations, when the brain stops creating any other thoughts or remembering and recreating imageries at random. Focused monitoring of a simple mental or bodily activity is the essence of all meditations, which would enhance the awareness of the mental activity or the bodily sensation. What is not clear is the possibility of any other outcome from meditation, other than the ability to focus attention, or if it is to be used only as a stress reducing method, which is indeed off a great value and a tribute to meditation as a method for positive health. Extensive meta-analysis by Cahn and Polich (2006) of findings of elecrophysiological studies of meditation in the last few decades has presented that several studies have uniformly shown increased theta and alpha activity in the EEG during meditation. This indicates that the blood supply to the brain may be reduced during meditation in some individuals and the brain steps into a non-processing default state. On the other hand, several of the neuroimaging studies (Herzog et al. 1990; Jevning et al. 1996; Lou et al. 1999; Lazar et al. 2000; Balkin et al. 2002; Khushu et al. 2000) have shown increased activation of the orbitofrontal cortex and anterior cingulate cortex in meditation compared to the control conditions they have used. The differences in the nature of meditation practice, whether it requires the individual to focus on a thought or breathing process may bring about a difference in the activation pattern. A few studies (Baerentsen 2001; Newberg et al. 2001, 2003; Azari et al. 2001; Ritskes et al. 2003) have shown clear indications of increased activation in the Dorsolateral prefrontal cortical areas in mediation.

Processing of internal information may or not take place in meditation depending on the type of focusing practised. Further, the focusing is a simple and continuous nonchallenging one, which does not engage any cognitive challenges in the brain. It is a base level mental state, which one needs to acquire through continuous practice. Staying in a state of attending to own mental or physical processes does not lead to any further problem-solving and one achieves the state voluntarily. Attaining this mental state may indeed has stress and anxiety reducing effects in the individual. Higher processing states in meditation can be demonstrated only by increased and synchronized gamma activity, which is demonstrated only in limited studies. Increased gamma activity and synchrony have been demonstrated in studies (Lehmann et al. 2001; Lutz et al. 2003, 2004; Faber et al. 2004) using Tibetian Buddhist and Zen meditations. However, its neurocognitive advantage is still not evident from these studies. What is not understood is its possible effects on enhancing the access of brain resources during thinking and problem-solving. Spiritual states considered higher than normal wakefulness have been claimed by all religiously oriented meditations, though this has never been demonstrated by any meditative and investigative procedure. On the other hand, all recent efforts have been to separate meditation from religion and allow people to practice it to benefit from its positive stress relieving effects. Music has equal or greater positive effects on brain functioning and it is easy to listen to and practice; hence music has been recommended and used as a rehabilitative measure in psychiatric and psychological disorders. The role of meditation as a stress relieving method is widely accepted today. However, true challenge for the brain is in using it at high drive levels and for extracting maximum information processing and problem-solving capabilities. This outcome is yet to be shown using these techniques.

Advantage Verbal Awareness

There cannot be an awareness of emptiness or void, when sensations are absent. Not having any sensations contribute to void and emptiness and not becoming aware of any sensation. There can be awareness of the body, if bodily sensations are monitored, even if nothing else is processed by the brain. Awareness in this sense is not different from perception. The brain must indeed be in a wakeful condition for it to become aware of its own processes. One becomes aware of having had a dream only when one comes out of the dream to a wakeful state. Hence, wakefulness is an essential requirement for the brain to become aware of its mental activities. Awareness is often equated to wakefulness because of this close association. Interestingly one can often remember several of the contents of a dream, when one is awake. One cannot become aware of a dream or its contents as dream occurs, as we dream only in sleep. We can fantasize such experiences by creating sensory-motor imageries in the brain, and then enjoy as well as become aware of the fantasies. Same emotions may be recreated in fantasy. Normal retrieval of all encoded information including that of experiences occurs automatically and almost mandatorily, when triggered by external or internal cue (Moscovitch 1992, 1994; Mukundan 2007a, b; 2008, 2010, 2011a). A stimulus or piece of information has a cueing value only when it is closely related, one way or the other, to the information stored. However, the neural activation patterns during retrieval of conceptual information and autobiographic episodes or experiences are significantly different (Mukundan 2007a for meta-analysis).

The speech-receiving centre directly monitoring the language activity of the thought/speech generating centre leads to the former centre knowing the language activities of the expressive centres. There is no evidence of such self-reflexive-awareness taking place in any other sensory-motor modalities. Child learns to monitor own speech and becomes aware of the words spoken and the thought. Awareness of own thoughts is equivalent to listening to speech made by others, except one knows the source or the origin of the thoughts. As one can semantically interpret the words heard or read and extract a meaning, one can analyse own thoughts as one can recognize them. As thoughts are created by the same brain using the language abilities commonly used for speech expression and comprehension, its recognition or awareness is equivalent to self-awareness. As thinking and becoming aware of the thoughts are closely interlinked, one can change words after thinking as it allows one to analyse the meaning created and then use appropriate words for creating a desired or self-approved meaning, which can be then expressed orally or in writing. By practice, one learns to carry out all these different levels of processing almost concurrently. Verbal awareness is equally important for knowing retrieved information, especially when the role of the retrieved information is not for generating a conditioned response. Every attempt to recognize an external entity including the words heard requires retrieval of internal models, and the transcoding of the nonverbal retrieved information creates its verbal awareness, which gives one opportunity to critically examine the retrieved information and approve the acceptability of the matching memory trace used for recognition. Somatosensory sensations, which bring about knowledge of body movements are precious for the experiencing person for their reality contact effects. One would focus on experiencing its pleasure and pain effects rather than transcoding the sensations, unless there is a specific need for communication. Those sensations have greater experiential value than merely knowing about their existence. When these sensations are not transcoded, there is no scope for developing their verbal awareness.

Awareness of the verbal transcoding of the retrieved information is different from the process of using it for recognition of an external entity, as one may recognize and respond without verbal awareness, if transcoding has not taken place. When words are retrieved for creation of a meaning, awareness of the words is important for creating specific meaning by assembling the right words. The relationship conceptualized using words and symbols may be exclusively at concrete, functional, or abstract levels, or at their combined levels. If the retrieved information represents a modality specific sensory imagery, then a verbal label or name may readily be used for naming the entity recognized. Blocks of verbal information are retrieved and used for large range of applications starting from naming, describing quality and intensity (adjectives and adverbs), and for creating meaningful relationships in thoughts and expressed speech. Awareness can thus be of a recognized entity, retrieved information, and/or verbally transcoded sensations and responses. During retrieval of transcoded information of autobiographical episodes, its awareness is further strengthened by the recreation of neural imageries of the perceived objects and/or the activities one participated or executed (sensory-motor imageries). They are retrieved using specific temporal and spatial coordinates which constitute their source memory. This comprehensive retrieval is what we call remembrance and we know that the neural activation pattern during remembrance is significantly different from the pattern seen during retrieval of encoded information without experiential components (for meta-analysis, Mukundan 2007a, 2011a). Information retrieved without accessing source memory and not accompanied by any experientially acquired sensory-motor imagery have a conceptual frame of reference. Non-auditory (visual, somatosensory, olfactory) recognition can take place without transcoding and we know that nonverbal type of encoding too can also take place. For example, one can learn to visually recognize a square without understanding the verbally transcoded details of a square, and one can use the same visual concept for creating a square. Transcoding allows one to make rational verbal relationships, which can be reality verified. Transcoding of the nonverbal sensory and motor participations help to make critical corrections and modifications of strategic plans, according to anticipated and actual effects of the actions, when one carries out actions to reach a goal. However, this may slow down actions and associated movements. Responses can definitely be made without thinking, when they are executed automatically, and they would then occur rapidly. One can remain aware of blocks of verbally encoded or transcoded blocks of information and conceptualize the action plans from them. These may be created within the brain, or received from outside, or retrieved from memory, and one can execute the action plans using the blocks of information carrying the action plans. This process has been studied under working memory operation. When planned actions are initiated and executed for arriving at a goal, several of the steps and processes involved in these acts need to be executed with self-monitoring. Verbal transcoding is essential for knowing or becoming aware of these processes and for analysing them, which help one to critically examine and modify them, ealier to their execution. Language ability of the brain allows one to document and store such endeavors. Nonverbal inputs and motor responses and actions can be readily transcoded and one creates detailed verbal account of the nonverbal experiences. Such account can be re-examined not only by the self but also by others, any number of times for understanding and verifying the various internal relationships created and proposed to be used.

As one is habituated to transcoding the routines almost online, one becomes often aware of the combined effects of the transcoded details and the original sensory motor effects. One may become aware of some of the associated sensory-motor processes, even though the main theme itself may not be retrieved, as they are not transcoded or encoded. Remembering an earlier awareness may often occur though one may fail to retrieve the contents of the earlier processing details. Verbal awareness, which is a self-reflection of the mental processes within, is only as real as a reflection is. Verbal awareness disappears just as all other recognitions vanish once the source is removed or not present. The emotional experiences, the transcoded, and the encoded details are stored and can be retrieved. Once retrieved, the awareness of all the retrieved information could be made all over again, which we call remembrance, which may not be qualitatively different from the orginal experience, except the latter has no components of reality contacts. This would mean that becoming aware of is a real process in the brain, which can be written into memory, even without encoding. Recreation of visual and motor imageries during remembrance, and remembrance of earlier attempts of remembering the same event are commonly encountered while extensively interviewing and testing participants for remembrance studies (Mukundan 2007a, b; 2008, 2010, 2011). These studies have shown that visual and motor imageries connected to experiences could be recreated, which would strengthen and validate the retrieved narrative. The meanings created from the sensory-motor signals may be equally important for all brains, which have learnt to share the meaning. However, if meanings are created from experiential interpretations, they may make significance only to the person who experienced it originally, and for others who can empathise with the former. Verbal awareness is unique and different from other forms of awareness or recognition as the creation of the meaning and relationships and their recognition or awareness take place in the same brain. Both creating and recognizing centers share the same knowledge base for interpretations and hence the meaning created is unique to the experiencing brain. Most important is the fact that the brain can assign meanings to auditory and orthographic expressions, as well as become aware of the meanings self-assigned. This unique ability to express the recognized meanings or become aware of the meanings self-created allows man to create them imaginatively and endlessly. We assign them the same meanings using the words and other creative methods as well as read (encode) similar meanings in the signals received from others. The brain learns to recognize as well as assign meanings in all physical expressions in the auditory, visual, and somatosensory modes. Learning the meanings created by others, and creating and recreating such meanings become the major functional capability of a developing brain. What the brain deals with is infinite number of meanings and the relationships expressed as ideas and concepts, designed and created by others and the self. This forms the major functional profile of the brain, which we have always called the mind. The verbal awareness of the meanings created in the signals expressed and received from the signals pouring from outside, is indeed different from the routine recognition or awareness of other sensory signals. The signals originating from external sources may not change significantly over time, but their meanings change from time to time, depending on the encoding methods used for their interpretations. Several decades back, a solar eclipse drove people indoor with fear and made them observes several formal routines, whereas presently, even children come out in the open with excitement, to view the same eclipse using their sunglasses. Learning to recognize a meaning or relationship is the major functional aspect of all perceptions, which we call recognition and awareness. Recognition of proprioceptive signals generated within the body is indeed different in significance from the signals received from outside, as one can easily block the signals from outside, whereas it is not normally possible to block those generated from within.

Awareness of the self can be therefore created by thinking about the body, its desires and pains, ambitions and adventures. However, the self is always represented by either the body image with several folds of sensory-motor effects, including language-thinking, and emotions. The self-awareness is always of a component or combinations of these. Creating such self-awareness is a process of conquering the self and its functions, as one has the opportunity to modulate the self and to decide the best action plans and execute them in strategic manner for achieving the best results. Verbal awareness can initiate a series of further thinking processes related to: (1) making judgments about the accuracy of own cognitive process; (2) making judgment about the goals one want to achieve and the appropriateness of the actions planned for achieving the goals, which direct and control one's behavior and navigational movements; (3) making judgments about the appropriateness of placing oneself in a situation where one is facing the challenges; (4) making alternate goals and program for the self, which will take one to a different destination. Mere sensory-motor effects in the brain do not initiate these entire complex sequential and parallel processing componets. These outcomes can happen only if one can monitor and become aware of the online sensory-motor processes taking place. Verbalization of the sensory-motor effects is an important requirement for developing verbal awareness, which can initiate further thinking and planning for the self-alleviation and achievements.

The brain is the storehouse of all the memory traces embodying information, which serve as the ever-expanding knowledge base of the complex and dynamic world, created using the knowledge base. This world with its multiples of emotions constitutes the mind in each brain. It is important to note that the neural signals and the processes carried out with them do not constitute the mind; it is the meaning and information embodied in the neural signals that constitutes the mind. The mind may be composed of information scientifically, experientially, and conceptually created and acquired. The mind has to be created by the brain by using its own resources. The meanings and the information banks are created and further modified all through, which reflect the dynamic, interactive, and evolving nature of the mind-brain. The development of the mind is often initiated and facilitated by the parents, and by all those who interact with the child during the developmental years. Once the child learns to build his own mind, the art he quickly learns, he has the choice and freedom to build it all the way, as he wants. The mind develops using the neurons as the building blocks, taking support of all other cells and their connectivities while creating the mind through the meaningful relationships.

Self-Image and Self-Awareness

The concept of self has largely moved out the fold of philosophy to psychology and cognitive neuroscience (Gallagher 2000). Gillihan and Farah (2005) strongly stated that "claims for the special status of self-related processing are premature", though the subjective references of self have never been ever lesser used by human beings. It is true that there is indeed no localization in the brain for the self, though the frontal cortex is the seat for self-related thinking and executive processing. On the other hand, Decety and Sommerville (2003) considered representations of self and others in the brain and proposed that the right hemisphere has a predominant role in connecting the self with others. They considered that the right hemisphere functions develop earlier than the left as reported by Chiron et al. (1997), and that the right hemisphere influences an infant's capacity to view others in an analogous comparison with the self (Meltzoff, Brooks 2001; Trevarthen 1979; Hobson, Lee 1999). Self has been a core feature of all philosophical thinkings, as it represents the individual as a unit in physical and spiritual forms. Development of the self from the monitoring of various sensory-motor effects has been studied from the stimulus-dependent and stimulus-independent points of view. It has been proposed (Mukundan, Ajayan 2011c) that self-image emerges in the early years of development from the feedback controls established between the sensory-motor systems. Such controls become the basic platform for the development of a body-oriented self-image in every person. The somatosensory nervous system represents all touch sensations produced from external contacts and sensations produced by own motor system. The somatosensory system is involved in the reception of diverse sensations of touch, temperature, proprioceptive and nociceptive sensations using diverse receptors all over the body. These sensations of external origin are produced by movements of the body parts initiated from the primary motor cortex. The primary somatosensory cortex is in the postcentral gyrus, where sensations from different parts of the body are registered and compiled. The anteriorly adjacent primary motor cortex directly controls the movements of the body and its parts and these movements are regulated by the somatosensory sensation produced during such movements. The motor skills needed for such movements are learnt through practice. The sensory-motor contacts made with the world are mostly voluntary and serve specific purposes for the individual. The sensory system directly controls the motor system and *vice versa*. It is posited that such direct interactive controls of the sensory and motor systems contribute to the development of a self-image, as verbal awareness is formed by the listening brain monitoring the processes of the talking brain. The self-image helps to differentiate own sensations and movements from those of others. The self-image becomes a complex phenomena, as sensory-motor effects alone are not that contribute to the self-image, but the semantic interpretations of the sensory-motor effects created from the frontal and temporal cortical areas are essential parts of the sensory-motor effects. The bodily contacts are often sought after with knowledge and intention, though they are indeed not necessarily for mere survival. That one can learn to produce movements with immense dexterity, coordination, and monitor them almost simultaneously, allows the creation of a body image, which one considers as the self-image. Tactile sensations are produced by own motor system or from the physical contacts with the external world, which include the touch sensations produced by other individuals. The self-image is a direct outcome of the brain representations of the sensory-motor activities within the body and hence it is indeed a product of the brain. The self is represented by the entire body and hence there cannot be a small spatial localization of the self in the brain. A child looking at himself in a mirror touches his own face and hair could be the beginning of the emergence of such self-image. The somatosensory and motor cortices may be considered the primary zone representing the self-image, further facilitated by other sensory inputs. The mutual monitoring and regulation between the somatosensory and motor systems may be considered to produce similar effects as the interaction between the talking and listening brain centers produce. As in the case of verbal awareness produced by the interaction of the two language centers, the sensory-motor interactions within the body produce a body awareness, which we call self-image and self-awareness. This is indeed facilitated by inputs from other sensory domains.

The diversity of somatosensory sensations makes them rich contributors of self-image. Sensations arise from the muscular movements used for chewing, rubbing, scratching, patting, squeezing, cuddling, movements of legs, hands, and the torso, etc. These movements are part of host of actions such as eating, writing, walking, bathing, dancing, playing, resting, muscular responses, responses and actions of sexual intimacy, etc. We move a part of the body and the somatosensory sensations produced during movements are monitored in the brain, and these perceptions in turn facilitate the coordination and harmony of the movements of the concerned body parts and positioning of the body. The brain in a body, held without movements may still be able to experience the passage of breath through the nostrils into the lungs while breathing in and out, giving rise to body specific self-image. The movements of the musculature and the sensations produced by those movements contribute to the development of another facet of the self-image. A fragmentary body sensation may initiate a self-image and become cumulative by participation of sensations from other parts of the body. The body is valued and accredited as the self, and the sensations monitored develop into the image of the self. Perceptions in other sensory modes may also contribute through movement controls to the wholesome self-image. A body image could thus become the core of a larger self-image leading to self-recognition or self-awareness in the individual. Self-image may be enriched by qualitative changes in the perception of the activities of the body. A body image must develop in the brain from birth and grow in strength and diversity until the child learns to identify it as the self. There is no reason to believe that such self-image may not be present in an animal brain. Self-image and self-awareness may facilitate each other, as transcoding of self-image may take place and contribute to self-awareness of the self-image. The owner of the image learns to verbally identify the self-image as "I", "me", and "myself".

Some of the major voluntary processes that take place in the brain are related to the search of the environment, recognition of entities, responding to them after or without perception, planning and execution of motor acts, verbal communication, creation of ideas, problem-solving, explicit and implicit learning, retrieval of information, and intentional and cued remembrance of the personal past episodes. Each brain has learnt to identify and differentiate itself from the realities around using the body image. The body-mind constitutes the domain frame for the self, as identified and demarcated by each brain. The self-image transcends the body domain as one learns to create values, consider those values important needs for existence, and start leading value dependent responses. What makes the self a powerful lobby is the verbal awareness of all encodings and transcoding carried out by the brain, which makes thinking and verbal expressions powerful tools for handling reality. The concept of self becomes more than a mere self-referencing method, as it embodies the values and principles one practices in life.

Stimulus-Dependent and Independent Processing

A stimulus-dependent processing occurs when the brain processes signals arriving from the external world. Brain may be said to be in stimulus-independent state, when the former is not happening, though the brain may be thinking, problem solving, remembering, or not engaged in any of these and apparently is in an idle state. Verbal awareness occurs, when the brain is encoding or transcoding. Stimulus recognition is the same as stimulus awareness. Verbal awareness is unique as it is the awareness of verbal expressions created from within either in the form of thoughts or speech. Interestingly neuroimaging studies have shown that such self-directed activation increases the neural activity in BA8, 9, and 10, chiefly representing medial prefrontal cortex. Castelli et al. (2000) pointed out that self-monitoring involves activation of medial prefrontal cortex, temporoparietal junction, basal temporal regions, and extrastriate cortex, based on which they suggested that the network of these regions process self-generated thoughts (McGuire et al. 1996) and emotional experiences (Lane et al. 1997). Lane et al. (1997) elicited significantly increased neural activation in rostral anterior cingulate (BA32) extending into medial frontal cortex (BA9), when the subjects selectively attended to their own emotions. McGuire et al. (1996) found that the same temporal regions monitor externally generated as well as self-generated speech and that monitoring self-generated speech additionally involves bilateral temporal lobe involvement. Differential activation of right dorsal and ventral prefrontal cortex was seen by Fletcher et al. (1998a, b) between internal search and external cueing in a search paradigm. Dorsal prefrontal cortex activation was greater when search demands were internal and it was greater in the ventral area when the search was facilitated by sensory inputs. Interestingly they could find similar disassociation within the parietal cortex between dorsal and ventral regions during the two search conditions. McGuire et al. (1996) postulated that MPFC is associated with stimulus-independent thoughts (SIT), which is different from externally cued stimulus dependent processing, and hence postulated that MPFC may be considered to represent a state of self. Gusnard et al. (2007) found evidence of increased neural activity in the medial prefrontal cortical (MPFC) areas when subjects attended to their own emotional responses. Gusnard et al. (2001) had made an earlier proposal that the default state is represented by self-referential mental activity and emotional processing and this state is associated essentially with the MPFC. They posited that their findings supported the earlier findings linking "self-referential" mental activity with the dorsal MPFC and this activity is the same seen in the default states, earlier suggested by Ingvar (1979, 1985). On the other hand, the ventral MPFC receives wide spectrum of somatosensory and external sensory inputs. Primate studies have shown that these inputs are sent via the orbital prefrontal cortex (Barbas 1993; Carmichael, Price 1995) to the ventral MPFC, which further receives extensive limbic inputs (Barbas 1993, 1995; Carmichael, Price 1995; Haber et al. 1995; Morecraft et al. 1992. The connectivity and the inputs received, render the ventral area especially suitable for engaging the external world. Gusnard et al. (2007) reiterated their postulation that MPFC is the default state which "instantiates functions that are integral to the self", whether one is or not aware of the state. Ingvar (1979) had reported 20-40% increased blood flow in the prefrontal cortex compared to other lateral and posterior brain areas in the resting default states when one is wakeful but does not attend or process any external stimuli. However, there are several types of stimulus-independent processing, and most of the working memory processing is stimulus-independent. Though the default processing state is a stimulus-independent processing state, it does not negate processing of internally held information, which may be present or absent in the default states. Thinking and problem-solving are stimulus independent processing, which may require intense cortical participation and alertness depending on the complexity of the internal subject, though the emotional arousal that may accompany cannot be labelled positive or negative. All types of introspective methods including meditations fall under this category of mental processing. Raichle et al. (2001) stressed on the importance of understanding the default mode as the baseline state of the brain and considered the MPFC as the main areas involved in the baseline control state, when there is no goal-directed and intentional processing takes place in the brain. Interesting findings have been also reported with EEG in such states. Another important feature of the non-processing default state is the readiness of the brain to start processing any new sensory inputs as well as initiate processing any new mental algorithm, which cannot happen in the non-wakeful conditions of sleep. Harmony et al. (1996) and Fernandez et al. (2000) demonstrated that awareness of internal processing was also associated with increased slow (delta) EEG activity. Robinson (1999) indicated that 4 Hz activity is related to behavioral arousal, which is negatively related to 10 Hz activity. Klimesch et al. (2000) suggested that synchronization of theta and alpha frequencies across distant neural areas is for specific processing of internal mental contexts during cognitive processing. Klimesch et al. (1994) indicated that theta oscillations represent hippocampal engagement required for retrieving from long-term cell assemblies in episodic memory recalls. Mukundan (2008, 2010, 2011a) has used increase in delta, theta, and high alpha activities as indicators of shift in attention to internal processing, and accessing source memory, when one remembers autobiographic episodes.

15 System Approach in the Mind-Brain

Human behavior is considered purpose driven, i.e., output or result driven, which needs a system approach for its understanding. A system may be considered a natural functional method. For example, we speak about the cardiac, respiratory, digestive systems in the body, with brain as the central controlling organ. Each system is maintained by several parts distributed across the body and working together for maintaining balanced activity within the system for supporting life. In similar pattern, human beings have created organizations and institutions for serving specific purposes, which contribute to the preservation of the human society and its growth. Human behavior and its varied manifestations can be explained only by "circular causation", in which a variable is both cause and effect (Karl Gunnar Myrdal, Nobel Prize winner 1974; O'Hara 2008). Action is controlled by its anticipated and actual stepwise outcome manifested during progression towards the goal. Reductionistic rational thinking is the foundation of science, which explains the sequential relationship between two variables within the closest time-frame, in which they are examined. Reductionist approach requires breaking down any phenomenon under examination to smallest possible particles separated with the least or minimal temporal interval and sequentially arranging the particles with or without change across the temporal intervals for understanding the relationship across particles over the predefined temporal intervals. The changes in the physical world take place in a predetermined manner, which can be predicted and the path outlined accordingly. However, such approach does not help to understand human behavior as most of human behaviors are goal directed and require navigational paths to approach the goals, which happen over large spans of time. Projection of changes or position to be achieved over large span of time, incorporating expected and unexpected effects from other human beings outside and effects from within self, give scope for defining purposes and goals for such navigation as one must reach specific goals despite obstacles and delays. The whole enterprise is conceptualized as a system. The need to define purposes and goals make it necessary to define roles people have to play and the need for personal mastery (Senge 1990) for role-playing and for achieving the goals. Such a system approach is not in conflict with a reductionist approach, but one cannot be a substitute for the other. Actions are intentionally carried out and one may create paths and take them in a strategic manner to reach the goal. What controls major parts of human behavior is not the biological need for survival, but their ambitions and wishes to create new economic and material realities, which form their emotional and intellectual pursuits in life. All these require highly goal oriented purposeful pursuits, which do not fall under the reductionist umbrella for explanations. Consideration of the development of value systems, which control and maintain manmade systems, is extremely important for understanding human behavior. Changes in social processes and social values continuously occur in all societies and the attitudes and reactions of the members of a society to such changes decide peace and harmony in the society. Absence of development of such value systems required to support the preservation of the society and their continued negation over long periods in the society result in alarming negative reactions. Social changes occur because of material needs, and greater enlightenment and improved knowledge base available to the members. When individuals oppose normal changes in social processing without debate and value judgment, they can destroy the social fabric and the positive controls that need to exist in the society. Preservation of a changing society requires cultivation of the value judgment in each brain, which cannot occur incidentally. Further, only through positive training in socialization, one would learn to examine critically such changes, and learn to respectfully accommodate or reject them at all levels of growth. Socialization is a process of training the individual learn to respect the legitimate rights of other individuals in the society, without which the society cannot be preserved. It is not part of any spiritual pursuit. It is indeed to be developed by practice at home, school, and in every sphere of human activity, where they gather and interact.

The brain functions as a system and man has indeed learnt and devised the same system approach for defining his presence and functional roles in the world. This is replication of devising a computer model of the brain. There is no way human behavior can be understood or explained outside the 'system' in which they live. It is apparent that the behavior of the members of a system cannot follow a simple rational approach for achieving goals for each. Mathematical models of the Game theory were proposed to explain human behavior under goal directed emotional and intellectual pursuits and under varying degrees of stressful challenges, which form the foundation of the manmade systems. Arthur W. Tucker's 'Prisoner's Dilemma' (Poundstone 1992; Cervone et al. 1995) was a revelation for biologists, social scientists, philosophers, economists, and politicians for considering human behavior from a larger system perspective. Systems are organizations or institutions created by human brains, in which they accomplish an existence beyond the biological survival needs, and progress in the various domains created by them. The 'Nash Equilibrium' and 'Nash Program' (Nash 1950a, b, 1951) were further examples of the need to consider the failure of rational thinking when outcome of strategies to be chosen by one depends on the strategies chosen by others, which are not known or available when one decides own strategies. Human beings have created several systems and they need to share them for their survival, emotional and intellectual development, and growth in all spheres. Each pursuing own goal disregarding the rights of other indviduals in the society may be a rational approach for each, but it fails the society. Individuals create strategies and execute them not for biological survival, but for pursuits, which are precious for the individual and for the team pursuing them, and for the members of the entire society. These needs decide the rules they make for their progress and achievements, and they adhere to them individually and as team. The systems created by the minds exist in the minds of people who have created them. We need to understand that (1) the human brain has the capability to indulge in such creative efforts and to accomplish them in a programmed and stepwise manner. (2) These brain efforts can be enhanced for achieving optimum efficiency in each individual. (3) Failures may occur in these processing steps, which deleteriously affect the individual's performance. (4) The brain performance can be evaluated and when deficiencies are present, they can be corrected fully or largely. The world created by the brain in which it lives, is indeed much larger conceptually and functionally than the physical realities that exist around and within him. Semantic interpretations are the biggest performing game of the brain, which has developed into unique capabilities to create new realities supporting and facilitating their life. The behavioral manifestations, their thoughts, and other processing capabilities need to be viewed and understood from a larger logistics than available by reductionist thinking. It is this capability to create systems and function within the system, which places human beings above other biological systems, which do not have such capability and hence go through routine survival needs. The human beings learn and employ various cognitive abilities, skills, and mold and deploy their emotional drives for achieving the goals they have chosen for themselves in life. Using the system approach, Peter Senge (Senge 1990) created the concept of 'learning organizations' and defined several important principles that he proposed could determine the functioning of a successful learning organization. Senge proposed that within a learning organization, individuals could enhance their capabilities and attain personal mastery, work in team, and reach higher levels of prosperity, creativity, and happiness. System thinking is one of the cardinal requirements of individuals for accomplishing their roles in the family, organizations, and society in general. One normally belongs to more than one system or group in the different domains of life viz., occupational, social, peer groups, political and religious inclinations. One is born in a social system and one grows in a social system. One indeed has the choice to select the social systems of choice, though it may seldom happen in an automatic manner. The systems influence one's personality, value systems, attitudes, and reactions. Democracy, political and religious systems are made by the people who share them, who may maintain the values or change them. Understanding the social processes and the responses of individuals to those processes are indeed very important for understanding human behavior, their mental health and related problems. However, if one is taken off from a system, the biophysical realities alone decide his existence.

The central theme of psychosocial development of a child is based on the cultivation of those functions in the brain, which help him acquire various cognitive abilities and psychomotor skills, and psychosocial etiquettes of behavior and responsibilities. The frontal cortex is the seat of psychosocial development to the best of our understanding. The frontal cortical development contributes to those capabilities, which help one to become purposeful and goal directed, learn to plan actions for navigation, and to initiate their execution for reaching the goals. One learns to create and adhere to such needs and purposes in life, learns to use drive optimally for personal gratification and achievements. Other than these, the frontal cortex is actively involving in encoding and transcoding by which concepts and ideas are created, all of which form the foundation of the human mind. The pattern of these developments decide how a growing child will use his emotions and cognitive abilities for overcoming distressing physical and biological conditions by creating new realities as Peter Senge (1990) proposed and how he will navigate in those efforts to create the new realities. Our knowledge of the brain shows the effects of extensive developmental pattern of the frontal cortex in the psychosocial development of a child. Yet another important regulation that originates from the frontal cortex is the control of various sensory and motor centres of the brain, which in turn control sensory inputs and motor outputs. The functional development of the frontal cortex accounts for the various controlled development of other functional capabilities, including language development contributing to thinking (encoding and transcoding) abilities under the umbrella of verbal awareness.

The concept of 'free will' has been always at the focus of debate and discussion in philosophy, religion, and to a much lesser extent, in science. It is indeed a concept, which has been greatly debated and misunderstood. The debate has been always between 'determinisms', and 'free will'. Determinism refers to the inevitable rule of the universe where everything progresses in time according to laws of the universe, and hence every change is determined by its antecedent state and the principle that governs the change. It is often argued that such deterministic change may not apply to human behavior, as human beings have the choice of "free will" and they can freely choose the change or a response. The concept of 'free will' is essentially applied to human behavior initiated from the human brain. William James (1842-1910), father of modern psychology and a great philosopher scientist, in his famous work "The Dilemma of Determinism" (James 2005), rejected determinism. In simple terms, according to him, determinism does not explain human judgments of approval and regret, and both approval and regret cannot be either good or bad. If there is no scope for deviation from predetermined path, there is no need for regret that one could have behaved differently or made a different choice. The scope for system thinking arises from the unique capability of the human brain for defining purpose for life and that each one can choose and set goals of life. The frontal cortex is considered endowed with this unique capability to define purposes, goals, and action plans for achieving the goals, and to navigate all the way over long spans of time lasting several years or decades, when necessary, for achieving the goal. There may be no reason to consider a purposeful action must be evaluated by using the same reductionistic principles applied for studying the changes, which we consider occur without any purpose. Even nonlinear approach and the "butterfly effects" may be the answer for some of the changes in the universe. There is no evidence for the existence of organizations and institutions anywhere else in the universe, except those created by the human beings. If there are equivalent life forms anywhere else in the universe, we have no option to think that they do not have similar abilities to think and create new realities. As human beings live within the systems they have created, most of their behavior and thinking have to be understood from a system perspective. The development of system approach has been explained even in animal behavior. Even the words "cause" and "effect" can be understood only when a change is explained and understood within a system model.

Experience of emotions and their expressions determine a large spectrum of behaviors in most individuals. Behavior could be manifested as part of emotional responses without perception and awareness of a stimulus, as discussed earlier. Several responses are released automatically by individuals, when they are conditioned to various socially relevant external stimuli as part of socialized behavior and when there are biological discomforts. The third category of behaviors is the one, which needs to be initiated from within, which depends on the drive or the need one has for executing the specific actions. There are responses made to various existing conditions and to new or recurring stimuli encountered during the execution of action programs already initiated and in progress. These behavioral components are spontaneously manifested as learnt voluntary expressions of emotional obligations. New actions are initiated and executed, when they are considered useful for further growth. The goals of the former would be already known to the individual as one is in pursuit of them, whereas one may be in the process of defining them in the second category. A third group of behavior may be exploratory and initiated purely out of curiosity and because of the novelty effects of the stimuli one receives. These are not conditioned responses, they are actions, one intentionally initiates and executes, so that a purposeful act is accomplished or they take the person to a certain new destination. One intentionally engages in social groups and seeks out opportunities for performance so that one finds opportunity to express oneself. One may receive appreciation or disapproval in such pursuits, and will further grow in those pursuits or give them up. For successful completion of the journey, one must know the goals so that navigation is well directed and controlled. One should also learn to anticipate the outcome or effects of planned steps of actions and the actual effects of actions executed, and must learn to self-correct using those effects. Developing emotional intelligence may be considered an important aspect of socialization as emotional intelligence allows control over drives so that actions and responses are made only after critical judgment. Anticipation of consequences of actions is an important aspect of emotional intelligence, which contributes to socialization and such judgments of anticipated effects help control negative and offensive behavior. Most of the social crimes committed by individuals belong to this category, as they cannot control themselves when drives throw them into actions. This ability to control oneself despite the force of drives or desires can only be developed through socialization in the early years of neurodevelopment. Whenever individuals engage in such actions, their actions indicate failure of socialization, which has a biopsychological origin. When the drive is developed because of own emotional and intellectual pursuits, they can be satiated only by wilfully indulging in activities which take them to such goals. We call them wilful acts or intentional acts, because they are not biologically propelled for survival needs. The human brain has the capability to conceptualize ideas by which it creates imaginary goals, and then strive to materialize them. These pursuits to goals, which are created through imaginative thinking and which exist in a future time point, are called volitional acts. They are wilful or volitional as the individual can survive without pursuing those goals. The goals are sought after as part of intellectual and emotional pursuits for personal or organizational gains.

Drives, Intentions and Actions

Intention to act is present when one is aware or has knowledge of the need to act. One may know the intensity, purpose, goal or objective and the type of the actions that are to be executed. Drive is the personal fuel, one has, which allows the release of actions, whereas the purpose or the goal can be expressed as an idea. Origin of action is identified as the expressed or manifested components associated with intention. Intention is the acknowledgment of the need and wanting to act and the acknowledgment occurs, when the presence of need or drive is transcoded and the person develops verbal awareness of the transcoded information. Intention itself may have an incidental origin, when it cannot be labeled intention, as the accompanying awareness has not yet developed. One may still act upon those unlabeled intentions. Action is initiated when the drive state reaches certain level of potentiation. We get to know or transcode the action only after it is initiated. However, action will not be initiated unless there is enough drive. Knowing the presence of drive is indeed different from acting upon the drive. Normally when we speak of intention to act, we refer to the knowledge of the presence of the need and the plan to act. Awareness of the action can occur only after action itself has been initiated. There cannot be awareness of an action that is not initiated. Generating a "go" signal in the brain does not automatically initiate the act. Action will start only when the drive needed for the action/response is released. There could be awareness of wanting to initiate an action and the presence of personal pressure or compulsion to start acting. Intention develops after entertaining an emotional state or listening to externally generated instruction or command to respond/act, when it becomes a need to act or respond. The individual becomes aware of encoded or transcoded details of the drive or the need, which makes one aware of the presence of intention or intentional state. Awareness of action can be generated only after the neural process needed for action has been initiated. Action is the end-result of a specific long neural process within the central nervous system. Absence of the drive can make a patient, with lesion in the anterior cingulate system, become devoid of initiation of actions and responses even in pain. The patient does not manifest the actions required for biological survival, becomes indifferent to the self and family, and shows total absence of actions and responses to environmental stimuli and personal needs. The question is what this drive is, which is used mainly in wakeful states. One can imagine running, playing, diving, etc. and the neural activation seen is the same as seen in real actions and is emotionally aroused. What is not present in imagination is the investment of energy, which is used by the body only for the execution of the activity, which makes them real activities. We know about the expenditure of energy in the concerned skeletal muscles during movements, needed for action and responses. We do also know about the emotional arousal required for one to engage in voluntary actions and responses. The emotional arousal is directly controlled and maintained by the limbic system and the anterior cingulate gyrus, with contributions from other areas in the frontal and temporal lobes. Emotional arousal is involved directly and indirectly in all actions, which individuals engage in everyday life. It is this emotional arousal or emotional need, which forms the major part of drive or need, which initiates actions and responses.

There are many simple examples given by individuals during interviews with the author about occasional instances of the absence of drive, though they wanted to act, in their lives. They wanted to carry out certain acts, viz., get up from a chair or bed and switch on the fan, close the door, switch on or off a light, etc., but they did not get up from the chair or the bed and did not carry out the act. Instead, they waited for someone to come around and then requested that person to do the said act. Similarly they felt that there were many instances in life when they were interested in carrying out certain acts, but never did them as they never felt up to doing them or felt that they did not have the drive to start working on it. They felt it was more of their personality, as they always needed more drive and needed someone to make them do even routine things. Similar to this are the statements made by young students who used to be excited by the set of textbooks they had bought for studies during the beginning of the year. Each wanted to read and learn from them all, picked up a book and started reading, and fell asleep within minutes. The same boys and girls could keep awake with hardly any sleep for weeks, before the examination and could spend all the time reading and learning. We speak about people with high and low drives. We know there were periods in life when the drive was low or not enough to do things, which made significant impact on the life. The emotional need determines the drive level and readiness to act. The "Inverted U curve" showing the relationship between drive and performance is an everyday example of the relationship between drive and performance in each individual. The drive to achieve may become intense and addictive as one keeps executing actions. In terms of biological need states of hunger, thirst, etc., we know the need means a disturbance in body homeostasis because of reduction in the energy levels and the consequent discomforts, which can be self-observed and examined. The need state simply disappears once it is satiated. However, human ambitions are not equivalent to the hunger for a one time meal. It drives them almost for the whole life. One may define a drive as a conceptual or concrete aim, where one wants to reach or acquire. The drive indicates only the psychobiological motivational state. These drives may not be easily satiated, as other biological needs are satiated by attaining the goal, though they recur frequently. Absence of drive puts down people. It is never the lack of physical energy that may stall pursuits in life. Psychological drives may become more intense propelling the individual to greater risks in life. The drive takes one through series of actions until one reaches the goal over time.

A need state may be considered different from a specific wanting expressed as intention, if the need is equated with a survival condition and intention with a state of drive for gaining or achieving prospective benefits. A button press task discussed in the Bereitschaftspotential paradigm of intentional acts is an elementary type of an action, and it is not directly elicited by a drive state to press the button, but indirectly because of a need to oblige an examiner or for a material gain, which can be temporarily helpful. Individual may normally have all types of drives under inhibitory control. Allowing a drive to grow within is often intentional, or because socialization has not inhibited the strengthening of the drive as it could trigger a person from indulging in antisocial activity. Therefore, one may have the option to keep away from such indulgence or nurture the drive and allow it to express itself. If the need or drive is allowed to grow in intensity and reach certain level, it facilitates the release of drive specific response or action. As one would habitually transcode such enhancement, one is indeed has the opportunity to become aware of the drive and to consider related actions as intentional. However, awareness of the action initiated by the drive state develops only after action is initiated. Intention is experienced and expressed by each in a specific manner, as it is always associated with a specific goal to achieve. Luria (1973) commented "Each human activity starts from a definite intention, directed at a definite goal, and is regulated by a definite program...." Action or sequence of actions is initiated because the individual has defined a purpose, and a specific goal for the action. There may be a plan of action already decided or one learns to develop the action plans through reasoning and experience. Such action is said to be intentional and the individuals are generally aware of the intentions as well as the goals. What is important to know is the fact that an action can be initiated from within only if there is necessary drive and it reaches the required level to trigger the motor response from the brain, which we call action.

Needs and drives are the two phases of the same condition. A need may be biological survival need or an emotional need to achieve a goal, and the drive the psychobiological force or fuel present in the individual to work for the satiation of the need. When the motor outputs are automatically initiated by need states or stimuli, then we call them conditioned responses. Similarly, we also respond to external conditions and stimuli after negotiations or their evaluations. Emotions too can initiate responses from within. However, when it is a thought created from a drive within, that initiates the motor effects, they are called actions. The drives initiate the motor effects, when it reaches certain level of strength, and it is considered voluntarily carried out, as the individual is aware of the presence of the drive and approves both the drive and the actions generated from it. The act is then considered intentional. Both require dispensation of energy for the initiation of bodily movements and responses, which are to be carried out by the motor cortex.

Having 'drive' is like being aroused and wanting to act. 'Drive' is the nomenclature used to describe energy available for deployment in the system. Energy is utilized in all movements, responses, and actions. Brain-mind is the control center for the release and utilization of this energy. Release of energy marks the initiation of all movements, which contribute to actions. Energy or drive in this sense is nonspecific, though its channelization as perceived by the concerned individual may be specific and as defined by him. Both socialization and creativity of the individual would play major roles in learning to define purposes and to set specific goals for materializing those purposes. Learning to label the drive is an important function as the biological state associated with all drives is always the same. Thus one has the option to choose and strengthen those drives, which are most beneficial and socially acceptable to each person. One learns to understand problems in the different spheres of life and learn to find solutions for them. One may acquire and spent enormous amount of valuable energy and time in this endeavor. All such behavior-actions/responses are at some stage called intentional as they are molded as per the purposes and goals defined by the individual. One channelizes the emotional drives according to the needs one has learnt to label by defining or encoding purposes, goals, action plans, and strategies for releasing and investing the energy, which result in achieving the goals. Defining purposes, identifying goals, and designing action plans may involve extensive verbal exercises facilitated by their awareness.

The neural effects of intention to act/respond are demonstrated by the Event related Potentials called the Bereitschaftspotential (BP) and the Contingent Negative Variation (CNV). An ERP paradigm in which the readiness to act can be directly measured is the Bereitschaftspotential (BP), which was first demonstrated by Kornhuber and Deecke (1965). The BP paradigms used are simple or complex self-paced button press paradigms in which the BP develops well before the voluntary response is executed by the subject (Deecke, Kornhuber 1978; Deecke, Lang 1996; Deckee 1987, 1990, 2000; Shibasaki et al. 1980a, b, 1993; Mukundan et al. 1986; Khanna et al.

1989; Singh, Knight 1990; Kitamura et al. 1993, Ikeda et al. 1992, 1993, 1994, 1995, 1996, 1999; Hamano et al. 1997; Rangaswami, Mukundan 1999; Sakai et al. 2000; Picard, Strick 2003; Soon et al. 2008). The subject is provided with a window to decide making the response. In our experiments, the subject was instructed to observe a horizontally moving visual trace on an oscilloscope and press the button(s) when the trace was anywhere between the two vertical lines drawn apart, with a choice not to press the button at all, if the subject did not wish. The negativity started developing 2-3 sec before the onset of the movement as seen from the EMG activity recorded from the palm of the hand, and the negativity reached maximum value at the vortex with bilateral symmetrical distribution (Mukundan et al. 1986) before the motor action potentials were initiated. This is the readiness potential proper or the early BP (BP1). It is a slowly rising negative DC shift prior to a voluntary motor act. There is an inflexion of the negativity about 500-700 ms prior to the movement and it is differentiated from the BP1/RP (Shibasaki et al. 1980a; Mukundan et al. 1986). The negative inflexion is called the negative shift (NS) or the late BP (BP2). The negativity becomes asymmetrical about 400-500 ms before the movement onset, with greater negativity seen in the electrodes contralateral to the side of movement. After reaching maximum negativity, the potential makes a positive dip for a shorter duration of about 80-90 ms, which is called premotion positivity. The negative deflection continues for another 50-60 ms and reaches maximum peak negative value when the movement itself is executed, when the motor potentials appear. Several studies have postulated the direct involvement of the Supplementary Motor Area (SMA) and the Anterior Cingulate Cortex prior to the onset of voluntary movements (Mushiake et al. 1991; Erdler et al. 2000; Huckabee et al. 2003; Cunnington et al. 2005; Colebatch 2007; Dirnberger et al. 2008; Matsuhashi, Hallett 2008; Soon et al. 2008). The SMA is considered the nodal center in the brain for the execution of complex motor programming based on which components of complex movements and actions are sequentially carried out. As the presence of DC shift in BP is a direct indicator of readiness to act, it has been discussed within the free will context by more authors.

Considering that the negative potential started well before the unfolding of the voluntary movement, Libet (1985) postulated that the negative shift indicated the cerebral initiation of the voluntary activity well before a person became aware of the conscious intention to carry out the specific activity (Libet et al. 1983; Libet 1985, 2001). He opinioned that one became aware of the intention to act only when one started unfolding the said act. He called the pre-awareness state an unconscious "urge". A person can become conscious of it only as the action is unfolded. The readiness potentials that were recorded by Libet showed that volitional process started at least 350 ms before the conscious wish to act is experienced by the individual. He reported that the potential showed conscious decision to act taking place about 200 ms before the muscles are activated. The word 'intention' used by Libet, therefore, has a highly context specific meaning than the commonsense definitions of intention, which refers to awareness of wanting to act for achieving an goal, target, objective or purpose. The subjects participated in the experiments with clear intention to carry out voluntarily the instructions given to them. It is true that the subject became aware of the voluntary response only when it was executed. He was indeed aware of the intention to take part in the experiment and carry out the voluntary act as instructed. Libet (1999) postulated that all mental activities which one considers conscious are "initiated unconsciously" and one becomes conscious of the mental activities only if the linked neural activity persists for sufficiently long and manifest into movement, which is captured as a conscious processes. The individual could opt to control the outcome of the volitional processes or the intended actions by vetoing or blocking the "urge" to perform (Libet 1985). He opinioned that the individual could use the "urge" for facilitating creative performances, such as thinking, artistic impulses, speech, music, etc. He considered that, "Rapid unconscious events would allow faster processing in thinking" (Libet 1985).

Mukundan et al. (1986) studied the BP potential using a button press paradigm in alcohol dependent subjects. Thirty-one ICD diagnosed alcohol dependent subjects with age-matched community controls were taken for the study (Fig. 9). There was a significant reduction in the mean negative latency of the BP in the patient group compared to the normal controls (–2.47 sec vs. –2.86 sec), which included BP1 + BP2 + Motor Potentials. This indicated that the alcohol dependency caused a reduction in the normal neural processing of the voluntary response and it became more abrupt in the patients, as though the patients have become impulsive. It has been proposed that awareness of an action can take place only when the act is initiated. The initiation of a button press is experienced when pressure is mounted in the finger kept over the button. The button moved down only when the pressure reached certain strength. Experience of the increased pressure in the finger is taken by the participant as indication of the initiation of the response. Interestingly participants who did not press the button experienced greater difficulty for not pressing than for pressing. The participants generally felt that pressing came almost automatically, as they had given consent to do the test and they knew they were expected to press the button, whereas occasionally they had to refrain voluntarily from pressing in between. They had to intentionally decide not to press, while pressing came naturally. The increase in finger pressure may be manifested slowly or abruptly according to the habituation pattern of carrying out such acts by a person or because of a certain situation specific need.

Khanna et al. (1989) used the same paradigm described above, in a group of patients with melancholic depression and found that the patient group had significantly reduced amplitude and onset latency, both indicating a frontal lobe involvement in depression, which was demonstrated by other contemporary studies (Buchsbaum et al. 1984 and Baxter et al. 1985) using PET scan in depression. Rangaswami, Mukundan (1999) used simple and choice movements internally and externally cued tasks, which required the participant to carry out a task in stepwise manner. The mean early onset average BP elicited in a

30 electrodes recoding in the simple and complex paradigms was at –1.99 sec. The participant self-paced the movements in these paradigms, different from the earlier tests in which the participant had to wait for the appearance of a slow trace in a vertical window on the oscilloscope screen. Interestingly several normal participants showed a greater BP onset latency in the externally cued task compared to the internally cued task. However, performance in the externally cued task was repetitive and predictable, which was not the state when the task was to be internally cued. Matsuhashi and Hallett (2008) showed that a mean 1.42 seconds existed before the conscious intention to move, as could be seen by a Bereitschaftspotential paradigm. They arrived at this time based on the presence of a real-time decision by the subject when a thought to move had occurred. However, studies have suggested that unconscious planning of longer duration may precede conscious intention to act. Soon et al. (2008) used a complex paradigm in which the subject had to make a 'motor decision' to press a right or left button and then press the decided button, followed by a choice of the point of time when the subject had decided to press the button. They found predictive neural activation using fMRI in frontopolar cortex and parietal cortex stretching from the precuneus into posterior cingulate cortex almost seven seconds before the subject's awareness of the motor decision. The study showed that decision to act reaches subject's awareness almost 10 seconds after the related neural processes started in the brain. The subject remains unconscious of the presence of intention to act until it reaches awareness. They found that the intention to make the movement has a frontopolar and parietal origin rather than of the SMA. This indicates that SMA is not the stage area where intention to act is consciously made. Another cognitive process, which indicates such negative shift in the scalp potential level, is that of expectation or anticipation, which is demonstrated by the Contingent Negative Variation (CNV) potential. The CNV is a slow negative shift that occurs on the scalp surface during states of anticipation. It can be demonstrated by presenting two stimuli at an interval with instruction that the first stimulus is a warning that a second stimulus will follow (2-3 seconds),

and he must make a voluntary button press response after detecting the second stimulus. The slow negative potential builds up immediately after the detection of the warning stimulus and the negativity reaches maximum levels before the onset of the second stimulus (Singh et al. 1986; Annet, Mukundan 1996a, b; Vandana et al. 1996). The response is made after the detection of the second stimulus. The negativity subsides after the subject has detected the second stimulus. The question is what triggers the slow DC change after the detection of the first stimulus. It has been the contention that it is the anticipation of the second stimulus initiated by the warning stimulus that produces the DC shift, as the shift neutralizes as soon as the expected stimulus is detected. The interesting feature is that the negativity does not build up if the subject does not make the response. It does not also build up if the subject does not have to make a response to the second stimulus, or if he does not know when a stimulus to which he must respond may occur. The need for response is introduced to make the person get into the state of anticipation waiting for the second stimulus to occur. The DC shift does not return before the next warning stimulus appears, it builds up only after its detection. The anticipatory change seen as the DC shift in the experiment may be considered to indicate the increase in the drive level required for the response, one wants to make. Expectancy and anticipation are important states, which animal species exhibit during biological threats. It does have a more socialized origin in human beings, though physical threats are part of living for all. Nagai et al. (2004) found in their fMRI and EEG study that increase in CNV amplitude was related to increase in activation in the anterior and midcingulate gyrus, SMA, and insular cortices and was associated with decrease in sympathetic arousal as measured by galvanic skin resistance. Chiu et al. (2004) found interesting relationship between CNV activity and anticipation of emotional attitudes, expressed facially and as prejudice in their subjects. The negative shift seen during anticipation may be considered to reflect the increase in attentional arousal or arousal required to meet the environmental demands of stimulus detection and response.

The orbitofrontal cortex is the largest cytoarchitectonic area in the brain, which contains Broadmann areas 10, 11 and 47 (Kringelbach 2005). Interestingly the functions of this large area of the prefrontal lobe are opined as not well understood (Ramnani, Owen 2004; Cavada, Schultz 2000) in terms of experiment-based knowledge base available about the functional systems of the brain. Most of the valuable information about its functional role is from clinical lesion studies (Luria 1966a, 1969; Cummings et al. 1995; Snowden et al. 2001), in which disinhibition plays a major role in forming the abnormal behavior patterns. It is often considered part of the limbic system because of its functional role in emotional regulation and expectations of reward in all decision-making instances and actions (Toplak et al. 2005; Paulus et al. 2002; Kringelbach 2005), other than touch and smell sensations. The area is connected to the anterior and the posterior cingulate cortex, and the retrosplenial cortex, amygdala, temporopolar cortex, and the anterior aspects of the superior temporal gyrus (Petrides, Pandya 2007; Ramani, Owen 2004). The connectivity allows the frontal area to engage in the integration of information originating from visual, auditory, and somatosensory systems at abstract and conceptual levels despite the mode specificity of the inputs. Clinical lesion studies clearly indicate how purposive and goal directed behavior is impaired in the patients suggesting the involvement of the area in strategic interpretation of information. That the area does not have connectivity with primary sensory and motor cortex further shows that the area is not involved in processes associated with sensory registration of external stimuli or direct control of motor responses, but is involved in strategic interpretation of information, which may be made use of in further sensory and motor controls of actions. Our current understanding of its functional roles is centered on the involvement of the area in strategic processing or decision-making, emotional regulation, and mental initiation and execution of actions.

Regarding actions, it is important to know that an action cannot be initiated without drive, and the drive has to reach a certain point of potentiation for the initiation of the action.

Drive is the task nonspecific requirement of all actions including mental processing such as thinking. Awareness on the one hand, is that of the presence of the drive, and on the other hand, it is state of becoming aware of the initiated action. However, a conditioned response or behavioral responses originating in preattentive emotions could be initiated without prefrontal lobe participation. Initiation of an action requires activation of the motor cortex, which has to receive the signals from the anterior cingulate and the orbitofrontal cortex through dorsolateral and ventromedial areas of the prefrontal cortex, and the basal ganglia. It is essential for one who intends to carry out an act, first take the drive to the potential level required for the initiation of the action, and not merely send a go signal for its initiation. The strength of the need determines the speed of the process, and the presence of the need is subjectively labeled as intention to act. A go signal cannot start action unless drive is built up for its initiation. Awareness of intention is the awareness of the need state or the drive. There cannot be a free-floating intention, which can start a specific action. In most normal situations, the person who intends to act would have already transcoded the need state and is in possession of verbal awareness of the state. One would readily transcode, a habit learnt from childhood, that one is hungry or thirsty well before looking for its satiation. Neural activation of an action never starts with its prior awareness; awareness can only follows the action. Verbal awareness of the processes taking place in the brain is indeed a great boon, as helps to organize execution of several of one's planned activities. It has contributed to the development of immense capabilities in the human brain, though awareness can come in handy only after a processing has started or a condition has emerged to be there. Once the strategies and program have been encoded and conceptualized, their awareness helps to modify the strategies, redefine goals and action plans, whenever required before or during the execution of the actions. Control of behavior can come only by controlling the development of the drive, which alone can initiate voluntary actions. If the drive is not kept under control, actions are initiated involuntarily. Action is indeed one of the most important expressions of drive. One must learn to generate drive and channelize them by labeling them and learn to keep the drives under inhibitive control, and learn to release them according to the needs after their critical evaluation. Socialization is the process when one learns to keep certain drive always control and never allow them to express themselves unless one approves their release. When the drive is released into an action, it is called a willful action, which is indeed one of the most important means for achieving predefined goals. Unlike biological drives, the secondary drives may not satiate by reaching the physical goals. There may be qualitative and meaningful changes than quantifiable goals that one aspires and strives to achieve, which cannot be physically realized. "Will" can be applied only if one has developed the controls on the drives. There are many folds or domains of socialization, and one has to acquire the inhibitive control in all those interfaces of human interactions. Sexual drive is one such drive, which requires immense inhibitive control, so that one would release the drive only when it is socially acceptable. The society expects that its members never develop drives, which may result in actions detrimental to the welfare of other members and the interests of the society. An asocial individual is prone to aggression and crime, as he has not learnt the art of response inhibition, which alone can keep those drives under control. Release of drives because of lack of control could result in restlessness and manifestation of irrelevant actions and responses. We have seen what happens in lesions of orbitofrontal functional system. Lesion studies have shown ample evidences of the material and processing nonspecific nature of involvement of prefrontal areas in cognitive processing and motor controls, except lateralization of language related processing methods. Neuroimaging experimental studies have further demonstrated that the medial and orbital prefrontal cortical areas are engaged in the processing of diverse mode and processing nonspecific cognitive demands and a common frontal network is the choice for diverse cognitive problems (Luria 1966a, 1969, 1973; Duncan, Owen 2000). These include large spectrum of higher mental functions viz., purposive goal directed activities, complex motor programming required for navigation of the individual, mental execution of thinking and problem-solving, interpretations of all sensory inputs, and cognitive control of emotions and drives in the individual. For example, areas in the frontal lobes may be considered the seat for psychogenesis and neurogenesis of several aspects of perception and actions. Increased and uncontrolled drive may manifest in several conditions and ADHD is one of the best examples of such phenomenon (Toplak et al. 2005; Willcutt et al. 2005). When an action is cued by external stimuli, there is bound to be additional neural mechanisms, which play roles in the initiation of the action. It is indeed different from initiation of action from internal sources. Response inhibition and voluntary release of inhibition for the initiation of action are skills to be learnt primarily through social conditioning by all in their early developmental period.

Temporal Binding Between Action and Effect

The most important feature of a voluntary action is the experience that it has been self-selected and executed. The temporal binding within the brain, between a stimulus and response, and between choice of internally initiated action or externally cued action, have been at the focus of several studies, which is considered the basis for the experience of voluntary origin of actions. An action-effect contingency is proposed to strengthen the temporal binding between the two (Wenke, Waszak, Haggard 2009; Moore, Haggard, 2008; Moore, Lagnado, Deal, Haggard 2009), giving rise to the experience of volitional origin of the action. Several studies have investigated the temporal binding effects of the selection of an action with its execution, when individuals have the opportunity to internally choose an action plan or when they are externally cued to choose a certain action (Haggard 2005; Haggard, Clark 2003; Haggard, Clark, Kalogeras 2002; Repp, Knoblich 2007; Sebanz, Lackner 2007; Astor-Jack, Haggard 2005; Obhi, Haggard 2004). Both the types of selections are indeed temporally bound though the binding was found stronger when the decision of choice of action is internally decided and carried out (Wenke, Waszak, Haggard 2009). The temporal action-effect binding therefore depends on the choice of action, and it may be strongest when action is selected internally than when it is externally cued. The neural binding in a conditioned stimulus-response association is also bound to be strong, which is the foundation for the automatic manifestation of response when the stimulus is detected in the brain, whether it has led to its recognition or not. Binding of the action-effects gives rise to the experiential interpretation of the act as voluntary. However, effects of actions need not occur instantly or immediately, they may occur temporally long distance away from the actions, and the individual would still consider them self-bound and self-attribute the responsibility for action selection and its execution.

Memory

16

Memory refers to the neural processes of storing and retrieving information in the brain. Encoded information is written into memory consciously or without knowledge. Retaining is generally long-term and it may be linked to already existing information or may make an independent and isolated storage. Storage of information is described as long-term and short-term storages. When information is stored in the long-term storage, it needs to be consolidated. Short-term retaining is equally important, as it is required for all working memory operations. Retrieval may be automatic or effortful with a conscious effort. All cognitive processing takes place at two levels in the brain. The first level is at the neural signal level. This is the physical level where neural signals represent information and the information is processed. A computer analogy is partly suitable for this. As information is digitized and stored in the computer, information is stored as neural signals using neurotransmitters and the associated processes in the brain. The brain learns to process these signals at another level, wherein we consider them to have information value; we call this level at which the signals have informative value the mental level and the domain is called the mind. The brain learns to use the signals for interacting with reality, for survival needs, and finally to develop a data bank which we call the mind representing all experiences and knowledge of the world and the self. Encoding helps to create real and imaginary worlds of information representing the real world, which forms the base of each human mind.

The individual may become aware of the retrieved information or it may be used automatically by the brain.

Retrieval of engrams/memory traces for recognition or identification of entities of the world is one type of retrieval from memory. Here, one may not be aware of the process of retrieval taking place, as one may only know that he has recognized the external entity. This is also called sensory memory. This takes place generally automatically and the retrieval helps the person to know the familiar objects or the entities of the world. One becomes aware of the need to retrieve only when one fails to recognize a familiar face, object, or entity. Memory is divided into different categories based on the type of information, states, and period of retrieval. However, one can pause, transcode the recognition as it takes place, and it contributes to the formation of verbal awareness of both the recognized entity and the process of recognizing or only one of them.

Memory Systems

Memory has been classified into different systems based on the process details and the type of information involved in storing and retrieval of the information.

Semantic Memory

1. Pure conceptual knowledge.
2. Acquired through semantic interpretation—encoding/ transcoding. Use of language important for creation and comprehension of information; acquired through thinking, reading and listening to others, books, media, and other modes of mass communication.
3. Information is essentially conceptual without requiring experiencing.
4. Conceptual Information Memory in the Knowledge Bank of the individual.
5. Recall does not require personal references of time and place (source) of acquisition.
6. Recall may require logical associations and knowledge of sequences.
7. Supported by extensive areas of Neocortex—temporal and frontal cortical areas.

8. The cortical areas in the brain can directly access the information.

Autobiographical Episodic Memory

1. Autobiographical episodic memory refers to memory for the events or episodes that took place in a person's life in which he participated. They constitute sensory-motor, emotional components of experiences and their temporal, spatial, and contextual references. During retrieval sensory-motor imageries are recreated which facilitate one to relive the experience (Mukundan 2007a, b, 2008, 2010, 2011a) and self-validate the original experience. It is important that the source memory related to the time and place of occurrence of the episode must be activated first for retrieval of the details of a specific experience. This memory is discussed in detail in the later section on 'knowing and remembering'.
2. Relevant external stimuli may also serve as cues for directly triggering or provoking the remembrance of the connected autobiographical episodes.

During retrieval of the autobiographical episode, referred to as retrieval of "experiential knowledge" (Mukundan 2007a), one must first access the source memory for accessing details of when and where a specific episode took place in the life of an individual. The source memory verifies the correctness of the episode retrieved as it provides the individual details of when and where the episode took place. Earlier clinical lesion studies (Tulving 1972; Schacter et al. 1984; Milner et al. 1985; Janowsky et al. 1989) showed that source memory has independent frontal localization as these patients with frontal lesions were found to have impairment in source recall during recall of personal episodic memory. Recall of experiential knowledge first requires accessing the source memory. Clayton and Dickinson (1998) proposed that 'when and where' behavioral episodic memory criteria were seen even in non-human animals. Further remembrance of experience is retrieved by the recreation of sensory and motor imageries of the original experience. During retrieval of experiential knowledge emotional responses may also be retrieved and all of which help to relive the experience.

Explicit Memory (Declarative Memory)

1. Develops later in life.
2. Requires conscious participation for acquisition and writing into memory.
3. During recall there is a subjective sense or acknowledgment of recall.
4. The stored information declares itself into awareness of the retrieving person.
5. The information encoded may be conceptually-semantically; or experientially acquired.
6. The recall is generally verbally or orthographically expressed or expressed in drawings.
7. Requires participation of hippocampus and medial temporal cortical areas.
8. Retrieval in both semantic memory and autobiographical episodic memory takes place into awareness.

Implicit-Procedural Memory (Nondeclarative Memory)

1. Present since birth, storage does not need conscious participation.
2. Conditioned Learning—learning emotional responses and automatic retrieval of emotional responses.
3. Learning psychomotor skills (riding, driving, cycling, skating, etc.) and habits.
4. Priming in the Neocortex.

Recent, Remote and Prospective Memory

Memory has been also studied classifying into memory for remote, recent, immediate, and prospective events in terms of the temporal origin of events. Loss of immediate memory and memory for recent past events are strong indicators of several neurological disorders viz., TBI, degenerative disorders, space occupying brain lesions, etc. These types of memory losses have been discussed elsewhere in different sections. Prospective memory is relatively less studied in the clinical settings, though it is indeed disrupted in several brain diseases (McDaniel et al. 2004; Thompson et al. 2010). Prospective memory is defined as the memory for intentions to act (Burgess, Shallice 1997; McDaniel, Einstein 2007). What is stored in the memory is the intention to act, which one must retrieve at the right time and place for its execution. It is not a concept or an imagery that is stored, which may need to be retrieved at any time if required, but an intended plan or a thought for a later execution, which should come up into awareness on its own at the right time. It is different from working memory, as processing itself does not take place. It is comparable to it as the person has to hold on to the intention or a plan of action until it is initiated. One may have several appointments in a day, and several such important appointments in the forthcoming days, and one must remember the appointment well before the schedule time of action. The need to hold intention prospectively arises only when one has plans of actions, which need to be carried out at different points in time. This is clearly indicative of an extensive frontal lobe involvement. Burgess et al. (2001) observed in their PET, neural activation of bilateral frontal poles (Brodmann's area 10) and of the right lateral prefrontal and inferior parietal regions plus the precuneus, during a laboratory simulated intention task. Information prospectively held may be reinforced by their frequent retrieval and indulgence or they may have not personal significance and may require only a onetime action. When there is personal significance, individuals find it easier to hold on to the intention, whereas if it is an impersonal intention, such as a causal appointment, they may often fail, unless it is there in their appointment diary. The neural mechanisms used for holding the information may be the same as in working memory, except the attention allocated to it may be very small, that it does not interfere with the other online processes. However, the method of holding the desired information is different from the method used in working memory operations, as the individual need not be continuously aware of the intention in the prospective memory. The individual could become aware of the intention according to its scheduled commitment time, as he could have been fully engaged in other activities, until he becomes suddenly aware of the prospective commitment. Creation or generation of intentions, their intensity, and the capability to release drive for execution of the intended actions are indeed more important than merely holding the intentions. However if intentions become weak and the weak intentions fail to trigger actions, it could be a normal process. In pathological states, intentions are neither generated nor acted upon by the individual.

Brain as an Indexing System

We do not any more try to personally store and remember all the conceptual information that we acquire in life as the volume of such information is too huge for one to encode into memory and retrieve. We have developed alternate methods of storage of such information, which are indeed huge storehouses of all vital information required for transactions in cultural, social, scientific, and business realms of life. We have stopped using the brain even for storing telephone numbers or doing even simple mental calculations as these can be carried out more efficiently with manmade machines. On the other hand, we keep an index or a "FAT table" in our brain, of all the information that we have stored in the computers so that we know about all the relevant data and we know where it is available. Knowledge of what we have has become more important than storing the enormous wealth of data in the brain. We use the brain for such indexing and storing the index rather than storing the data itself. Professionally the highest uses of the brain are to formulate hypotheses, solve problems, and create new realities and learn from and through those experiences.

Declarative Memory

There are two types of memory systems based on the nature of retrieval. In one mode, the stored memory need to be retrieved to awareness, or the person becomes aware of the selected information retrieved from the brain. This is called declarative or explicit memory. If the stored information can be directly retrieved and used in an online processing, the retrieval is called nondeclarative or implicit. One does not have to become aware of the retrieved information for making use of it in an application that one is engaging. For example, an experienced person can retrieve the skills needed for driving or riding, playing certain games, automatically and apply the skills. Declarative memories are the semantic and episodic types (Tulving 1972; Ullman 2004). One system represents the knowledge bank of the individual, which is used for recognition of the world and knowing the world. The other represents experiences of the individual, which have specific source memory in terms of place and time of occurrence. Writing information into declarative memory requires conscious participation and must be aware of the information encoded, as the retrieved information is retrieved into awareness. This does not happen in the nondeclarative type of memory as the process of storage or learning itself does not require awareness of the details of the skills, but one needs to practice and learn the skills. The relevant skills and responses may be directly retrieved and used in their execution. A major route of storage and recall for the declarative type of memory is through the hippocampus in the temporal cortex. Hippocampus provides the connectivity for the retrieval of time and place, and context specific details of the episode or event stored. All information transcoded from experience is written into long-term memory through this structure. A dual memory system was proposed (Eichenbaum et al. 1994) in which the hippocampus proper takes in relational representation to long-term storage. In this type of storage, the new information is linked to an existing stored cluster of information. The same route is used for their retrieval. The parahippocampus controls isolated independent memory, which cannot be transferred into long-term storage because of lack of links or relationship to information already in store, and hence they remain isolated. Once the hippocampus establishes the connectivity with the long-term storage, relevant information may directly be accessed then after. A meta-analysis of the findings of neuroimaging studies by Lepage et al. (1998) showed that rostral parts of hippocampus is involved in episodic memory encoding, whereas activation of the caudal hippocampus was seen in retrieval of episodic memory.

Consolidation

Consolidation is an important aspect of declarative memory, which helps in the long-term storage of information in the brain. It has been widely suggested that consolidation of the newly learnt information into long-term storage takes place during sleep. The first 3.5 hours of sleep, often categorized as Slow-Wave-Sleep or deep sleep (SWS consists of stage 3 of non-rapid eye movement sleep, AASM) is considered the most important (Iber et al. 2007) as consolidation occurs during this stage. The stabilization does not occur during the later stages of sleep. Consolidation is the process of neural stabilization of the memory trace acquired through (McGaugh 2000; Dudai 2004) semantic interpretations. Consolidation may occur at synaptic level or at a system level. Synaptic consolidation is conserved to occur within hours, whereas system consolidation is dependent on the hippocampal activation. Without consolidation, the interpretation or the meaning cannot be recovered, even if the person is aware that he had acquired a specific knowledge or information. The information is considered consolidated as a physical or neurochemical memory trace or engram. Semon conceptualized in 1921 the engram as representing memory and Karl S. Lashley considered that engrams could be distributed all over the cortex (Darryl 2001) and they could be retrieved together to constitute a wholesome memory of the original entity. Consolidation is a neurobiological process of stabilizing the memory trace in the brain cells. Meaning or interpretation can be stored only if the same is written into a physiological or biological substrate. Whenever information is retrieved, the information is straight called back. There is no evidence to indicate that another interpretation or encoding of the stored signals need to be carried out, whenever information is retrieved. What is retrieved directly is always the encoded or interpreted information, whether the retrieval is in the explicit or implicit modes. One becomes aware of the meaning or the stored knowledge straightaway. The writing system has interpreted the meaning and it can directly read the meaning when it retrieves it from the neural signals. However, this would mean that the writing/reading system must be equally capable for writing and reading, as the storage system is capable of only storing the signals. If the writing/reading system becomes defective, it will not be possible for it to recreate the original meaning written from the signals, even if they are available. It is found that sleep stages with sleep spindles have a positive effect on consolidation of declarative memory (Gais et al. 2002; Schabus et al. 2004). Though the declarative memory is facilitated by consolidation, the memory related performance does not change. Interestingly later stages or total duration of sleep does not seem to have any effect in improving the consolidation process (Tucker, Fishbein 2009). Persons with insomnia and sleep disorders have poor deep sleep, which prevents/interferes with memory consolidation resulting in poorer declarative memory in them (Backhaus et al. 2006). Presence of emotion or emotional arousal is considered a significant facilitator for memory consolidation (Sharot, Phelps 2004; Hamann 2001). What is meant by emotional arousal here is the alertness and the intensity of the need/drive state and not the presence of positive or negative emotions.

The hippocampus and the parahippocampus have major roles in the consolidation of declarative memory (Eichenbaum et al. 1994; Eichenbaum 2001; Gabrieli, Kao 2007). Eichenbaum (2001) proposed three processing roles for the hippocampus, viz., mediation of the recording of episodic memories, identification of common features between episodes, and interlinking the episodes using their common features. Information that declares itself into awareness is both conceptual and experiential types of information. One remembers the entire theoretical formulation or the details of a document, which one can further organize, alter and reproduce. This is called "semantic memory" of the individual. Such information may have no personal relevance to the person who has memorized it and there may not be any experience associated with it. Each brain may carry huge repertoire of such knowledge base, which may have no personal relevance, but is important for the professional life. Quality of intellectual life of each person may be decided by the knowledge bank one has carefully acquired, as one may use that knowledge base for interpretation all new incoming signals into the brain. Autobiographic episodes constitute another spectrum of experiential knowledge base, which one has acquired in life and may remember intentionally or when cued by external stimuli.

Effects of Emotions on Memory

Information is acquired though cognitive efforts purely conceptually or experientially or both combined. Conceptual learning and storage are generally carried out intentionally as the possession of information created or recreated enhances knowledge base in specific areas, which can be used by the person at various competitive and challenging occasions in life. On the other hand, information acquired through experiences (experiential knowledge) may be considered cherishing or disturbing and may be remembered all through in life (Mukundan 2007a). Penfield's (1975) brain stimulation experiments demonstrated that under such stimulation, one would retrieve information that one could not otherwise remember in normal circumstances. However, several of the daily activities are routine requirements of life and are not retrieved later, even if they may be stored in the brain. Thus, one does not remember what one ate for breakfast or lunch every day, after a day or two. On the other hand, one remembers a dinner one had with a certain person, even after decades. All experiences with cherished emotions are remembered. Presence of emotions in an experience indicates the personal significance of the event. Thus, one would readily recognize one's date of birth, if a list of several similar dates are presented in a cluster. One would recognize own personal belongings even if they are kept along with those of others. Personal significance does not necessarily origin from positive emotions alone. It could be associated with need for self-preservation rather than any positive or negative emotions. Emotional arousal indeed is a basic requirement for all neurocognitive performances and hence it has facilitating effects on both storage and retrieval of experiences and information. There have been several scientific efforts to understand the role of emotional mediation on both declarative and nondeclarative types of memory, from the medial temporal lobes and specifically from the amygdala (LaBar, Cabeza 2006; Sharot, Phelps 2004; Phelps et al. 2004; Hamann 2001; Zald 2003; LaBar, Phelps 1998; LaBar et al. 1998; Anderson, Phelps 1998). These studies revealed the effects of emotion on encoding, consolidation, and long-term retrieval. The role of the frontal lobes has been a cardinal issue of investigations related to emotion and memory, as frontal evaluation determines the emotional valance and magnitudes of the sensory inputs and somatic conditions, which in turn have direct effects on both storage and retrieval of the associated experience and information. Emotional arousal has a direct effect on all psychological and physiological functions controlled from the brain. Emotional arousal is primarily a physiological state, mediated by internal and external conditions. It can be aroused by external factors, which produce variety of sensory inputs with positive and negative valances. Many of these external conditions and objects are indeed beyond the spectrum of survival requirements in human beings, as they are associated with self-generated need states.

Emotional arousal supplies the fuel necessary for the brain to drive itself in various activities that lead to performance, navigation, and achievement of goals in life. Emotional arousal beyond an optimum level can become a hindrance for performance including cognitive performance, as well established by the inverted U relationship between the two. Both emotional arousal and its valance affect recognition, encoding, transcoding, consolidation, and retrieval. Presence of an emotional component in an experience may render the experience memorable for life. On the other hand, activities, one may engage routinely are readily forgotten after lapse of limited time. The nature and the strength of the emotional component determine the importance of experience. However, there may be no such emotional arousal associated with encoding, storage, and retrieval of conceptual information, except the need to accomplish in various tasks, which one may consider non-personal. Storage of such information may depend on the strategies used for encoding and organization of information during memorizing and retrieval. Such conceptual information, though they may have emotional and experiential value to the individual, form the major body of the knowledge base in the brain.

Presence of intense traumatic emotions may not only block and interfere with encoding but also block the retrieval of such information. Psychoanalytically the process has been identified as repression. The most significant aspect of repression is that the affected person is not aware of the occurrence of the episode or the action committedly by the self. The affected person will deny the action and may not attempt to retrieve the action, which he believes was not committed at all by him. On the other hand, intense emotional need may force one to imagine false experiences. Presence of such repressive effects were frequently encountered with person who indulged in certain types of criminal acts, which were encountered in their BEOS investigations (Mukundan 2010, 2011b) by the author and his team (personal communication). Though the concerned individuals' involvements in the acts were confirmed through confessions and other primary evidences, they did not have remembrance of the specific details of highly traumatic acts committed by them.

Knowing and Remembering

Mandler (1980) differentiated between two types of retrieval of information, one for knowing various conceptual types of information, and the other for remembering autobiographic episodes. Thus, all may recognize a famous monument as they have seen its pictures and read about it, though a few may remember visiting the place. The differentiation was supported by several later studies (Tulving 1987; Gardiner, Java 1990; Tulving et al. 1994a, b; Lepage et al. 1998, 2000; Henson et al. 1999, 2000, 2005; Smith, Jonides 1999a, b; Aggleton, Brown 1999; Fletcher, Henson 2001; Burgess et al. 2002; Schnyer et al. 2004). Moscovitch and Winocur (2002) have reported that recognition by knowing elicited dorsolateral prefrontal cortex activation, whereas remembrance elicited activation of the anterior cingulate-part of ventromedial prefrontal cortex, and related limbic structures. Studies by Tulving et al. (1994a, b); Lepage et al. (1998, 2000), Henson et al. (1999, 2000), and Fletcher and Henson (2001) using mental tasks involving remembrance reported activation of the anterior prefrontal cortex.

Retrieval of conceptual information for recognition of entities and semantic understanding of ideas and concepts is considered the process of knowing. One knows the capital of India, the US and many other countries, may know that $2 + 2 = 4$, and $15 \times 5 = 75$, knows $(a + b)^2 = a^2 + b^2 + 2ab$, and may possess large spectrum of conceptual knowledge, which help in their recognition and applications. Recognition of external entities necessitates attention to be directed outward, whereas retrieval of semantic information may require attention to be directed inward or within. Recognition always involves retrieval of names, if present, though the names are retrieved without any effort to shift attention, as in the case of retrieval of other semantic information, which may require shift in attention. If one remembers a semantic idea or experience for speaking out, then attention needs to be also directed to the process of expression. All learn to shift attention rapidly accordingly to the needs. While driving, one attends to the traffic and movements outside, and one may also engage in conversation with fellow passengers, which may require focusing attention on conversation and frequently shifting attention in and out. One learns to attend to several mental and sensory-motor exercises simultaneously so that multiple tasks can be carried out as efficiently as possible. Aziz-Zadeh and Damasio (2008) in their meta-analysis of the work in this area found that sensory-motor areas used for producing actions also represent their semantic conceptualization. If remembrance is essentially a mental exercise, then attention needs to be directed inward, whether the remembrance is that of an idea or an experience. Retrieval may take place automatically and attention must be deployed for making use of the retrieved information. If remembrance is semantic and is that of an idea, one has to recreate the idea as thoughts and then only one can becomes aware of the idea. If remembrance is that of an experience, one may transcode it or relive (fantasize) the experience. Knowledge may be acquired not only through conceptual exercises but also through experiences. One knows that a steel bucket is heavier than a plastic bucket, light travels faster than sound, a car has a better balance on the road than a two wheeler, and hundreds of other things, acquired through experiences in life. An experience could be as simple as reading a newspaper or watching a match or a movie, travelling in a car, eating breakfast, meeting a friend, making a presentation, walking, running, visiting a holiday resort, attending a dinner, getting married, spending time with a loved one, and so on. One of the major differences in the two types of retrievals is the amount of information or experience that is recalled. Most of the semantic recalls have highly specific and focused information and the brain resources used for this may be minimal. Remembrance of experiences have a different format, as one often remembers the source—the time and place of the occurrence of the experience, and the details of the experience, which may be accompanied by sensory-motor imageries and proprioceptive activation, including emotional arousal all over again. Remembrance may therefore demand higher level of brain activation compared to retrieval of a semantic information.

Neuroimaging studies have shown significant differences in the brain activation patterns of knowing and remembrance. Remembrance of autobiographic episodes or experience may be associated with activation of large spectrum of the brain viz., orbitofrontal cortex, anterior cingulate, and temporal cortex and other sensory areas depending on the modality of imageries recreated (Steinvorth et al. 2006; Vandekerckhove et al. 2005; Umeda et al. 2005; Naghavi, Nyberg 2005; Moscovitch et al. 2005; Cabeza et al. 2004; Giloba et al. 2004; Horiike et al. 2004; Turriziani et al. 2003; Luu et al. 2003; Graham et al. 2003; Markowitsch et al. 2003; Fletcher et al. 2001; Aggleton, Brown 1999; Smith, Jonides 199a, b; Tulving et al. 1994a, b; Gardiner, Java 1990; Tulving 1987). Remembrance of past personal events would further require activation of the source memory, which provides the time, place, and contextual links for the remembered episode. Source memory has independent localization, mainly in the anterior frontal cortex (Cinel et al. 2002; Marsh et al. 2002; Hicks, Marsh 2001; Jones et al. 2001; Cycowicz et al. 2001, 1997; Troyer, Craik 2000; Lepage et al. 2000; Janowsky et al. 1989; Milner et al. 1985; Schacter et al. 1984; Tulving 1972). A frontal activation and judgment becomes imperative for remembering (ecphory) and associating the specific source and episode that happened in life. The stage of ecphory occurs when brain areas are activated producing the remembrance of the actual episode (Roland, Gulyás 1995). Source memory provides the index details of when and where for all the autobiographic episodes, which help one self-verify the remembered episode. Activation of bilateral middle temporal lobes including hippocampus and medial frontal regions have been reported in remembrance of autobiographical episodes (Graham et al. 2003; Maguire, Frith 2003; Haist et al. 2001; Leveroni et al. 2000; Reinkemeier et al. 1997; Nyberg et al. 1996b; Evans et al. 1995; Harris, Kay 1995). Pure semantic recall produced activation of left frontal and temporal activation, whereas person identification was found to be associated with bilateral frontal and temporal engagement (Steinvorth et al. 2006; Reinkemeier et al. 1997; Nyberg et al. 1996a, b; Evans et al. 1995; Harris and Kay 1995). Gilboa (2004) obtained a left ventromedial prefrontal cortical activation during autobiographic recalls, whereas a right mid-dorsolateral prefrontal activation was seen in the recall of familiar words, pictures, and faces, differentiating between routine episodic recalls and recall of autobiographical events. Cabeza et al. (2004) reported that autobiographical recall produced greater activation in the medial prefrontal cortex, visual and parahippocampal region, and hippocampus, representing self-referential processing effect, visuospatial memory effects, and recall effects respectively. A comparison of recent and remote autobiographical information with remote semantic information showed that recent and remote autobiographical remembrance elicited activation of large bilateral neural network (Steinvorth et al. 2006). They found that the neural activation elicited during remembrance extended across the anterior and posterior parts of the middle temporal gyrus spreading into superior temporal sulcus, temporoparietal junction, middle and superior frontal gyri, anterior paracingulate and cingulate gyri, and left inferior orbital frontal gyrus. On the other hand semantic retrieval produced activation in the bilateral supramarginal and inferior frontal cortices, left insular cortex, and inferior temporal gyrus. Motor imageries could produce neural activation in the motor and premotor cortex (Amick et al. 2006; de Fiorio et al. 2006; Nyberg et al. 2006; de Lange et al. 2005; Rodriguez et al. 2004; Solodkin et al. 2004; Ross et al. 2003; Rosen et al. 2001) as if the brain is really activated during remembrance. Such recreated motor images are often part of remembrance of experiences of participation of activities (Mukundan 2007a, 2007b, 2008, 2009, 2010, 2011a), which further supports that no differences exist between the neural activation between imagined and real movements. These studies also have revealed the extensive use of EEG coherence technique for the detection of visual and motor imageries, when individuals are cued to remember experiences. A verbally transcoded or encoded detail would be sufficient for one to recreate the associated imageries, which straightaway validates the remembrance. Thus, when one thinks of dear ones, home, or office, one recreates the respective visual imageries. One cannot recreate the relevant imageries, if one does not know the person or he was not in the place referred. However, one may not normally recreate the imageries of the persons, objects, and places if one is very familiar with them, as one can use the transcoded detail for routine applications. The results of various studies show that the extent of neural activation in the brain during remembrance is indeed a function of the complexity of the details of remembrance decided by the individual's preoccupation with the components of the activity participated.

The source details of time and place are not either written or retrieved from the brain as absolute information. They are relative information and in comparison with the episode that took place immediately prior and they are arranged in sequence, which the individual can retrieve and personally verify. The source details are therefore often retrieved more easily in comparison with other important details, unless the episode has an extraordinary importance for the concerned individual. Remembering the place of occurrence of an episode is found to be always easier than remembering the time of its occurrence, as place is associated with several other features of the episode remembered. Thus, one remembers a party, which one celebrated in a hotel. One may more easily remember an encounter, discussion or argument one had in a place than its specific occasion. Remembrance of the temporal aspects occurs only slowly and one has to often remember the antecedent and precedent activities, before one can confirm the occasion of a specific activity. This is true of all other remembrances of time, as the brain does not have subjective sense of time. On the one hand all of us depend on external estimation of time and it is always used as a reference point for the brain. Each brain estimates time from its own engagements or participation in activities. Time of occurrence is fixed by identifying the activity in a sequence of the activities that took place during a particular period for which there is an external reference of time. One remembers a certain day as the one, which fell two days after a certain particular incidence and one day before another incidence. The time stands subjectively still, while the whole world and the body pass through continuous changes from which a time estimation is made. One can experience visiting the same place repeatedly at different points in time. Objects around and places become as real as the body, whereas the self continues staying in the present forever as it emerges as a self-referencing reflection of the body and its sensory-motor processes, without ever being able to visit the past or the future.

Memory relates to complex functions related to storage and retrieval processes of information, as known to the person who created them, as well as those not understood by him, which one has consciously learnt and acquired without knowledge. What is stored in the brain is indeed a neural signal carried by the neurotransmitters or equivalent neurochemical substances. Billions of neurons make several trillions of connections and these connections carry information created at an extraordinary and unique mental level and we call the information domain created in the brain, the mind. The information stored in the connections can be directly read (?) by the brain in a different occasion, and this process marks the retrieval phase of information. The emotional state of the brain is indeed different from the domain of meanings, even though emotional states may also be transcoded and stored. Presence of emotions indeed affects the meanings created, their storage, and retrieval. Hence, it is indeed appropriate to think that the brain has its own equivalent digital system for carrying information created. We believe that the trillions of connections form patterns carrying the meanings or units of information created in the brain and they are equivalent to the familiar digital patterns. We have developed the concepts of cell assemblies, engrams and memory traces, which represent this system that carry information. It would mean that there is a cell assembly for each unit of information and cell assemblies may represent several such engrams representing multiple units of information. There is no reason to consider that all signals received in the brain through sensory inputs are saved or stored automatically and permanently. What can be recalled are only those, which have been converted to information. Mere recognition of an external object involves the process of retrieving a stored memory trace and matching it with the external model or the sensory image formed by the external stimulus, and identifying the external model as the matching internal model or memory trace. It may be more appropriate to consider that all sensory inputs trigger retrieval of matching memory traces automatically and the source of stimulation is directly identified. The brain continuously acquires new internal models and redefines them if needed. During recognition, one readily recognizes the object or makes efforts to remember or retrieve the matching engram. One is normally not aware of the processing of the neural signal or retrieval taking place. When recognition does not automatically happen, one may retrieve part of the source and even have notion of familiarity, and the source may or not be finally recognized. The conversion to neural signals and from neural signals, are normally beyond any voluntary control of the individual, and the brain becomes aware of only the sensory effects and the converted equivalent or the information. Not only the interpreted units of information, that are stored, but also their sensory and motor images, if present. Information acquired through conceptual exercises and experience may have different storage mechanisms, as the latter do not have experiential (sensory-motor) components. A unit of conceptual information can be retrieved in isolation, without any interlinking details. However, experiences always have their source details of time, place, and other contextual details, without which one cannot personally ascertain that one is retrieving a self-acquired experience. This is also true of recognition of most of the entities one makes. Thus, one may readily recognize the building or an object in a picture, without ever having visited the place or handled the object even once. One may have information about an entity without ever experiencing the same. One can create a concept even if it is imaginary and without having any reality verified composition of its components. However, if one has visited the same building or handled an object even once before, one readily remembers visiting the place or handling the object, and the associated visual and motor imageries may be readily recreated, which substantiate the experience. Presence of mental imageries is readily accepted as indication of having done reality verification, because the brain activation pattern in imagery is as good as online recognition or participation.

When semantic information unconnected with any experience is stored, it could be stored in isolation even though one may link up several such ideas. However, several of the semantic units of information may not have any such links though we may repeatedly retrieve such isolated blocks of information for various cognitive applications. Thus, we learn arithmetical tables and the definition of several concepts and keep retrieving them for use in everyday life. Such pieces of information remain isolated and we learn to retrieve them with least effort. The recall is always automatic and needs least conscious effort, and can be generally accomplished without shifting attention and interrupting another ongoing mental processing. This is not possible when the semantic information recalled is complex and has strategic importance and is to be used for critical decision-making. During complex decision-making, attention needs to be withdrawn from the external world and directed to the thinking process and its contents. The brain-mind resources used will increase in such attended mental processing and the increase can be expected to be proportionate to the complexity of the processing.

Repeated retrieval of the same idea renders the idea familiar. Even a single repeat recognition of the same entity, person, or idea may help develop the notion of familiarity, though the notion of familiarity may be week and not long lasting. Knowing that one has seen the stimulus before creates the notion of familiarity. The N-back test is a common ERP tool that is used to elicit this neurocognitive effect. Familiarity could be conceptual as well as experiential. Significant morphological and amplitude changes in the P300 potentials (Fig. 7) may be the neurocognitive effects (Mukundan, 1999) seen, whenever one notices a stimulus has been already seen in the immediate previous trial (n-1). It could be more complex as shown by Curran et al. (2006), where they found a negative potential followed by a positive potential when familiar words were recognized along with new words in a study for determining the adverse effect of a pharmacological agent Medozolam on familiarity. Such negative potentials followed by positive peaks were also reported in BEOS profiling (TIFAC-DFS report 2008) and it is used as a measure of familiarity in this test. Familiarity can arouse emotionality if the original experience or the stimulus had indeed elicited an emotional response.

Failure of retrieval of engrams easily result in failure of recognition, which are called Agnosias. In visual agnosia, patients with posterior brain lesions fail to recognize common objects like fan, pen, wristwatch, book, etc. Similarly, with left hemisphere lesions, patients may fail to recognize words from auditory images and to recreate words by retrieving them from the lexical system. These deficits manifest neuropsychologically as receptive and expressive aphasias and their variations. The patients who are unable to retrieve the internal traces respond as though they have never seen those objects or heard the words ever before, when they are presented to them by the examiner or others. Agnosias occur in all sensory modalities and their cause could be loss of the memory trace, which is required for matching of the sensory image of the external object and its identification, because of neural degeneration or damage, or the neural assembly carrying the memory trace remains inaccessible because of blocks or loss of connecting networks. Visual agnosia, simultanagnosia, prosopagnosia, impairment in getting names, recognition of meaning of words are because of difficulty in retrieving the internal models. The fact that the patient's ability to recognize the sensory model is restored sometimes within a few days or longer periods, clearly indicate that the impairment can occur even if the memory trace itself is not lost, and difficulty in accessing the meaning produces the same difficulty.

Recognition is a basic survival need and hence each brain learns to recognize various stimuli in the environment automatically, whenever and wherever they are encountered. As already mentioned, response from the brain can occur even without recognition if the sensory source has survival threatening value. However, if there is no survival need or threat, one may be able to thwart or block the automatic response and an object, or person may go unrecognized. Study (Mukundan et al. 1999) using hypnosis clearly shows that recognition of a stimulus can be blocked or altered, even if sensory registration of the stimulus has taken place. This is proposed to be a frontal lobe phenomenon (Mukundan et al. 2013), which interferes with normal stimulus interpretation (recognition) process under suggestion. The P300 ERP associated with recognition was blocked mainly in the frontal and central areas. Hypnotic suggestion induced a person to hear a weak tone (40 dB) much louder than a louder (80 dB) tone, and it produced a P300 potential of significantly greater amplitude than the one produced by the 80 dB tone in the same participants in normal testing condition. Comparison of the memory trace and acceptance of a trace as matching with an external stimulus can be influenced by suggestions and a prevailing mindset of an individual. Under external or personal influences, one may not recognize or recognize what one wishes to see or hear and accept that as the reality. Critical decision-making has to be intentionally practised for overcoming the suggestive and inducing effects influencing decision-making.

Retrieval Mechanisms

Two different processes have been identified for the retrieval of any information from memory, based on the type of information stored in the memory.

1. Automatic Retrieval—cue dependent, recall is mandatory and effortless.
2. Strategic Retrieval—voluntary, recall is intentional and effortful.

Retrieval required for recognition of external stimuli (persons, objects and other entities). Retrieval is also required for applying stored information from the knowledge bank, in various cognitive processing tasks, and skills required for execution mental and other motor tasks, etc. Most of the data retrieval requires the use of languages. Another category of recall is of autobiographical episodes, which may be cued recall or intentional recall. A cue can be a person, object, or a place visually perceived, or heard or read in verbal statement heard, which makes one remember a related past personal episode. When the episode is personal, it is called autobiographical episode. The stimulus, which provides the cue need not necessarily be directly related to the episode recalled, but must have an incidental or contextual relationship. A stimulus serves as cue for provoking or triggering the recall of the stimulus-linked experience. The appropriateness of the experience or autobiographical episode remembered is assured by the contextual validation from the source memory, i.e. when and where the episode took place. Examples: The pen reminds one of the birthday party when it was presented by a dear friend. Reference to a person (X) during a conversation with a friend makes one think of him (X), and the violent argument that took place between the two a few years ago. One remembers not only the incident, but also the experiences of visual and motor activities are recreated in the brain as imageries, which validate the remembered experience.

Recall of episodes is different from the recall of strategic information. Autobiographic information or episodes are retrieved with cues or intentionally. The person may remember the episode with their source and recreate the imageries of the original sensory-motor experience.

Autobiographic recall of recent episodes may become weak during ageing, though remote memory may become more prominent. Studies (Belleville et al. 2006; Ball et al. 2002; Stigsdotter et al. 1995; Verhaeghen et al. 1992) have shown improvement in serial and episodic recall after memory retraining in ageing adults with and without mild cognitive impairment. Cued recall is automatic, mandatory, and effortless and the retrieved material may be a conceptual information or autobiographic episode. When autobiographical episode is remembered, the individual is suddenly filled with the recreated sensory-motor imageries, emotional arousal if present and these are accessed through source memory.

Strategic recall, on the other hand, requires organization in the retrieval process, as the stored information has an original sequence and the various parts of information need to be sequentially retrieved or at least organized after retrieval. Retrieval may require logical-sequential links, which have to be mentally provided for the retrieval of relevant and linked pieces of information. Such retrieval may also require close monitoring to assure the relevancy/appropriateness of the retrieved information, both totally and in the time slot where it is recalled. Examples of strategic retrieval are recalling information for answering a question in the examination, recall required for preparation of an article or document, recall required when one wants to present a point of view in a discussion, or delivery of speech. Both retrieval of the information and the inclusion of the retrieved information as appropriate are intentional. However, such strategic recall may be difficult for persons who have not practised and built the ability for the application of strategies for recall purpose.

Retrieval Strategies

Strategic retrieval consists of several steps as given below:

1. Intention to retrieve and setting a mental set of retrieval mode.
2. Evolving a Strategy to Retrieve—sequence of recall, semantic/conceptual organization.
3. Hold the Strategy in working memory.
4. Engaging in monitoring the retrieved contents—Evaluation of the accuracy and appropriateness of the retrieved information. This requires working memory operation.
5. Correction of retrieval process as well as retrieved information needs working Memory.

Need for retrieval of large data banks of information does not exist anymore, as such data banks are stored in computer. Therefore, the major task is to decide the composition of the document rather than retrieval of the information. Though one may habitually learn strategic recall ability, construction of complex and strategically important documents will efficient retrieval of complex pieces of information for strategic applications will require learning and practice, and need to be mastered with great amount of practice and critical feedback. Careful evaluation of each stage of strategic retrieval is important, which one must personally carry out or obtain as feedback from competent others, and learn the strategy of the retrieval process.

Retrieval from memory takes place automatically. Writing into memory is an art, especially when the encoded information does not have personal significance and may not have any significant contextual reference. Information, which cannot be retrieved, is as good as nonexistent to the brain, which has stored it, unless it has a potential value to influence thinking and actions at a non-conscious level. The importance of such contextual reference or the need to link up the stored information with a piece of information is experienced only when one knows that some information is stored, but one is not capable of retrieving it. The following are examples of typical difficulties encountered by individuals, who could reveal their difficulty in interviews on remembrance (personal communication):

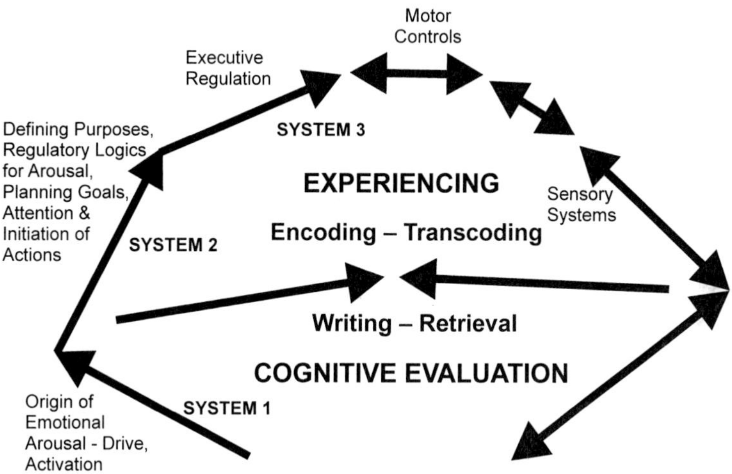

Fig. 11: The Brainmind

"While trying to sleep, I tried to recall the movie that I saw the previous night. Surprisingly I found that I could not remember anything about the movie. I remembered sitting in front of the TV and watching the film, but absolutely no idea about the movie that I watched. I could not visualize a single scene or the face of the actors. I tried to remember the sequence of events in the evening before watching the film. I remembered changing the movie channel to Star Channel in which the movie was shown, and swapping channels in between. Still there was no clue of the film or even a minor detail of the movie, its contents, or theme. I made all the efforts to recall a scene from the film. I even knew that I had watched the same movie once before. Then, it happened. As I was making efforts to recall, two faces emerged and the scene of a train. I could even remember the name of the movie—'Narrow Escape'. I recognized the characters, the scene and entire film was unfolded in a second.

"I was driving back home from the vet's clinic. I have to take a right turn to get into the main road. I was tired. I drove ahead straight. I did not remember that I should have turned right. I did not remember noticing the cross where I should have turned right. Then my son said that I should turn back. It is then I knew that I had not taken the right turn. In fact it is then I remembered that I was driving back home. Earlier I was not aware that I was driving back home for some time. In fact, I did not know where I was going. I was just driving. It occurred to me only when my son told me I should turn back that I remembered that I was to reach some place.

"I was trying to recall the name of the famous Tabla player. I could not. It was not the first time I had difficulty to recall his name. At least thrice before, I have failed to recall the same name. I know that he has two names. I can even visualize his face, his hair! He is young, the son of the famous tabla player Alla Rakha. I know he composed the music for a film in which 'so and so' acted. He has played tabla for several classical recitals. I have some of those cassettes and CDs. I struggled to recall his name, but without any success. I know if check one of my CDs, his name is there. I thought of several names and I know his name is none from them. At last, I checked the CD on which his name was printed. It was there! I knew that name all the time, but could not recall. I know I may not recall his name again. I decided to find an association for his name. I found that one of the Presidents of India had the same name, so next time I will recall the President's name for remembering the name of the tabla player. It worked exactly the same way. I could not again recall his name in another occasion, and I knew that I must recall the President's name first. Alas! I got it without difficulty."

Memory Deficits

17

There is scope for using complex forms of tests in clinical neuropsychological assessment of patients with focal brain lesions, as many of the tests will show normal functioning whereas some will be affected by the lesion. Diffused brain lesions in the two hemispheres affect all functions including attention and comprehension in all modes, rendering testing patient beyond these limits difficult. Verbal as well as visual tests are to be used for testing patients for detecting impairment of encoding. The NIMHANS battery (Mukundan et al. 1979a, b; 1991; Mukundan 1996) consists of a verbal and visual learning and memory functions test, in which the same learning (stimulus) material (verbal or visual) is presented in three consecutive trials and the patient is instructed to recall what he heard or saw immediately in each trial. The verbal test is a narrative passage, which is read out to the patient by the examiner with instruction that he must recall the passage immediately (immediate recall) after the presentation. Immediate recall is possible only when the encoded information is held on, which is a working memory operation. The three trials are given one after the other. In the visual test, the stimulus material is a complex figure presented on a 6″ × 4″ card and the figure on the card is shown for 15 seconds each time, and the patient is instructed to draw the figure shown from memory immediately. A fourth trial is used in both the tests, and the patient is asked to recall from memory (speak and draw) the same material 10 minutes after (delayed recall) the third trial immediate recall. During the 10 minutes of delay, the patient is engaged in conversations instead of taking any test. In the visual form, a fifth trial is used when the patient is asked to copy the same design by looking at it. For scoring the recall performance, each passage is divided into several units or blocks of information. Instead of verbatim reproduction, if the patient recalls the central word from a block, which can indicate the meaning of that part of the sentence, the patient is considered to have reproduced it. Similarly, the complex visual design is divided into several small and independent sections and the patient's drawing is scored using this pattern. The test findings in frontal and nonfrontal focal lesion cases are presented here to discuss the role of these specific cortical areas in the performance on the tests and specifically encoding. A profile of rate of learning of each test material is thus obtained in different frontal and nonfrontal brain lesion groups and these mean scores are shown in the tables 11 to 14. The improvement in the scores normally seen in individuals in each trial is considered to indicate the learning made through repeatedly listening or seeing the same stimulus material (Mukundan et al. 1991, Mukundan 1996). The passages discussed here have 20 units of information using 53-60 words. Each block has 1 to 4 words. The scores on these tests are compared with the scores on tests of (Mukundan 1996) Sentence Repetition Test (SRT) for the purpose discussion. In the SRT, the patient need to reproduce the sentence verbatim and omission of any word is considered an error. The purpose of giving this test was to make sure that the patient was capable to repeat words after hearing them. The scores of all the tests are provided in the same tables. The SRT has 20 sentences; each to be repeated by the subject verbatim after it is read out by the experimenter. The number of words in the sentences increases from 3 to 17, in the increasing order. The score on this test is the number of sentences correctly repeated. The visual design has 23 blocks of components including the gestalt. The major categories of visual impairment are related to micrographia, macrographia, distortion, fragmentation, spatial disorientation, visual neglect, closing-in-phenomenon, exploded copying, and simplification. Several of these are the effects of right parietal lobe involvement. Only when the parietal lobe deficits are not present, and the drawing is still incomplete mainly because of missing figures, one may think of encoding (transcoding) deficits because of lesions in the left frontal and temporal lobes and that the patient probably failed to retrieve the transcoded detail instead of retrieving the detail from visual memory.

The three consecutive trials on the tests of Verbal (VLMF) and Visual Learning and Memory Functions (VSLMF tests) provide the encoding profile of an individual. The units of information in the passage are words related to (a) names of persons, places and objects, (b) emotions, (c) intentions and (d) actions related to specific persons, places, and objects. They are so arranged to provide (1) a sequence of events involving the above, (2) and association between any two successive sequences, and (3) an emerging theme. During encoding, one must take into consideration all these aspects. The encoding on this test is essentially that of semantic comprehension. The listener must comprehend the organization structure of the narration and the different components in each sequence of the event. The recall process reflects the existence of these organizational structures and their utilization from trial to trial. The three trials of VLMF test show how a subject improves performance in terms of details, over the repeated exposure to the same test material. It is very important that the subject understands the meaning and the logical associations in the story as he is expected to recall the events with the correct associations and sequence. In contrast to this, what is expected on the SRT is a phonologically correct recall. Example of the easiest sentence is "The wind blows" and the most difficult is "Mahatma Gandhi who won freedom for the country from the British is called the Father of the Nation". The emphasis in the test is on the words being recalled without mixing up or missing any. We do not test if the subject has understood the meaning of the sentence or not. The educational status of the patients is an important determinant of the scores they make in the three trials. However, the rate of increase in the score from trial 1 to trial 3 is not really affected by the educational status of the individual. This increase in the score over repeat trials is an indication of the learning ability of the brain and the score indicates the rate of learning in each individual.

In SRT test, all patients could repeat sentences with 10-12 words without any mistake. Difficulty was seen in the subsequent trials, when they started missing words. Words from the middle section were missed more often than words from the front or the end. Often they could reproduce the meaning of the sentence in their own words, though they could not repeat the same sentence verbatim. For example, though a patient could not repeat correctly the sentence—"Mahatma Gandhi, who won freedom for the country from the British is called the father of the nation", could say, "Mahatma Gandhi is called father of the nation. He got freedom for the country from the British." Though this response will not fetch the subject a score, it is apparent that the patient could understand the meaning of the sentence, which is suggestive of the presence of adequate encoding. Despite the fact this flexibility was allowed in the recall of the passage in the VLMF test, patients had difficulty to recall details and connect them. Though several patients could repeat 10-12 words in a sentence correctly, they could not recall more than 4-5 units of information even using single words in the units. Therefore, the difficulty in the SRT is to recall the sentence structure than the contents of the sentence. This is significantly different from the difficulty seen on the VLMF performance, in which patients have difficulty to recall the contents. The right frontal and left nonfrontal patients have difficulty to recall encoded material, whereas, it is the left nonfrontal patients who have maximum difficulty to repeat the sentence structure. The purpose of discussion at this stage is to understand how we improve performance in immediate recall during repeat presentation of the same test material.

Table 11: Showing the mean scores and SDs (in parenthesis) scores of patients with lesions in the left and right prefrontal, and left and right nonfrontal areas of the brain, and of normal control group (NC) on SRT and Verbal Learning & Memory Functions (VBLMF) tests in Trials 1 to 4

Group	SRT	(VBLMF) Passage 1							
		T-1	%-Tot	T-2	%-Tot	T-3	%-Tot	T-4	%-Tot
LPF (n=30)	16.2 (2.8)	5.9 (5.3)	30%	8.8 (6.4)	44%	9.8 (6.5)	49%	6.5 (5.3)	33%
RPF (n=30)	17.5 (2.6)	11.4 (4.9)	57%	13.9 (5.1)	70%	16.7 (5.6)	84%	14.3 (6.0)	72%
LNPF (n=11)	15.1 (2.7)	9.5 (4.9)	48%	11.5 (4.1)	58%	10.7 (4.2)	51%	5.6 (4.2)	28%
RNPF (n=11)	17.6 (2.5)	11.1 (3.4)	56%	14.8 (4.5)	74%	18.1 (4.9)	91%	17.1 (4.9)	86%
NC (n=30)	19.0 (1.1)	11.6 (3.6)	58%	15.6 (3.8)	78%	19.4 (4.4)	97%	18.8 (4.4)	94%
P	<0.05	<0.01		<0.01		<0.01		<0.01	

(LPF - Left Prefrontal Cortical lesion; RPF - Right Prefrontal Cortical lesion; LNPF - Left Nonprefrontal Cortical lesion; RNPF - Right Nonprefrontal Cortical lesion; NC - Normal Control Group; n - number of patients; %-Tot - Percentage of the Total Score. The normal group is age and education matched with the patients groups.

Table 12: Showing the mean scores and SDs (in parenthesis) scores of patients with lesions in the left and right prefrontal, and left and right nonfrontal areas of the brain, and of normal control group (NC) on Visual Learning & Memory Functions (VSLMF) test

Group	(VSLMF) Complex Figure							
	T-1	%-Tot	T-2	%-Tot	T-3	%-Tot	T-4	%-Tot
LPF (n=30)	3.9 (4.2)	17%	4.5 (4.1)	20%	4.6 (4.5)	20%	3.3 (3.3)	14%
RPF (n=30)	4.1 (4.5)	18%	5.4 (4.6)	23%	5.8 (5.2)	25%	4.6 (4.5)	20%
LNPF (n=11)	8.3 (5.1)	36%	10.5 (4.6)	46%	12.7 (5.2)	55%	6.4 (4.6)	28%
RNPF(n=11)	3.1 (3.4)	13%	4.7 (4.3)	20%	4.6 (4.2)	20%	2.1 (4.1)	9%
NC (n=30)	8.6 (4.6)	37%	10.6 (5.7)	46%	14.6 (4.2)	63%	15.1 (4.1)	66%
P	<0.01		<0.01		<0.01		<0.01	

Table 13: Showing information gained (learnt) in the 3rd Trial recall and lost in the 4th Trial Delayed Recall shown as Percentage of 1 and 3 Trial recall scores in the Verbal Learning & Memory Function (VLMF) Test.

Groups	T-1 Recall % of Total Passage Score (20)	T-3 - T-1	T-3 Recall % of Total Passage Score	% of Increase in Trial 3	T-4 - T-3 Loss in Delayed Recall	% of Loss in Trial 4 DR
LPF (n = 30)	30%	3.9	49%	20%	3.3	34%
RPF (n = 30)	57%	5.3	84%	27%	2.4	14%
LNPF (n = 11)	48%	1.2	54%	6%	5.1	48%
RNPF (n = 11)	56%	7.0	79%	35%	1.0	6%
NC (n = 30)	58%	7.8	97%	39%	0.6	3%

Table 14: Showing information gained (learnt) in the 3rd Trial recall and lost in the 4th Trial Delayed Recalls shown as Percentage of 1 and 3 Trial recall scores in the Visual Learning & Memory Function (VSLMF) Test.

Group	T-1 Recall % of Total V Design Score (23)	T-3 - T-1	% of T-3 Recall Score	% of Increase in Trial 3	T-4 - T-3 Loss in Delayed Recall	% of Loss in Trial 4 DR
LPF (n = 30)	17%	0.7	20%	3%	1.3	5%
RPF (n = 30)	18%	1.7	25%	7%	1.2	5%
LNPF (n = 11)	36%	4.4	55%	19%	6.3	27%
RNPF (n = 11)	13%	1.5	20%	7%	2.5	11%
NC (n = 30)	37%	6.0	63%	26%	+0.5	+ 2%

Patients whose results are shown in above tables were selected after the sites of the brain lesion were identified by CT scan, which was confirmed later in the neurosurgery, each patient underwent. The size of the lesion was not controlled. The different groups of patients with specific brain lesions were as shown in the tables 11 to 14. There were seven patients with temporal lobe lesion in each of the nonfrontal lesion groups and the remaining had parietal lobe lesion. None had clinically significant speech problems that could interfere with the administration of the test. They all could perform on the visual drawing test.

The results are indicative of significant left and right lateralized impairment in verbal and visual and verbal learning and memory functions respectively, indicated by their immediate and delayed recall profiles. The learning and memory impairment is most significantly present in the prefrontal lesion cases compared to the non-prefrontal lesion cases. Analysis of the data shows that the left prefrontal lesion groups had significant impairment in the verbal learning test in the first and subsequent trials, whereas the performance of the right lesion groups on the same test was comparable with that of the normal control group. On the other hand, visual learning and memory functions were significantly impaired in both right and left prefrontal lesion groups. With regard to the non-prefrontal lesion effects, visual immediate and delayed recalls were impaired mainly in the right non-prefrontal lesion group. The mean immediate recall of the left non-prefrontal lesion group was comparable with that of the normal control group in the first and second trials. The mean third trial performance of this group did not reach the level of recall of the normal group, though the difference between their means was not statistically significant. However, the mean visual delayed recall of the left-nonfrontal group showed very significant impairment in comparison with that of the normal control group. The mean delayed recall score of these patients was indeed better than that of the other two prefrontal lesion groups, and especially better than that of the right non-prefrontal lesion group. However, it was very significantly poorer than that of the normal control group. The visual delayed recall of the right nonfrontal lesion patients was the worst. What is not apparent in the present results is the effect of visual search on the visual learning and memory functions test. Visual search could be impaired if the functions of Frontal eye field area (Brodmann's area 8) is affected by the lesion. Visual search may be considered a part of the visual attention and impairment in the visual search can contribute to poor encoding and consequent poor retrieval. Encoding and retrieval processes themselves may not be impaired in these cases. However, both left and right lesion groups and right nonfrontal lesions groups have performed poorly on the visual learning and memory functions test.

The percentage of loss of information in the delayed recall is insignificant in the normal control group in the verbal test, whereas they have shown a minimal insignificant increase in the performance in the delayed visual recall. The verbal loss of verbal information in the delayed recall is very significant in the left frontal and nonfrontal lesion group. The left frontal lesion group could learn only 49% of the passage by the third trial and it reached 54% in the left nonfrontal lesion group suggesting the role played by the left frontal area in verbal learning. The profile is significantly different in the right lesion group with regard to verbal learning. These patients showed significantly higher verbal learning ability compared to the left lesion patients, even though they did not reach the normal level of rate of learning. Their loss of information in the delayed recall is also very high compared to the right lesion groups. There was hardly any significant loss of verbal information in the right lesion groups and it was comparable with that of the normal control group. With regard to visual learning, the right hemisphere lesion groups and left prefrontal lesion group show very significant impairment in learning ability. The left nonfrontal lesion group could perform significantly better than the other lesion groups. Loss of visual information in the delayed recall, compared to their third trial recall, was not much in the right lesion and left prefrontal lesion groups as their third trial learning itself was very weak. The left nonfrontal lesion group did better than the other lesion groups on immediate visual recall test, but showed severe loss of visual details in the delayed recall test. Interestingly, the delayed recall of normal participants was as good their third trial recall. The mean score of the group showed a marginal (insignificant) increase in the delayed recall compared to their third trial recall.

The findings clearly support the role of the left prefrontal area in modality nonspecific encoding function. Interviews with normal and patients had shown that almost all of them verbally transcoded any non-familiar visual material, especially in a test situations, and tried to remember the verbal details of the non-familiar visual stimulus material during their later recalls. This is found to be all the more important when the visual stimulus material or the task is complex. Remembrance tests using EEG parameters have clearly supported (Mukundan 2007a, b, 2008, 2010, 2011a) the presence of visual imagery during the recall of visual information triggered by verbal inputs, which activate left prefrontal areas. The time allotted to the participants to examine the complex figure was only 15 seconds, which was too less to make a visual pattern which could be stored in memory. Even the normal control group could recall only 63% of the total units of visual information in their third trial of the test, whereas their mean delayed verbal recall was 97% in the third trial. In the visual test, it was easier for the participants to recognize and think of the different components, and later recall the verbal information for their visual reproduction. Several neuroimaging studies have revealed the role of the left frontal cortex in using verbal information for recreating visual and other imageries of experiences (Babiloni et al. 2006, Kosslyn et al. 2005, 1999, 1997; Ganis et al. 2004; Beck et al. 2001; Mellet et al. 2000; Buckner et al. 1999) during their remembrance. The encoding dysfunction associated with left prefrontal lesion produced the impairment in both verbal and visual tests. This effect is not seen in the left nonfrontal lesion group of patients. The right hemisphere lesion, whether it is in the frontal or nonfrontal areas, has a severe detrimental effect on visual learning and recall, as seen by the scores of these groups of patients. Both immediate recall and learning through repeated exposure to the same visual stimulus were poor in these patients, indicating that learning may be severely impaired in frontal lesions and to lesser extent in nonfrontal lesions. Learning in the tests used here is the ability to recognize and hold on to more units of information, when exposed to the same information matrix, which can be consolidated if required. Their recall is the indication that they have taken in more information from trial to trial.

Most important indicator of the effect of lesion is seen in the rate of learning over trials of both verbal and visual materials. Normal controls could show 39% and 26% mean increases in their verbal and visual recall through repeat learning from trial 1 to trial 3, and they could learn to recall 97% of the passage and 63% of the visual pattern. They could also retain what they learnt and present the entire material during the delayed recall. These aspects were severely impaired in the frontal patients indicating the important role played by the frontal areas in encoding as well as retaining the material in short-term or working memory. What the patients could not learn despite repeatedly listening to the same passage are the details of the events and their sequence, including the details of the persons involved in the narrated events. Interestingly, it was seen that many normal individuals tend to forget the verbal and visual material totally or near totally when asked to recall the same after a day or two, whereas some (20%) do remember 70-85% of what recalled on these later occasions. What is recalled is what one has learnt, and therefore recall has to be used as an index of learning. Recall can occur in various contexts, as seen in the present tests. Visual learning is tested by measuring the number of units of visual information one has been able to reproduce while drawing memory. However, one cannot recall what is not learnt and one may not recall all that one has learnt.

Effect of Age on Learning

The three factors that may have effects on the capacity for learning are age, education, and occupational background. Performance is indeed improves during the developmental years and there is hardly any difference because of age since then. The tables 15 and 16 below show the mean scores of normal controls of age groups ranging from 16 to 40 and 41-55 years of the literate and illiterate categories. Literacy does have a definite effect on the performance on the learning and memory functions test as shown in the table below. Despite this, it is not uncommon to find in the clinical situation, that some patients with poor formal educational backgrounds perform reasonably well on those tests, which may be facilitated by their occupational proficiency.

Table 15: Showing the mean scores on VBLMF tests (Passage 1) in the normal controls

	GROUP I (n=60) Normal Literate Community Control Group				GROUP II (n=60) Normal Illiterate Community Control Group			
	A (16-40 Yrs) MA = 27.6 Yrs		A (41-55 Yrs) MA = 46.5 Yrs		A (16-40 Yrs) MA = 28.6 Yrs		A (41-55 Yrs) MA = 48.6 Yrs	
	MEAN	SD	MEAN	SD	MEAN	SD	MEAN	SD
Trial I	11.8	4.8	10.7	4.6	6.4	3.7	7.2	4.1
Trial II	13.3	4.1	12.5	4.2	4.6	4.6	9.5	4.8
Trial III	16.6	3.8	17.4	4.1	12.5	3.9	13.5	4.1
Trial IV	15.6	3.5	16.8	4.3	12.3	5.1	12.5	5.9

MA - Mean Age

There is a significant difference in the mean trial scores of the two age groups in the literate and illiterate normal control groups. The (41-55) year illiterate group has done better than the (16-40) year group in the Trials 1 and 2 verbal recalls compared to the Trial 3 recall. However, the two groups have shown significant increase in the performance from Trial I to Trial III in both verbal and visual recalls and the loss in the delayed recall is not affected in the illiterate group of community control subjects in either mode of presentation. Despite absence of formal education, the brains of the individuals of the second group have shown remarkable learning ability, which reaches a heightened level of ability through formal education, as seen in the first group.

Table 16: Showing the mean scores on the VSLMF Figure tests (Visual) in the normal controls

	GROUP I (n = 60) Normal Literate Community Control Group				GROUP II (n = 60) Normal Illiterate Community Control Group			
	A (16-40 Yrs)		A (41-55 Yrs)		A (16-40 Yrs)		A (41-55 Yrs)	
	MEAN	SD	MEAN	SD	MEAN	SD	MEAN	SD
Trial I	10.8	4.6	10.7	4.6	4.4	3.7	6.2	4.1
Trial II	14.3	4.5	14.1	4.8	7.6	5.6	9.5	5.8
Trial III	16.6	6.8	16.8	7.1	10.5	5.9	10.5	5.1
Trial IV	16.1	6.5	15.8	6.3	9.8	6.1	9.5	6.9

Encoding is a cognitive process used in each human brain for converting sensory signals from outside and those generated within the body into information based on stored knowledge base, as well as for creating new units of information. Encoding allows constant expansion and enrichment of the database, which may be purely conceptual or experientially verified. Encoding may occur at simple to complex levels for creation or recreation of meaning or information. The need to encode and learn by repeated efforts is extremely important and complex cognitive ability, which is employed for facilitating performance to optimum levels. Encoding takes place at multiple levels for creating diverse and complex ideas, which may be formed in a hierarchical and sequential manner. Normal individuals show significant improvement in their immediate recall from trial to trial, when they have chance to read or listen to the same complex verbal material or examine visual inputs. This is an extremely important cognitive asset, in which every person may want to excel. It is true that listening or reading a text once may be enough to understand and reproduce most of the information in the text, when the text is simple and familiar. Repeat practice is important for learning and mastering various skeletomuscular movements and motor skills. Repeat practice is the method used by all for learning and remembering all verbal materials. Left frontal cortex is the core brain center, which develops the encoding ability. The left non-frontal cortical areas support the encoding process of verbal inputs, whereas right hemisphere carries out the processing of visual inputs. Encoding involves semantic interpretation of parts of the inputs and interpretation of the parts into a total to extract a final and ultimate meaning. The same may be carried out with visual inputs also though the primary task is to transcode the visual segments into verbal equivalents. Thus in the VSLM, the individual sees "a large rectangle, with diagonals, and another rectangle inside and so on...". Prior to semantic processing, the verbal inputs pass through processing at phonological, lexical, and syntactic levels. The left prefrontal cortex works with the auditory cortex for semantic interpretation, which would include determining the word meaning and logical/sequential associations. Lack of language skills affected the performance of the illiterate groups as was elicited from their interviews. They held on to the same visual designs, which they could identify separately for the immediate and delayed recalls.

There was also no evidence of utilization of any particular strategy during the recall in the left lesion patients. What most of them have produced are unconnected events or sequences, which would not, or only partially, add up to the total theme or the narration in the passage. Earlier studies have revealed that lesions of both prefrontal cortex and medial temporal cortex impair performance on memory tasks (Squire et al. 1996; Squire 1992). They cited evidence from several animal and patient studies to show that medial temporal lesion has caused partial and total loss of new experiences, though other cognitive function remain relatively normal. Similarly early Pet studies (Jones et al. 1978; Fletcher et al. 1995, 1997; Haxby et al. 1996; Cabeza et al. 1997) have consistently demarcated the prefrontal cortex in encoding and retrieval tasks. However, there is no evidence to suggest that temporal areas are actively involved during encoding. They do appear to have a major role in the consolidation of information. The hippocampal and parahippocampal areas interact with the frontal lobes through cortico-cortical connections (Clarke et al. 1994). Buckner et al. (1999) put forth the hypothesis that memory formation takes place only when the medial temporal cortex mediates the new information processed by the frontal lobes. They suggested, "The medial temporal lobe may then function to bind together processed information from frontal and other cortical regions to form lasting, recollectable memory traces." Normally, encoding occurs in an incidental manner, though most of encoding carried out by one may be intentional as there is a need to encode.

Clinical Memory Disorders

Several etiological factors have been identified which cause memory impairment in individuals. Some of these are (a) degenerative disorders of the brain, (b) space occupying lesions in the brain, (c) traumatic injuries to the brain, (d) deficiency disorders, (e) neurological disorders (e.g. epilepsy) affecting memory specific areas in the brain, and (f) functional traumatic conditions. Clinical memory impairment has been traditionally classified into (a) Progressive Amnesia, (b) Focal Amnesia, (c) Global Amnesia, (d) Transient Global Amnesia, (e) Anterograde Amnesia, and (f) Retrograde Amnesia. Amnesia has been identified as a specific symptom of alcohol dependence. All progressive diffused pathology of the brain produces dementias of which amnesia could be an important feature. Brain traumatic conditions inflicted in head injuries can cause anterograde amnesia and Transient Global Amnesia. Lesions affecting the axial structures (mainly hippocampus and thalamus) cause the progressive type of amnesia (Eichenbaum et al. 1994; Eichenbaum, 2001; Paller et al. 2003; Milner 2005; Gabrieli, Kao 2007; Kopelman et al. 2009). The different types of amnesias clinically identified indicate the complexity of writing into memory and strategies required to retrieve the stored information. It is important to differentiate between storage of information and its retrieval, as difficulties at both the processing sites may manifest as memory problem. The inadequacies in the two phases of storage and retrieval occur because of brain pathology as well as functional inadequacies in the brain. A brain lesion can directly interrupt the storage process of information, whereas presence of anxiety and emotional factors affects both storage and retrieval functions. Encoding information and its storage must be conceptualized as the activity of a complex functional network rather than as a localized brain function. However, when encoding is not affected, but there is problem in the consolidation and retrieval of information, it is identified as a memory problem, and clinically as amnesia. A differentiation of problems that arise during consolidation and storage and retrieval would help to identify and focus on the real problem of amnesia in a patient.

Progressive Amnesia

Progressive amnesia is the most common clinically encountered memory problem, when individuals fail to retrieve all newly learnt information, even though they have no difficulty to remember information or knowledge acquired prior to the onset of an illness or lesion of the brain. The characteristic feature of the amnesia is the progressive loss of all newly learnt information, which may occur within a few seconds to hours, after acquiring a new piece of information. However, the actual neural problem is that of poor or absence of storage of information than the difficulty for retrieval. The progressive amnesia becomes severe as the disease progresses. It becomes worse as the patient keeps forgetting his recent past and thereby loses touch with the recent activities one has engaged in. The patient's ability to recall events and conceptual information learnt prior to a specific period may be found intact. This particular amnesia was called the "axial" amnesia by Barbizet (1971), as it was noticed that the axial structures of the brain are responsible for the memory deficit. The typical memory deficit of progressive nature was detected in Wernicke encephalopathy, which alcohol dependent patients develop. The neurotoxicity caused by thiamine deficiency affects the diencephalon and the frontal cortex, and the thalamic and hippocampal involvement manifest as a disorder known as Korsakoff's syndrome, with memory disorder (Shimamura et al. 1990; Joyce, Robbins 1991; Paller, Acharya 1997; Kopelman et al. 2009). Patients with bilateral temporal lobe damage may develop memory impairment for experiences and knowledge acquired in daily life, whereas their previously acquired knowledge remains preserved (Milner 2005, Kopelman et al. 2009). Frontal lobe pathology has a special effect on cognition and memory, as the affected patient may lose his ability for critical judgments of activities of daily life. However, this would depend on the extensiveness of frontal involvement, as the diffused and global impairment do not occur if the lesion is highly focalized. Lesions directly and indirectly affecting bilateral hippocampus produce progressive amnesia to all newly learnt information. Lesions in medial temporal lobe lesions and various fronto-temporal lesions that affect the functions of hippocampus directly or indirectly are responsible for this type of memory disorder. Severity of the effect of the lesion determines the progression of loss of information in the patient. Some patients forget what they newly learnt within seconds whereas some may take time like a few hours or a day. Some of the typical cases are the following:

1. The examiner told a young patient his name and made him repeat the name a few times. The examiner waited for 10 seconds and then requested the patient to speak out the name and the patient had forgotten the name. The patient had not only forgotten the name he did not also remember that the name was given to him and he was made to repeat it.
2. 80 years old female patient forgot that she was introduced to the guests, who were visiting her. Within minutes after such introduction, she went back to each of them requested them their names and other details. In the clinical examination situation, this was repeated six times when the examiner decided to call it off.

3. Patient used to ask for tea/coffee or any other drink, a few minutes after drinking a cup and wondered why he was not given the same by his family.
4. Patient forgot that he was already examined, and forgot the tests administered to him, though the patient did not show any other deficits in tests using visuospatial perceptual and performance functions.
5. Patients may live without realizing and acknowledging that their living conditions and surroundings have changed for several years.

However, some of these patients show normal emotions in routine life situations (Douglas, Wilkinson 1993; Paller, Acharya 1997), whereas some may become apathetic. The patients may also show confabulations (Kessels et al. 2008), in their conversations as a mechanism for compensating for the memory loss and may respond to such confabulatory ideas. This has raised issues of impairment of source memory in these patients as the confabulatory ideas have never taken place and hence may not have any source memory. This further supports the involvement of the frontal lobes in these patients. The rate of loss of newly learnt information could be acute and rapid or gradual depending on the severity of the lesion. Simple clinical examination can often confirm the presence of this type of amnesia. Presence of amnesia and the consequent results on the patients and their family are generally major complaints from the patient's informants. For example, asking the patient what he had for his breakfast or lunch or asking him to repeat a simple postal address after allowing him to repeat it several times may often bring out the amnesia. In more pronounced conditions, the patient is likely to forget a new unit of information even after a minute or so, and at times it can be so severe that the amnesia leads to disorientation in a new place. The patient generally has normal memory for events that took place before the onset of the lesion. This is an indication that the impairment is in writing into memory and holding in the working memory. The patient may perform well on other tests of higher mental functions as long as their performance does not involve memory for newly learnt information. Lesions of the hippocampus, focal amnesia—a material specific amnesia produced by unilateral lesions in the right or left cerebral hemispheres, global amnesia—combination of both axial and focal types of Amnesia associated with diffused cerebral lesions and transient global amnesia—loss of selected events or information seen in recovering head injury and temporal lobe epilepsy patients. On the other hand, Korsakoff's amnesic patients may have intact implicit type of memory (Oudman et al. 2011).

Semantic and Episodic Amnesias

A major difference between the memory systems depends on the nature of acquisition of the information and experience. When it is merely conceptual information that needs to be stored and retrieved, it is considered semantic memory. However, if it is the experience itself that it stored, it is indeed a lot more complex and dynamic as experiences may have several components in the sensory-motor domains, and associated proprioceptive and emotional components. Even if not all these components are present, it is an autobiographical episode, which gets stored and requires later retrieval. All episodes of life have sensory-motor components and source details, which have been already discussed in the section on remembrance. The differences between episodic memory and semantic memory have been already discussed in an earlier section. In episodic amnesia, what is encountered is the inability of a person to remember events or episodes that took place in his life, recently, which can become so acute that a patient may not remember that he met and interacted with another person within few minutes after the episode, took place. This could create acute difficulties in everyday life and affect interpersonal relationship and credibility of the affected person with other individuals in the family and in the occupational sphere. Its effect on the personal life is indeed a more acute and devastating than the difficulty produced by semantic memory disturbances. The affected person ceases to exist as what he used to be, in the awareness of other closely related individuals. On the other hand, semantic memory is a product of the intellectual capabilities of individuals, because of which immense individual variations exist in this capability across individuals. Retrieval of semantic information depends on other cognitive factors other than its mere input. Semantic memory can also be affected by emotional factors. Semantic forgetfulness is therefore accepted as a normal phenomenon across individuals. On the other hand, none expects to forget significant autobiographic episodes, whether they have taken place recently or remotely. Even if we do not remember details of the several of the routine activities and related information, like what we ate for breakfast or dinner after a day or two, we remember several other episodes for longer periods in life after they take place. Amnesia for such episodes soon after they take place does not normally occur or expected. Therefore, when someone develops episodic amnesia, others notice it immediately.

Identification of individuals with loss of memory for episodes of life is of paramount importance for early detection of degenerative disorders of the brain mainly when other neurological signs are absent. Episodes are events in which a person experientially participates. Experiencing is the only method of establishing subjective or personal contact with reality and verifying reality. Remembrance of autobiographic episodes occurs intentionally or when they are cued by external stimuli. Remembering the past allows one to play one's role in the present and project oneself into future. External stimuli that cue remembrance may generally consist of verbal references to an episode or visual cues. Remembrance of autobiographic episodes normally takes place automatically, when externally cued. Even normal forgetfulness of episodes can occur. We invariably remember even a forgotten episode when someone else gives specific details of the episode. Many elderly persons who lead retired life do complain of difficulty to remember episodes that took place in their recent past. However, if they are reminded of the same with details, they do come around and start remembering the events. Yet another difficulty often seen in patients with early episodic amnesia is in remembering the sequence of major episodes. This would mean that do have some remembrance of the two or more episodes, but makes mistakes in remembering which occurred first. When the difficulty is not part of a degenerative disorder, the individual can correct by checking back and once corrected, then may not forget. If the amnesia is a normal phenomenon occurring because of preoccupation of the individual with other matters, then the individual can be helped to remember and he will not forget it later. On the other hand, in patients with degenerative disorder, there is no way that they would remember whether the sequence of episodes and the episodes themselves, despite any amount of efforts from others to make them remember the episodes. The outcome is that the patient may gradually lose his past and will not know how to design a future as well, and will not know what to do with the present.

In degenerative disorders causing dementia, a diffused lesion of the brain is considered, and the accompanying memory disorders are considered part of global amnesia. Focal lesions may cause memory impairment mainly because encoding functions or other specific abilities may be disturbed. Dementia is a degenerative disease and can be caused by several diseases primarily affecting cortical and subcortical areas of the brain. They are generally classified (DSM-IV) as dementias of Alzheimer's disease, vascular dementia, HIV disease, head trauma, Parkinson's and Huntington's diseases, Creutzfeldt-Jakob disease, substance induced dementia, etc. Though amnesia is the most disabling condition of dementia, there would be other accompanying functional deficits depending on the site of the lesion. Some of these deficits are disinhibition, impulsiveness, apathy, indifference, irritability, impulsiveness, aggression, suicidal tendencies. The severity of the psychological and personality deficits depend on the extensiveness and the severity of the lesion affecting the brain. Amnesias and personality changes are most prominent symptoms of various frontotemporal disease conditions. Amnesia may be also associated with deterioration in encoding ability, working memory impairment, as well as there maybe clear progressive deterioration in cognitive speed, frontal executive functions and other neuropsychological deficits related to attention, cognition, and response controls. Frontotemporal dementias caused by cerebrovascular diseases, Pick's disease, Creutzfeldt-Jakob disease, and other degenerative conditions invariably produce typical deficits of functional systems associated with anterior cingulate, orbitofrontal and dorsolateral prefrontal cortical areas (Cummings 1995) discussed earlier.

Hodges et al. (1999) found that Alzheimer's dementia patients had predominant episodic memory difficulty whereas patients with semantic dementia of frontotemporal origin have naming and word comprehension impairment. They forget to cat their food and even if they are fed in time, they may forget that they have had their meals. Extreme memory problems cause disorientation in the sense, they forget where they should sit and eat their food, use toilet facilities, etc. The frontal dementia is thus different from sematic dementia in which the patient has normal phonology and syntax, but difficulty in naming and word comprehension (Hodges et al. 1999; Mummery et al. 1999). Occasionally, they may fail to recognize even close relatives. Extensive and severe loss of cognitive functions may robe the individual of all mental assets and will require continuous help and support to engage in everyday life (Olney et al. 2005). Absence of inhibition may result in excessive and uncontrolled motor activities and may result in 'frontal release signs' (Schott, Rossor 2003) or manifestation of primitive reflexes, which are reflexes seen in infancy and very early childhood and which get inhibited as the frontal lobes functionally develop. Personality changes are either the direct or the indirect effects of brain pathology that causes dementia. Focal lesions also may be associated with personality alterations. The marked personality alterations following orbitofrontal and medial frontal lesions have already been described. Patients with Wernicke's aphasia are often suspicious, demanding, aggressive, and irritable. Preliminary studies of adults with right hemisphere lesions suggest that they may exhibit alexithymia with reserved expression of emotions and a tendency to forego symbolic thought. Right hemisphere damage sustained in childhood may result in a schizoid type of behavioral pattern, perhaps because the inability to perceive or execute emotional cues limits the child's ability to engage in interpersonal relationships.

Impairment in memory may or not be noticed by a patient himself depending on the nature and the severity of the lesion that causes it. Even if a patient has not identified its presence, relatives and those who work with the patient are sure to notice the deficits, even when they are mild. This is important when the presence of the memory deficit is almost exclusive and when the patient and the relatives are not able to identify any other symptom, or when the deficit is not associated with any known illness or traumatic incidence in the patient. A major early symptom of Alzheimer's dementia is the loss of memory for recent events in life. The reason for neurodegeneration is still to be understood more precisely, the brain of the affected patient becomes a battleground of neuritic plaques and neurofibrillary tangles (Miller et al. 1984; Arnold et al. 1991; Petrovitch et al. 2000; Tiraboschi et al. 2004; Galvin et al. 2005; Rapp et al. 2010). The neuronal death and the consequent decline of all mental functions take place in a progressive manner in these patients. Patient and his relatives may often notice in the early stages, that the deficit is particularly of loss of memory for recent events, whereas memory for remote events of life may be seen as normal. It is reported that cognitive deficits including semantic memory deficits other than episodic memory loss are present even before memory deficits are detected, during the early stages of the longitudinal course of the AD (Storandt et al. 2009, 2006; Storandt 2008). Impairment of attention (Balota, Faust 2001), planning and sequencing (Chen et al. 2005), associative memory (Celone et al. 2006), and semantic memory (Koenig et al. 2007), mild personality changes (Duchek et al. 2007) were some of the neuropsychological deficits already reported in the early stages of AD. However, these deficits often described as mild cognitive impairment may not be clinically evident as episodic memory loss present in these patients in the early stages, and they may be seen only when neuropsychological assessment is carried out. As the disease progresses, patients may have greater confusion, mood swings, irritability and aggression, and difficulty with language use. Interestingly the relatives would notice that the remote memory or memory for remote events, especially episodes of childhood and early life becoming sharper, in the sense the patient becoming more preoccupied by remembering those events of early life events, which he has never attempted to either remember or narrate to others earlier. The individual has difficulty to remember recent events, which others clearly remember. Gradually increasing recent memory loss is often considered to indicate the presence of a degenerative change in the brain. The deficit need further neuropsychological examination and confirmation, when presence of other cognitive impairment, and behavioral and personality changes may be elicited. The affected individual would soon develop other symptoms and the severity of the impairments seen would keep increasing affecting the daily routine of life of the patient.

Transient Global Amnesia

Transient Global Amnesia (TGB) is an isolated memory problem when a person develops sudden profound loss of memory lasting for a specific duration and disorientation (Hodges, Warlow 1990a, b). TGB has a sudden and unpredictable onset. The affected person may wonder how he got to the place, where he may go after the start of the TGB. Generally, the duration is never more than for 24 hours. The affected person has normal cognition—remains alert, recognizes and name familiar objects and persons. Personal identity of the person is not lost (Shekhar 2008). As the person forgets the recent past, he would not know where he is and how he got there, etc. Disorientation may result from the fact the person does not remember his past and hence cannot relate to the present and present whereabouts. This causes anxiety in the patient, as he is generally aware of the immense mental block that he is suffering from (Noel et al. 2008). There is no evidence of seizure during the transient attack and normal memory is gradually restored in the person with TGB. The underlying cause of TGB is still unknown (Kirshner 2011; Berli et al. 2009), though the condition has been reported in persons who have had strenuous physical activity, medical procedures such as angiography, mild head trauma, etc. Quinette et al. (2006) observed that TGB episodes are more common in women, who have a history of anxiety and personality disturbance and it occurs after an emotional trauma in them, while intense physical activity precipitates it in men. Possibility of hippocampal involvement has been suggested for the genesis of TGB by some authors (Adler et al. 2012; Bartsch, Deuschl 2010). TBI has been defined as a self-limiting disorder without any late consequence (Forman 2012).

Two cases were seen in the study discussed above (Mukundan et al. 1987), who had totally lost memory of their stay in the hospital after admission. After regaining consciousness, the patients were in the hospital for a period of one week, when they came to know the doctors, nurses, and other staff who were looking after them. During their follow-up visit, both did not have any memory of staying in the hospital and they could not recognize the doctor who had treated them. They were taken to the wards to find if they had memory of staying in the ward and if they could recognize any of the staff who had looked them after. Not only they had forgotten the whole event, they did not also have any memory of the accident, which were not anyway elicited from them during their stay. Interestingly the patients gradually recovered their memory after one year and could remember about their stay in the hospital. This indeed looked like Transient Global Amnesia, but there was no particular incidence, that could be identified after their discharge from the hospital, which preceded the sudden occurrence of TGB in them.

Memory Disorders in Traumatic Brain Injury

Brain injury may be caused by physical trauma (Traumatic Brain Injury—TBI) to the brain or it may be acquired (Acquired Brain Injury) because of diseases like tumors, stroke, infection, poisoning, ischemia, encephalopathy, and the effects of substance in the brain. Sharp blow to the head causes movement of the brain inside the skull causing shock and damage to the brain. Prevalence of concussive effects is reported to be greater (Cassidy et al. 2004) than the effects of contusion and cerebral laceration. Younger persons have more frequent concussive injuries than the same reported in older people (Ryan, Warden

2003; Ropper, Gorson 2007). The site of impact or blow may receive maximum injury. The force of impact may travel diagonally opposite to the site of the impact and cause neural damage in the opposite site, called the counter-coup effects (Shaw 2002). The counter-coup effects and the consequent cognitive dysfunction may often be more severe than the deficits caused by the injury at the site of impact. Axonal shearing and neural damage in the counter-coup effect may be greater in severity and cause equally severe functional deficits in the patient. Bruises and cuts on the brain caused by direct blow to the head cause cerebral contusion. Laceration or tears in the neural tissue are caused by a foreign object or fragment of pushed-in bone from a skull fracture.

Patients with Traumatic Brain Injury (TBI) may suffer from disorientation, confusion, and amnesia for the events that occurred after the head injury (Lee 2007; Gilbertson et al. 2008; Mukundan et al. 1987). Storing new information may turn out to be difficult for these patients as long as the initial amnesia remains and some may have islands of memory during this period (van der Naalt, 2001). Both retrograde and anterograde amnesia may occur in these patients, though the latter type may be more common (Shaw 2002; Cantu 2001). Anterograde amnesia was observed to develop only after certain delay after the injury being inflicted (Binder 1986). Severity of the trauma is measured in terms of duration of unconsciousness and Glasgow Coma Scale and these scores are used to classify TBI into mild, moderate, and severe categories. The range and the magnitude of neuropsychological impairment in TBI depend on the severity of the injury. TBI patients may report persistent symptoms for weeks or months and some may report them for years after the injury (Millis et al. 2001; Hillier et al. 1997; Pelczar, Politynska 1997; Ponsford et al. 1995, Hilton 1994; Zwil et al. 1993; Hugenholtz 1988). When impairment of attention and encoding are present, it always leads to poor memory as found in retrieval trials. There could be additionally expressive and receptive language disabilities, visuospatial impairment, and several focal deficits like prosopagnosia, anomia, dyscalculia, dysgraphia, etc. in the patient. The site and the severity of the injury determine the nature of the deficits in a patient. There is a short period of spontaneous recovery, when several of the symptoms that appeared after the TBI may disappear and only more severe deficits, if present, will persist for longer periods (Petchprapai, Winkelman 2007; Anderson et al. 2006; Mukundan et al. 1987). They may also present impairment in the areas of attention, learning, and memory (Mukundan et al. 1990, 1987). Severe TBI patients may have difficulty in initiating movements and actions, impairment in planning, problem-solving, thinking, and may present dissociation between thought and action, communication difficulties, and poor self-awareness. Personality changes with poor motivation, socialization, and disinhibition may be indicative of extensive frontal and temporal lobe deficits (Malia et al. 1995; Max et al. 2001), though language functions and visual and spatial functions may remain relatively less affected.

A study (Mukundan et al. 1987) conducted during the years 1984-1986 on 42 road traffic accident victims (mean age 33.2 years and SD-11.2), who sustained TBI and who were admitted in the hospital in unconscious condition were followed up for a period of more than one year. These patients did not have the benefit of cognitive retraining or any specialized rehabilitative help (as the same was not available) after sustaining the head injury revealed the neuropsychological recovery pattern over a period of one year. The patients were neuropsychologically assessed 1 month, 3 months, and 12 months after the initial admission and their performance was compared with that of a normal control group (n = 26), matched for age and education (Table 17). On the Glasgow Comma Scale (Teasdale, Jennett 1974), 24 patients had scores in the 6-8 range, 16 had scores in the 9-11 range, and 2 had scores of 4 and 5 during admission immediately after sustaining the injury. Of these patients, 76% were neurologically normal during the third month assessment. Thirty-two (76%) patients attained neurological normalcy one month after the injury and 18 patients could not tested at that stage. Thirty-five (83%) patients were neurologically normal at the end of third month and all patients could be subjected to neuropsychological assessment.

Table 17: Showing results of neuropsychological tests administered to TBI patients (n = 42) and normal control group (n = 26). Patients were assessed three months and one year after the TBI

	Control GP		TBI - 3rd Month			TBI - 1 Year		
TESTS	M	SD	M	SD	P	M	SD	P
Visual Scanning 1 —seconds	46.0	9.3	114.1	85.44	<0.01	76.6	55.3	<0.01
Visual Scanning 2 —seconds	116.0	25.7	435.8	216.3	<0.01	265.41	29.1	<0.01
Ideational Fluency	8.5	3.4	7.1	4.6	NS	9.8	3.7	NS
Working Memory	8.6	0.8	3.2	26	<0.01	5.8	2.1	<0.05
Verbal L T1	11.4	4.6	8.0	6.5	<0.05	12.0	6.3	NS
Verbal L T2	13.6	5.8	10.8	7.4	NS	14.1	5.8	NS
Verbal L T3	16.8	5.6	12.3	7.7	<0.05	14.7	6.0	NS
Verbal L T4	11.6	4.9	11.9	8.6	NS	15.2	6.5	NS
Visual L T1	12.6	4.6	4.5	3.8	<0.01	7.0	3.4	<0.01
Visual L T2	14.8	4.8	5.7	5.4	<0.01	7.5	4.1	<0.01
Visual L T3	19.7	7.8	6.9	6.0	<0.01	10.6	5.1	<0.01
Visual L T4	16.4	6.5	7.2	6.4	<0.01	11.6	5.4	<0.05

Visual scanning scores are in seconds, all other scores are correct responses.

Neuropsychological tests showed significant impairment in the tests in the third month assessment except a few as shown above. In the one-year assessment, the patient group showed comparable performance with the control group on tests of ideational fluency and verbal learning and memory functions. Significant impairment persisted tests of visual scanning, working memory and visual learning and memory functions. The tests of verbal learning and memory functions have been already discussed in detail in earlier sections. Comparison of the patient group with normal controls at the end of one year continued showing significant impairment in visual learning and memory functions, visual scanning, and working memory tests. Majority of the patients (69%) continued expressing difficulties in social adjustment and had emotional problems even one year after the trauma. Event related potential tests (Mukundan et al. 1990) on the same patients showed that process of sensory registration was normal in these patients, but there was significant delay in the arousal of attention as seen by increased latency of the N1 component, and the subsequent P2 component. Significant differences in the recovery pattern of verbal and visual memory pattern may be considered an indication of the presence of differences either in the processing or material specificity of the task engaged in. As seen in the earlier results left prefrontal, and right nonprefrontal lesion patients have maximum impairment in the immediate and delayed recalls, as well as in rate of learning only in the visual tests. Immediate and delayed verbal recalls and rate of learning are impaired maximum in the left prefrontal and in the left nonprefrontal lesion patients. The working memory was tested using a verbal test involving arithmetical operations (delayed response ability test), which indicates that material specificity was not that contributed to the continuance of impairment.

Table 18: Showing the visual search time in seconds per number (Sec/Number), for marking in the two Visual Scanning tests by the TBI patients, in their 3rd month and 1 year assessments

	NORMAL	TBI PATIENTS	
	Sec/Number	3rd Month Sec/Number	1 Year Sec/Number
TEST 1 (20 Nos.)	2.3	5.7	3.8
TEST 2 (48 Nos.)	2.4	9.1	5.5

The performance on the visual scanning test (Table 18) provides important indications of the true deficits that persisted in these over the year. The visual scanning test administered to detect their speed of detection of numbers presented on a sheet of paper. Interestingly the patients did not make mistakes, but were extremely slow in their visual search. Normal subjects took average 2.3 sec and 2.4 sec per number, for searching and cancelling them in sequence in the 20 and 48 numbers formats respectively. In the 3rd month assessment, the patient group took average 5.7 sec and 9.1 sec per number respectively for the 20 and 48 number formats. In the one-year assessment, the patient group took average 3.8 sec and 5.5 sec per number respectively for the two formats of numbers. Though the patients have shown marked increase in the speed of visual search from the third month to one year, it is still far behind that of the normal group. In the visual learning and memory functions test, the visual figure was exposed to them only 15 seconds and obviously, they could have detected only much smaller number of details of complex visual figure compared to the normal subjects, during that exposure time. Obviously, their immediate and delayed visual recall was significantly inferior to that of the normal controls. This does not happen with regard to the verbal learning and memory functions test and the comparable immediate and delayed recall of the normal and patient groups in the one-year assessment clearly supports this. In the third month assessment, the patient group had lower scores on two trials of the verbal test and they performed as good as normal subjects in the ideational fluency test. The working memory performance continued to be poor in the one-year assessment also in the patient group. Both verbal learning and memory functions test and the working memory test need encoding. In the learning and memory functions test, encoding helps to build up a meaning sequentially, whereas in the working memory test, unconnected blocks of information need to be held on and one must switch sequentially across those blocks and plans of actions and execute the plans. The slow visual search may be because of the lack of control required for visual search, which must emanate from the frontal eye fields, which (area 8) is adjacent to the dorsolateral prefrontal cortex (area 9) involved in working memory. The study (Mukundan et al. 1987) has not considered the exact sites of traumatic lesion and hence, this cannot be concluded from the findings. Himanen et al. (2009) have reported that TBI patients may have persistent deficits of complex attentional processes even 3 decades after acquiring the head injury, though slowness and attention deficits may later be related to symptoms of depression.

The above test results indicated a differential recovery status for verbal and visual functions. Even one year after the TBI, working memory and visual learning and memory functions did not recover, whereas verbal learning and memory partially recovered within 3 months and fully recovered one year after the injury. None of the patients had dyscalculia and they could carry out arithmetical calculation using large numbers on paper. A significant shortcoming of group comparisons is that such comparison does not allow patient-to-patient changes in the recovery pattern (Dikmen et al. 2003; Millis et al. 2001; Francis et al. 1991; Chu et al. 2007; Till et al. 2008). Millis et al. (2001) reported that 22.2% of the TBI patients improved, 15.2% declined and 62.6% of the patients remained unchanged in their neuropsychological profile in a 5 years follow up study. Higher standard deviations of the comparable mean scores of the patient group are indication of some of the patients having either very high or low scores, whereas some having scores comparable with the control group participants. These studies have reported marked differences in the recovery patterns of TBI patients. As evident from the above results, the long-term difficulty of the TBI patients was the absence of recovery even after one year in working memory functions, visuospatial scanning, and visual memory functions. As far as working memory is concerned, the persistent difficulty appeared to be that of holding and sequentially switching rather than semantic processing. This is supported by the fact the patients have performed remarkably well in other verbal recall tests. Himanen et al. (2006) found that good recovery of semantic memory is a most convincing finding in long-term TBI patients. Visual scanning was also impaired, but the difficulty was the slowness in scanning and the consequent longer time, the patients took for the completion of the test rather than mistakes they committed in the test. Slowing of visual search ability could also have impaired the visual immediate and delayed recall performance as the stimulus material was presented only for a brief duration (15 seconds) to a subject in each trial and this duration was not adequate for the TBI patients to search and recognize the different components of the figure. Therefore, the visual immediate and delayed recall impairment seen in the above study could have been caused by input difficulties rather than true memory impairment. This has been also supported by other researchers (DeLuca et al. 2000; Fisk, Schneider 1984) who found that impairment of memory could be caused by initial acquisition deficiencies rather than deficiencies in the retrieval process. Several earlier studies (McKinlay et al. 1981; Levin et al. 1984; Richardson, Barry 1985; Brooks et al. 1986; Wechsler 1987; Levin 1990; Kapur 1990) have identified memory deficits as the most significant impairment in TBI. Even a 7-year follow up study (Oddy et al. 1985) has indicated memory disturbance as a core deficit in TBI patients. Barker-Collo, Feigin (2008) opined as memory is the outcome interrelated sequential processes of paying attention, encoding, storage and retrieval, deficit of processing at any of the levels could affect memory performance. Levin (1990) reported that approximately in one third of the survivors of TBI, encoding and storage deficiencies could have been the main source for creating subsequent memory problems.

A reexamination of the results of the study (Mukundan et al. 1987) indeed has helped to understand the role of attention deficit because of slow visual search as the possible core reason for visual memory problem persistently seen in the TBI patients studied over one year. This has been further supported in our cognitive retraining study (Christina et al. 2009) of TBI patients, in which the patients showed significant increase in the visual immediate and delayed recall after they were trained using Brain Function Therapy (BFT), a computerized cognitive retraining program (Christina et al. 2009; Mukundan, Hemalata 2011; Mukundan 2012) over a period of 4 weeks. The patients also showed normal performance on the 4 trials of verbal learning and memory functions test. An important and preliminary retraining module of BFT is attention retraining. It is a common observation in BFT retraining that performance on working memory and other cognitive modules start improving only when the patient shows improvement in the attention retraining modules. We seldom observe persistence of memory problem as a general phenomenon in TBI patients over long periods, as cognitive retraining programs are easily available to all brain disordered patients. The effect of the TBI on memory could be varying. What is detected by neuropsychological tests may be only part of the effects on memory. Memory impairment would cause increase magnitude of disabilities impairing their quality of performance and life in general. This has been strongly indicated in several other related studies of neurorehabilitation of TBI and other patients with memory disorders (Kessler et al. 1992; Robertson 1993; Wilson 1996; Barker-Collo 2000; rmid Vaz, Heinrichs 2002; Prigatano et al. 2005; Barker-Collo, Feigin 2008).

Remembrance in Posttraumatic Stress Disorder

Posttraumatic Stress Disorder (PTSD) has been defined as a debilitating anxiety disorder acquired by being exposed to psychological trauma at interpersonal levels or to disaster caused by accidents. Even witnessing a traumatic event could induce trauma and the person may later suffer from PTSD. DSM-IV has considered traumatic event as one caused "actual or threatened death or serious injury, or threat to the physical integrity of self or others", and "the person's response involved intense fear, helplessness or horror". PTSD must consist of persistent re-experience of the trauma for more than a month. The re-experience consists of continuous remembrance of the thoughts, imageries, and the emotional disturbances experiences by the person during the traumatic event, the affected person may behave as if he is going through the event all over again and emotionally react to it. Persistent remembrance of the original traumatic event and reactions to the contents of remembrance are therefore the core feature of PTSD. Three major syndromes of PTSD are related to "reliving the event", avoidance and arousal. Re-experiencing the original trauma is indeed the major distressing component of the disorder. One who has participated or witnessed intensely the traumatic event can develop the PTSD and have intense negative feelings of "fear, helplessness, or horror" (Mayo Clinic staff). The PTSD patient relives the memory of the original participation or witnessing the experience of physical or sexual assault, accidents, drug addiction, illness, or medical complication (Fullerton et al. 2004). PTSD is considered less frequent, though more enduring compared to posttraumatic stress (Rothschild 2000). Continuous remembrance of the traumatic autobiographic episode and the inability to differentiate the past from the present are the essential features of disorder, because of which the patient may react repeatedly or continuously to the remembered experiences. The re-experiencing is so acute and real for the patient, that he is unable to differentiate it from the original experience and fail to look upon it as a past episode. Remembrance of the episode causes recreation of visual, proprioceptive, motor imageries, and the emotions causing intense fear and anxiety in the person.

The somatic responses to the fear and anxiety contribute to another dimension of distress, rendering the entire experience stunningly disabling and bullying to the individual. Presence and absence of such imageries may be considered for the diagnosis of false memories in the patient (Conway et al. 2000). Recreations of visual and motor imageries are important features of remembrance of experiences (Mukundan 2007b, 2008, 2010, 2011a) in normal individuals also.

Emotions for Survival and Growth

18

The most stunning discovery in the area of emotions was the discovery of the presence of emotional experiences and expressions elicited by stimuli unconsciously and without their perception (Ledoux 1996, 1998; Morris et al. 1998; Whalen et al. 1998; Soars, Ohman 1998; Windmann, Kruger 1998; de Gelder et al. 1999, 2005; de Gelder, Rouw 2000). The emotion experienced and expressed was essentially that of fear. This came to be called the 'preattentive emotion' occurring as a result of neural hijack (LeDoux 1996, 1998), indicating that emotional responses and experiences relayed fear, anger, flight and freeze have independent origin from the amygdala. A stimulus can elicit these responses directly from the amygdala, even if the stimulus has not reached the primary sensory cortex. LeDoux found that the small direct path from the thalamus to amygdala and hippocampus elicits the survival related emotional responses directly, based on familiarity of memory, provided by the hippocampus, instead of the complex perceptual analysis that may emerge from the sensory-frontal decision-making circuits. Emotional experience and expression in the preattentive state would appear as impulsive as it is not preceded by conscious thinking or decision-making. Several further studies showed interesting involvement of amygdala in deciding interesting features of emotions. Kim et al. (2003) noted that negative interpretation of facial expression was associated with activation in the right ventral amygdala, whereas positive interpretations were associated with activation of ventral medial prefrontal cortex. Vuilleumier et al. (2002) reported that despite visual neglect because of a parietal lobe lesion, a patient could respond to a visual emotion provoking stimulus and the response was associated with activation in the amygdala and the orbitofrontal cortex. Supported Pessoa et al. (2002) in their first study reported the need for adequate attentional allocation for eliciting emotional response from the amygdala, though they supported in the subsequent study (Pessoa 2005) the possibility of a preattentive emotional response from the amygdala. Interestingly studies by Batty et al. (2005) and Phillips et al. (2004) did not find supportive evidence for the preattentive emotion in their studies. There is also further possibility of the presence of preattentive emotional component in all emotion provoking stimuli in real life situations, though this has not been yet demonstrated. It is apparent that only a few types of emotion provoking stimuli can elicit response from the amygdala, which happens even if the stimulus is not perceived by the individual. The neural network responsible for preattentive emotion may be considered the structural basis of experiences, which the individual cannot consciously report. The fact that a permanent sensory input path to the amygdala through the hippocampus exists shows that the hippocampus must always receive all sensory inputs, though fear or anger provoking stimuli alone are recognized by the system, which in turn activates the amygdala for generating the preattentive type of emotional response. There may be fear or anger provoking element in many stimuli, though they may not be finally judged so by the perceiver, but a partial fear or anger related emotional response might be provoked by this system as soon as it is detected. This might explain some of the incomplete fear or anger, often displayed by people in challenging situations. However, this needs further investigation for mapping the response and its etiology.

Emotion has been studied and documented ever since man made efforts to explain behavior. Religions have placed very important role in explaining the needs to control emotion as well as invest emotions, as emotion has been always identified as the central force for generating explicit behavior. People in general considered emotion as a weakness rather than strength, unless the emotional attachment was a supreme power. Many have considered emotion of devotion and love to a supreme force or power as the noblest of emotions. All forms of arts have immense expressions of emotions. Without emotions or emotional arousal, none can act in pursuance of a goal in life; emotional gratification has been always considered the index of true achievement of various pursuits in life. Scientific explanations always focused on the need to explain emotional arousal as an experience different from emotional expression manifested as specific types of behavior. Emotional experience mould feelings, moods, and affective states of the individual, whereas expressions generally considered are three folds manifesting as flight, fight, or freeze phenomenon, expressions vital for the survival of the living being. Charles Darwin proposed in 1872, from an evolutionary perspective, that emotion was essential for communication as well as survival (Darwin, Paul, Philip 1998). The earlier theories of emotions were influenced chiefly by the need to differentiate physiological responses from psychic experiences and deciding the sequence of occurrence of the two components, as cause effect was stipulated between the two. James-Lange theory postulated that perception of bodily (physiological) changes leads to emotion. Thus, emotions of fear, anger, crying, sadness, etc., and follow responses like running, striking, trembling, etc. The theory aimed at postulating a cause and effect relationship between various bodily responses and emotions and thereby emotion was always the result of the perception of a bodily response. However, the theory does not adequately explain how such bodily responses are learnt and expressed in the manner they occur. The entire focus was to decide the sequence of the two components and explain how emotion could only follow a bodily response.

The Cannon-Bard (1929, 1927) theory approached this issue in a more comprehensive manner and based on the thalamo-cortical neural circuits involved in perception and responses, postulated that both emotional experience and expressions must take place simultaneously. None of the theories examined the arousal value of emotion, and emotional arousal as a prerequisite for initiation of action, learning, and performance. The emotions examined were intense emotions associated with flight-fight-freeze behavioral responses. Their contention was that the richness of emotional experiences cannot stem from poorly differentiated bodily responses and cognitive appraisal of the source is important for developing such rich emotional experiences, and hence both must occur simultaneously. These were far before the discovery that some of the emotional expressions and experiences could be triggered by certain types of stimuli even without their perception or awareness. There have been attempts to postulate a reverse order reaction, in which the cognitive appraisal of an event or external entity triggers physiological responses and emotional experiences. The postulations and the works of Lazarus (1991) and Mandler (1984) emphasized on the importance of understanding the role of cognitive appraisal in triggering physiological reactions and consequent emotional responses. The Polyvagal theory proposed by Porges (2001, 1998) considers three branches for emotional regulation with specific effects on the autonomic nervous system. The first stage is characterized by depression of metabolic activity and behavioral freezing, and the second stage leads to increased sympathetic activity and flight or fight behavioral expressions in life-threatening environments. He proposed a third phylogenetic approach for environmental engagement through socialization, managed through facial expressions and speech. The physiology of the fight-flight models of emotions does indeed explain animal behavior and the animal in man. However, some of the human behavior could be the manifestation of very different forces in which fight and flight needs are encountered with compassion and love. This does not stem from a larger need for socialization, but stems from the thoughts created in the minds of individuals, who consider the need and possibility of higher levels of existence than offered by nature. However, we know responses have always happened and are happening; it has taken several men to levels of existence beyond the 'tooth for tooth' principles and domains of human interactions. The elementary components of these experience and expressions are probably present in all, though they are never activated and expressed in normal circumstances, unless they are consciously nourished and allowed expression.

Socialization is a process of conditioning and absence of this ability during developmental years has significant impact on the neurodevelopment of personality, which make them vulnerable to criminal behavior (Yu Gao et al. 2010; Lorber 2004; Patrick 2006; Raine 2008, 1993). Blair et al. (2005) hypothesized that poor functioning of the amygdala could result in poor fear conditioning and it could increase the risk for criminal offences in individuals. Yu Gao et al. (2010) examined the effects of absence of early childhood fear conditioning in the very early years (3 years) of neurodevelopment on precipitating criminal behavior in the adulthood. They reported the findings of a longitudinal study in which 137 adults, who were convicted by courts as criminal offenders at least once by the age of 23 years, had failed to show conditioning responses when they were 3 years old. The conditioning effect was recorded using auditory tones as the CS and unpleasant noise as the UCS. The conditioning effect was recorded using galvanic skin responses. The authors explained their findings by implicating the absence of functional involvement of the amygdala for the poor fear conditioning, seen in them during childhood. They proposed that failure of fear conditioning was responsible for weak socialization and the resultant criminal behavior in the later life. Birbaumer et al. (2005) found that the neural activation seen in the amygdala, orbitofrontal cortex, insula, and anterior cingulate in normal subjects during delayed fear conditioning was absent in the male psychopaths, they investigated. Studies (Arseneault et al. 2000; Pine et al. 1997) have implicated the presence of a marker of limbic neural maldevelopment namely 'Cavum septum pellucidum', in persons with antisocial personality, psychopathy, delinquency, and criminal offences. It is indeed a matter to be considered seriously if we are to accept that ability to abstain from crime has to be cultivated through fear of punishment only. However, in the absence of positive socialization, individual may not have the option to stay away from criminal responses when aroused by drives, which could easily release criminal responses, unless controlled by fear of consequences. There are also strong indications of dysfunction of ventral prefrontal cortex and orbitofrontal cortex in persons with psychopathic behavior (Blair 2007; Raine, Yang 2006; Blair, Cippoloti 2000). Skeem et al. (2011) reported in their recent review that individuals with high scores on Psychopathy Checklist, Revised (PCL-R) have indications of involvement of amygdala, hippocampus and parahippocampal gyri, anterior-posterior cingulate cortex, striatum, insula, and frontal and temporal cortex. Yet another review by Weber et al. (2008) of neuroimaging studies revealed the involvement of prefrontal, temporal, and limbic areas in psychopathic individuals. A psychopath has variety of abnormal affective and behavioral traits, such as impulsivity, lack of remorse or empathy, irresponsibility, etc. whereas antisocial person's chief character is the pervasive disregard for the rights of others in the society. Socialization of the individual is important for preservation of society, and the development of this ability can occur in natural manner only in the early years. Aberrations of socialization could occur because of dysfunctional brain or the absence of opportunities for socialization in the early years. Members of a society who fail to preserve the values of the society would never be able to transcend the fight-flight-freeze rules of the society to higher horizons emotional interactions. The process of socialization could be impaired because of functional anomalies of the brain areas associated with the development of the functional process or the absence of the process being provided during the developmental period. Marking the presence of developmental milestones of socialization is equally important as that of intellectual development in children. Socialization provides the skills required for the deployment of emotional arousal for actions and responses in life.

Emotional Arousal

The continuous efforts to separate physiological responses from the cognitively appraised emotional experiences either as antecedent or precedent factors have only masked the true understanding of the complexities of emotional arousal and emotional expressions. Physiological activation is linked to emotional arousal, especially when they are related to emotions aroused in survival threats. Cognitive appraisal of emotion consider components related to the individual specific context of the arousal, survival threats if present, and the nature and magnitude of the physiological activation. Emotions associated with fight-flight-freeze responses indeed have extremely singular cognitive modulation, one of fear, anger, helplessness, etc. Sexual arousal is associated with physiological arousal, the need for intimacy, gratification, and extensive cognitive effects of the personal state and the source of the arousal. However, there are emotions, which are sublime and complex, and difficult for clear cognitive labeling, as they are not linked to survival needs and hence not associated with any predefined physical or physiological responses. Emotions of happiness, love, affection, compassion, appreciation, confidence, hope, patience, regret, guilt, distress, etc., are of those categories, which may be associated with behavioral expressions resulting in individuals joining and sharing the rewards and distresses, instead of taking recourse to merely self-preservation. Manifestation of sharing and self-sacrificing behavior, instead of deploying fight and flight for self-preservation indicates the presence of a new dimension of emotion and self-preservation, not hitherto seen in the animal world. They could be considered different from the protective behavior shown to offspring by parents. These emotions and the associated behavioral expressions are helpful for the preservation of the society and its values, rather than self-preservation. These emotions with varying levels of positive or negative cognitive modulation effects, may still contribute to variety of performances and learning to take place. The endeavors may be contributed by a performing individual, who may seek out or create a context for performance, rather than encountering them in the nature. These actions take individuals to heights of achievement and satisfaction, which may become the foundation for the aspirations, hopes, and endeavors of members of a human society. This emotional arousal is a necessary precondition for performance or learning to occur. Performance is dependent on such emotional arousal, which may be experienced as interest, dedication, achievement and excitement. Performance and learning cannot take place without such emotional arousal. As mentioned in the earlier section on drives, one cannot carry out even simple motor act without drive, or the drive reaching a certain level of potentiation.

As the cognitive modulation is sublime and expansive in these contexts, the emotional arousal has been called just arousal or the drive. The cognitive modulation may be merely that of 'wanting or needing' to act, and the need is not because of a biological deprivation. The need is created by aspiring for certain anticipated effects or results, and the need must initiate the relevant actions, which can take the individual to specific goals. The goals are always in a different temporal-spatial location, and hence one has to learn to anticipate the effects of performance and alter the performance according to the discrepancies between the anticipated and actual effects. Arousal in this sense could be considered a psychophysiological state representing psychological and physiological components of the need to act, without any external threat. These are self-initiated activities maintained through self-motivation and perseveration. The emotional arousal in these contexts causes the necessary alertness of the brain for engaging in simple to complex sensory-motor processing and problem-solving with highest levels of efficiency, until the goals are achieved. The emotional arousal in such conditions could be best labeled as that of anxiety to perform and accomplish. Anxiety is a state of anticipation of positive or negative effects, and its intensity may have positive or negative effects on the ongoing cognitive and motor performances. Excess of anxiety impairs performance, whereas its absence or inadequate level brings down the level of performance. According to the most acceptable Yerkes-Dodson law, higher levels of drive enhances performance when the task complexity is weak, whereas it may impair performance when the task complexity is high. Normally, one learns to adapt to a drive level accordingly to the perceived or known needs, so that one functions at the most efficient or predefined levels. One may always attempt to function at the optimum drive level, as over and under emotional arousal does not contribute to the best psychomotor and cognitive performance.

The need to pass through the streams of positive and negative emotions is a regular feature of normal life, though one learns to pass through or come out of these emotional states with satisfactorily or unsatisfactory consequential effects.

The effects of emotional arousal on the biological system vary according to the experiential states produced, which is a function of the perceived discomforts or comforts one encounters in the various contexts. The cognitive strategy used for appraisal of emotion provoking state is a learnt ability and decides the psychological effects interpreted and generation of the associated emotional arousal state. Unlike fight-flight responses, in which emotional responses precede their perception, the cognitive appraisal of one's performance and achievement may easily trigger secondary physiological responses, and influence behavior, speech, and have the potentiality to affect other cognitive processing, unless the effects are critically isolated and handled. The psychosocial origins of expressions of emotions form an extended domain for scientific pursuits of social behavior and shaping of individual personality from these effects. Learning control of emotions or response inhibition controls from the core of socialization process in each growing child, and the failures in the acquisition of this control may find adverse expressions in them, throughout their lives. The disability may not only affect individual's behavior and performance, but it may fail preventing emotional expressions against other members of the society, which may be easily labelled antisocial and criminal. Every human being experience and express emotions and the various social customs they practice are generally expressions of the cherished emotions of the members of the society or the social group. These expressions become complex depending on the channels used for their modulation and expressions. One experiences its presence within the body as subjective mental state affecting thinking and behavioral expressions. We observe, study, and comment upon these experiences and expressions, both scientifically and artistically though understanding the subjective mental states is always a complex and difficult process. The related experiences could easily affect the physiological functioning even though others do not directly observe them, unless emotions have affected behavioral expressions including speech. We learn to control emotional arousal even in intensely challenging situations, so that performance and behavior are not adversely affected. The experiences and expressions of emotions are always labelled by each according to the interpretations of the subjective context of the experience and using subjective criteria.

Drive for Performance

There would be no movement, without emotional arousal, even if ample energy were available in the body. The body energy is engaged and utilized only when emotional arousal propels and directs the physical energy. Manifold expressions and experiences of emotions, which trigger various forms of behavior-responses and actions, are well understood. It is also established and accepted that emotions provide the psychic energy required for living for each biological being. Animals throw themselves into responses when there are biological need states like hunger, thirst, sexual urges, and external threats. The need-states automatically propel the animals into responding for their gratification and similar other survival needs. However, biological need states related to survival may form only a small spectrum of such drive states in human beings, which propel them into spectrum of behavioral responses and actions leading to satiation of the drives. Most survival threats from the nature are handled efficiently with minimum loss of lives, though this would not have been attempted at the best of efficiency in all such threats. The mental states of emotional arousal contain the larger spectrum of forces, which propel them into varied responses and actions. These mentally or psychically created arousal states are often the outcome of needs produced through creative/imaginative thinking. These driving forces are experienced and expressed as emotional drives and they shape their pursuits in life. The physical energy utilized in all responses and actions are the same and available all through on self-initiation, unless the body is diseased and cannot deploy the energy. The need for developing emotional drive for pursuing various goals in life is inevitable, and all these pursuits make use of the same bodily or physical energy. Though the physiological components of the drive may be the same, the psychological labelling varies, and there may be several drives or psychological needs in every individual. Desire indeed is the common word that is associated with the psychological state. However, desire or psychological need alone is not enough for actions or responses to occur. The physiological arousal associated with the psychological desire is a necessity for responses and actions to occur. The psychological and physiological states are interrelated and contribute together for behavioral expressions. Presence of psychological states or desires, which fail to switch on the physiological state for making use of the physical energy for movements, can only make one fantasize the desired effects.

Performance is an outcome of the drive/arousal level in the individual. As drive increases, the level of performance-learning increases and reaches highest efficiency at the optimum drive level. Any further increase in the drive levels brings down the level of efficiency as shown in the inverted U curve. This is known as the famous Yerkes-Dodson (1908). Performance is a function of the interaction of complexity of the task carried out at a given time and the accompanying drive level. If the task

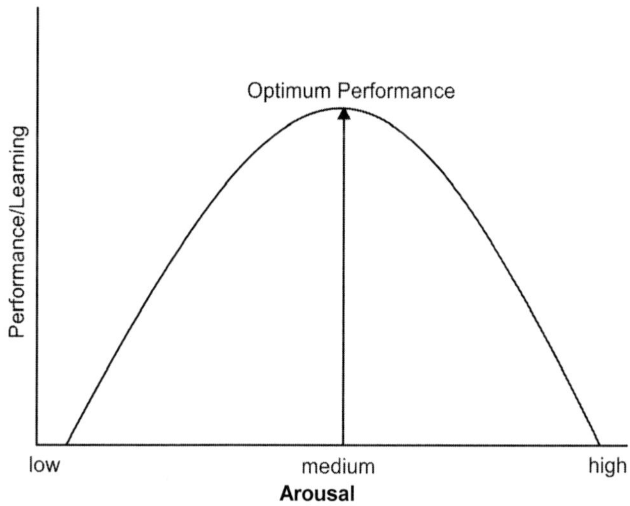

Yerkes-Dodson Law

complexity is high and the drive level is also high, it is expected to adversely affect performance. If the task complexity is high, the drive level must be proportionately lesser, for achieving best of efficiency. On the other hand, if the task complexity is low, performance improves only if the drive is high. It is often left to the discretion of the individual to maintain the right drive level so that performance is always at the highest level. Absence or reduced drive is often the complaint with many individuals for unsatisfactory performance, and this is often the result of one being unable to find the work carried out interesting, challenging, and rewarding. Attitudes can play a major role in defining interest and one may perform at the peak level even if the task demands are not personally exciting. One would find higher purposes for giving the best, especially when one is part of a team and the team has to achieve specific goals. Hence, finer control of attitude would play an important role in helping a person to raise or adjust the drive level to optimum conditions for achieving highest efficiency in performance. Reduced and lack of initiative resulting from very low drive levels is the biggest hindrance for good performance and achievement. Loss of drive may be primarily because of the involvement of the Anterior Cingulate Cortex system that controls the creation and release of drive. ACC as the source of emotional drives for the DLPFC to carry out online processing has been the model of the executive system developed (Lezak et al. 2004; Alvarez et al. 2006; Chan et al. 2008; Rolls et al. 2008; Clark et al. 2008; Banich 2009). Reduced drive level in a person could be because non-cultivation of the drive and the poor availability of the drive for high levels of performance. Excessive drive is also a hindrance as in ADHD disorders. Rubia et al. (2001) observed that reduced right prefrontal activation was associated with response inhibition deficits resulting in the presence of hyperactivity in adolescents. Right inferior prefrontal involvement was also proposed in disinhibition by Konishi et al. (1999). Meta-analysis by Mostofsky and Simmonds (2008) has revealed the importance of pre-SMA circuits in response inhibition-selection process. What is important is for the person to cultivate the ability to keep the drive under control, so that one can release it or reduce its release according to the perceived needs or inner needs. Inner needs are determined by the strength of purpose one has cultivated or defined and identified for the self, and the ability to decide specific goals to achieve and the action plans designed, which can be executed by the release of appropriate levels of drive. Once these are available, one can release the drive according to the needs of the situation for navigating oneself for achieving those goals over the predefined time schedules, whether it is in minutes, years, or decades. Learning to be aroused to the appropriate levels for performing to achieve the goal for satisfying a need is possible only if the person has the primary capability to be aroused and has the controls to organize the drive as per the exigencies that may arise during the navigation to the goal. However, release of drive for actions, which are not part of those approved by the society, can become a hindrance to one's personal growth and acceptability in the society. Some of these actions are indeed antisocial as well as criminal. Actions displaying disrespect and aggression to women, children and elders may reach such criminal dimensions. Ability to control and release the drive is part of socialization of each member of the society, which one acquires in the neuropsychological developmental stages of growth. Fear conditioning is often considered an important index of early socialization taking place in individuals. Fear could be a factor that prevents the development of drive and the release of aggressive actions and responses in many individuals, whereas some may have positive thoughts and feelings and they will never entertain negative actions, rather than having fear as the controlling factor. They never drive themselves to such offensive behavior. Absence of fear in the early developmental years may have detrimental effects in the adult life (Yu Gao et al. 2010) in some individuals, as it may become the foundation for the manifestation of criminal responses, as the related drive may not be controlled because of absence of early socialization process in them. Fear conditioning may therefore, have important role in socialization of individuals in some societies unless socialization process has alternate refined positive components, which can take care of release of such drives.

Acquiring Positive Drives

Acquisition of drive for positive performance is not the same as meeting life threatening exigencies or survival related external threats. It is not because this drive is physiologically different, but because the responses are for satiation of positive psychological needs, which do not pose any biological survival need or threat to the individual. This is an entirely different dimension of human behavior as the responses are not in the form of physical fights or fleeing. Human beings engage themselves in variety of nonthreatening and intellectually or emotionally stimulating positive tasks with positive attitudes for achieving their goals. Therefore, to be aroused by an idea for pursuing a path of actions needs tremendous self-initiated and self-nurtured emotional arousal, instead of the type of emotional arousal seen in natural threats. Survival needs train the animals learn to be emotionally aroused with associated fight-flight responses in natural manner. There is no such natural manner in which human beings can learn to be aroused for setting goals and then for working hard to achieve the goals after long and enduring struggles, and finally realizing or materializing the ideas, which they created. The capability to be aroused in this stream of realization, one must acquire the drive to be persistently aroused as a child, and learn to preserve it throughout life.

Emotional arousal takes place because of sensory inputs and during remembrance of autobiographic episodes. It happens during and after creation of new ideas, which one may want to accomplish. The components present during emotional arousal within normal perceptual contexts are a pattern of physiological activation and psychological experiences. The emotional arousal generates motor acts in the place of the flight or fight components manifested during threat to survival. Socially approved responses and actions do not have such emotional contents. The former types are emotional responses, also associated with equally severe emotional experiences, whereas the latter are socially approved responses representing the value systems of the society, which the individual share, and which may or not provoke unwarranted emotional experiences. Responses may also be in the form of speech expressing the emotional components as prosodic changes as well as semantic contents. The psychological need may be considered the most volatile and significant, as it is the driving force for initiating responses and actions in each person's life. Physiological arousal is present in varying magnitudes in living system, which is easily associated with emotions. However, only when the psychophysiological activation associated with a specific need becomes strong, related responses would be released. In the animal world, these are perceptions related to survival, which produce appropriate responses instantly. However, in human beings, the physiological activation is decided by the psychological need one creates and nourishes, and the manner the responses are released from the system. Psychophysiologically, it is a state of the mind-brain; when the arousal becomes sufficiently strong, it impels one to act. The state is indeed similar to other biological need states viz., hunger, thirst, and sex. One knows that one has to act and achieve satiation when the need is recognized and the drive is being built. One has the opportunity to consider the advantages and disadvantages of entertaining a need, and can voluntarily nourish it to reach levels, when it can release behavioral responses. One also has the opportunity to think, plan, and navigate to achieve the goals, which will finally satiate the need. Acceptance of a need may also help to constitute anticipation of failure and an anticipated deprived state, and one learns to build the drive in a positive manner, to succeed in the pursuit of need satiation and avoid failures. These need-drive combinations are called the motives, yet another word used for conveying the presence of the propelling force the drive in the individual. Thus, one needs to be motivated to act and achieve survival unrelated needs, often built with passion and hope. They motivate people to set goals, act, and achieve the goals. Unlike biological needs, the psychological needs may not always be fulfilled, if one does not have sufficient drive to get into sustained actions for achieving the goal, and/or does not have the competency to achieve it. It is also possible that the goals are unrealistic. The goals set may be to propagate an idea, a social practice, which can bring in more harmony and peace to the members or to an organization. Unlike biological drives, these needs are the products of human imagination and intelligence, and the goals and methods vary across huge spectrum of choices. Unlike biological needs psychological needs do not produce a direct survival threat, if the drive is not gratified, though some of the failures may result in despair and suicidal wishes in individuals.

Psychological arousal is always accompanied by physiological activation, and hence it is appropriate to consider them as psychophysiological. There are no alternate solutions for biological drives, whereas one can always come up with alternate solutions for psychological drives, as one can compromise on the needs themselves. Biological drives normally require almost immediate gratification, though delayed gratifications have been attempted by some exceptional individuals. One may not survive for more than 10 days without fluids. Mahatma Gandhi stayed without food for 21 days during the freedom struggle of India. Psychological wishes and associated drives can be the result of positive or negative thinking and hence may have equally impelling goals, which may be constructive or disastrous to the self and others. Yet another important aspect is that one always knows what would quench a biological drive and one learns to seek them out. With respect to psychological needs, one normally has ample time to ponder over the choice of needs, the actions, and the goals to be achieved. When the drive becomes intense, the response is automatically released or initiated. These are actions generated from within as one has cultivated and nourished the need or the drive. Normally the drives may remain under inhibitive controls, until it surpasses the personal limits of control. When the drive reaches certain level of potentiation, it overcomes the inhibitive controls and the responses are released, which we call actions. Response inhibition takes place depending on the social acceptability and strategic appropriateness of the response and inhibitive controls one has acquired during the brain developmental stages. As one has to learn to develop the inhibitive control, its strength, and applicability are bound to show marked individual variability. Inhibitive controls are learnt and used for the management of responses in various contexts, viz., social interactions (Eisenberg et al. 1996; Kochanska et al. 2000), all realms of movement management (Konishi et al. 1999; Braver et al. 2001; Rubia et al. 2001; Mostofsky, Simmonds 2008), thinking and decision-making, (Bechara, Damasio, & Damasio 2000), and motivational-emotional regulations of behavior (Rodriguez-Fornellsa et al.

2002; Ochsner et al. 2002; Phan et al. 2005; Walcott, Landau 2004; Leotti, Wager 2010). Once the inhibitive control is weak or not present, the response is easily released. However, the proposition here is that the true control one exercises is by learning to hold back the release of the drive, rather than giving a go signal to a response. One holds back the drive when it can lead to socially unacceptable or strategically incorrect responses. One has no direct control on the initiation of a response or action, as the neural processes are initiated well before one becomes aware of the occurrence of the response. However, one can indeed control the development of a drive, learn to keep it under control, and thereby, in turn learn to control the initiation of various responses from the brain. This ability has to be acquired primarily through socialization process and by practice, which are hazardous indeed, as many do not get adequate exposure and the privilege of acquiring the mind to brain controls. In appropriate releases of responses enhance the arousal and the associated physiological activation contributing to stress responses in the individual.

The presence of arousal can be cognitively appraised and its recognition would take place almost automatically, whether it is acceptable or not to the individual. The labeling is influenced by the reinforcing effects of the presence-absence or increase-decrease of the arousal as one imagines or contemplates on the need or the desire. The gratifying-distressing and approach-avoidance effects decide the cognitive labeling used in the specific emotion. It may produce positive effects like joy, happiness, elation, love, achievement, approach motivation, appreciation, satisfaction, confidence, or negative effects like apprehension, sense of failure, anger, frustration, sadness, depression, apathy, hate, guilt, uncertainty, etc. The mutually exclusive nature of each of the above two categories and the over inclusive effects influence the cognitive resourcefulness available or made use of for explaining the specific context, and the nature of each emotional experience. These experiences are also embedded in thoughts and speech, in their semantic and prosodic interpretations. On the other hand, when it is a matter of expressions of emotions in terms of actions, they are expressed as creative actions or adapted from the basic fight-flight-freeze alternatives. The creative actions form the foundation of multiple pursuits in arts and science. The short, and long-term cognitive appraisals are indeed more important than the long-term physiological and the psychic arousal, as the immediate consequent effects of the emotion are decided by the associated cognitive appraisals and the consequent effects of the responses, which may have constructive or disastrous effects on the individual and the society. Emotions and their effects on the individual are the best example of the effects of mind over the brain. The origin of the human mind from the brain is indeed a mystery and the reverse effects of the mind on the brain are more difficult to understand. The psychological drives propel human beings to sustain and extensive variety of psychobiological responses, most of which do not have direct biological survival value. Value based emotions have immense positive reinforcing effects on the individual and the society. They encourage value based adaptation effects, which foster and make living glorious, thrilling, and challenging. These emotions may propel responses or actions in the form of playing games or musical instruments, singing, giving speeches, writing fiction, researching for discovering the mysteries of the nature, critically thinking and creating new relationships based on the results, documenting and publishing the results, starting a coffee shop or a star restaurant, establishing social-political institutions and organizations for carrying out socially relevant works, and establishing institutions for the creation of new products for fostering working and living standards. No action will be self-initiated unless the drive reaches the critical level of potentiation, which may vary (?) from individual to individual. Holding and building up the drive, so that the action is initiated only when one is ready, is an important skill, which one has to acquire from the early years of upbringing, normally acquired as part of socialization, during the developmental years. The movements, actions, and responses of a person are indicative of the presence of emotion. Experience of emotion may be best regarded as a psychobiological state originating from the brain and spreading all over the body and the mind. Both the domains are equally important and contribute to the genesis and spread of emotions. When there is extensive lesion in the Anterior Cingulate Gyrus and the limbic system, origin of this drive state is found missing, which is needed for the individual to make movements and responses, or even experience pain. There are indeed other forms of prefrontal cortical participation in emotions, which control the responses and actions. There may be no dearth of physical energy, but if the psychic or emotional energy is absent, then the physical energy is wasted. Having fuel in the vehicle is not enough, there has to be a dynamic mechanism—the driver, who wants to move and can release the fuel for supplying the energy for movement as well as navigate the vehicle. This mechanism has to navigate the vehicle to unknown destinations and take unknown routes. The 'Mind' creates the destinations and the routes, and supplies the details of the destinations and the GPRS map of the routes. The brain-mind interface is a two-way path; the brain creates the mind and allows the mind to work on it in return. The fight-flight-freeze is a poor model of emotion for explaining the internally generated drives and the consequent initiation of actions, which embody the variety of pursuits of semantic programming and their actualizations by man.

Emotional Arousal for Navigating into Future

The externally directed response elicited by an external stimulus from a living organism is what came to be called the behavior. Many of these responses have pure survival value to enable the organism to overpower or withdraw from the threatening source. There are responses directed by hunger, thirst, and sex, which enable the animals to move around for drive gratification. These behavioral expressions were described as conditioned reflexes, and they develop because of stimulus generalizations or because of positive rewards. Perception of the stimulus is important for eliciting the unconditioned as well as conditioned responses. Occurrence of preattentive emotional responses produced by fear evoking stimuli without their perception was discovered much later, and is discussed elsewhere in the book.

Burrhus Frederic Skinner (Baum 1994; Thorndike 1901) demonstrated learning taking place when responses were reinforced positively or negatively by reward and punishment. Reward strengthened the occurrence of a behavior whereas punishment reduced or stopped its occurrence. This is called operant conditioning. Different neural circuits have been found which support reward and punishment in the brain. Release of acetylcholine is activated in the presence of a reward. Similarly, the dopamine release is activated in the frontal lobes of the brain in the presence of reinforcements. When a certain behavior is reinforced with reward, the brain learns the behavior quickly so that the dopamine is released which produces rewarding and gratifying feelings to the individual. Operant conditioning is also called instrumental conditioning and this mode of condition of behavior is widely accepted by the society and is the basis of social conditioning or socialization. Operant conditioning principles are used to help individual learn social and institutional norms for the preservation of the society and its institutions. In this model, behavior is essentially reinforced and elicited by external factors. Behavior is also generated from within, without the presence of such instant rewarding and punishing conditions. This is said to be motivated behavior and the neural programming responsible for behavior has been referred to as complex motor programming (Goldberg 1985). The essential characteristic of a conditioned behavior is that it is a response to a stimulus or stimulus condition. On the other hand, when an individual initiates behavior on his own, without any compulsions of instant reward or punishment, it is called an action. However, an action can be initiated only if there is a need experienced by the individual. This need serves as drive for the initiation of actions from within. Drive is the psychic fuel required for starting the action. The drive is generated from the early years of growth. The child goes through routines, which have been well defined by the grown-ups in the society and work within the system created by them and gradually learn the purposes of the system through the mental drills. The system grows within each member, and he learns to live within the system, by abiding and accepting the goals and the laid out action plans.

They learn to understand the purpose of the goals they are made to accept and set for themselves, and learn to plan actions for reaching the goals. The goal becomes a need within, which one has to achieve. The need or the drive serve as motivation, or they motivate the person to act. Generally, free societies offer opportunity to each to think independently and make changes in the system or create new ideas and prove their worth. This enhances the strength of the system, as one joins and works within the system with conviction, instead of having to accept the system values forcefully. Freedom to think allows all to create new ideas and experiment with life.

Behavior of the individual is a complex mixture of responses and actions. Responses strengthen and preserve the social system, whereas planned actions take one to the goals set for the self. Execution of actions may need continuously monitoring and regulation so that the respective goal is finally achieved. None of these comes under the phylogenic model of fight-flight behavior. The whole process consists of series of actions based on complex motor programming and their execution. The functional systems of the frontal lobes already described elsewhere play the magic role of the 'executive system'. A complex motor programming system deployed in the human brain has several unique features. Some of the most important features of the internal regulator controls used in the system are summed up here, though the same have been discussed in detail elsewhere in the book. First, the system accepts a purpose for the actions and sets the goals, which can be achieved by the actions. The goal could be a physical one or a semantically interpreted idea, or a process of acquiring the capabilities required to play a role in life. As most of the goals are in a forward spatial and temporal location, one has to learn to navigate to that location. This would make it necessary that one must have plans of actions, so that they can be executed in steps to take one to the goal. This would further mean that one must learn to anticipate the effects of the planned actions and must compare the anticipated effects with the actual effects for resolving discrepancies, if they arise. The planned actions may require one to learn the skills of body movements by simultaneous participation of different body parts. The movements may have to be executed in predefined sequential manner, which one needs to master. All decisions may have to be internally made according to the strategies drawn for the navigation of the individual or the organization to reach the goals. The goals may be defined semantically, before one starts the navigation, though they may need to be achieved both physically and conceptually. The navigational control one learns during the development of the programming abilities allows one to strive forward with strategic plans and arrive at the goals through the perusal of the planned path, even though the goal itself may never be in sight until it is reached. One learns to predict the outcome at various steps in the strategic pursuit, and hence anticipate their occurrences. One even learns to alter the goals, if the goals pursued are unattainable because of unexpected obstacles and difficulty in overcoming them. Such long and tedious pursuits in life are possible only if one is emotionally aroused and has the ability to remain so through the journey. One needs positive emotions for these pursuits as the journey is for not escaping from threats. One learns or could learn to counter threats with love and sacrifice instead of adopting the normal fight-flight-freeze behaviors used by other living species in the nature.

Annexures

ANNEXURE 1

CLINICAL NEUROPSYCHOLOGICAL EXAMINATION

Clinical Methods

Clinical neuropsychological examination is carried out on patients with suspected or confirmed brain damage due to neurological disorders, presence of neoplasm, head injury, etc. The changes that occur in the brain due to neurochemical imbalances, vascular pathology, structural changes, and trauma result in the impairment of cognitive and emotional functioning of the brain. This affects psychological, social, and occupational abilities of the affected individual. Earlier views of the brain and behavior considered specific psychological functions as associated with specific areas, which gave rise to functional localization theories of the brain. Some of the eminent scientists of the 19th century, whose work contributed to the understanding of brain-mind relationship are Franz Josef Gall (1758-1828), Alexander Bain (1818-1903), Herbert Spencer (1820-1908), Paul Broca (1824-1880), Hughlings Jackson (1835-1911), and David Ferrier (1843-1920). Their postulations implied that each structure in the brain has an independent function and various functions are distributed over the different structures of the brain. A distinct departure from this line of thinking is seen in the works of Luria (1966a, b) in his publication *Higher Cortical Functions in Man*, in which he describes the different functional analysing capabilities and the interfaces between different lobes of the brain for supporting functional integration across systems. This work is the culmination of two decades of clinical investigation by the author. He described the Gnostic system, the visual analysing system, the auditory analysing system, the memory system, etc., which incorporate functional interaction of different areas of the brain. The advent of systems research theory and concepts and application of neural network systems strongly supported the application of systems approach for understanding the evolutionary origin of mind in the brain.

As opposed to extreme reductionism, which lays emphasis in breaking down any issue or matter into smaller ingredients and studying them in parts, the systems approach lays emphasis on how different parts interact with each other to produce a total effect and how a function emerges from such interactive processes. As every conceivable psychological function is an outcome of complex interactive process, the systems approach is the most suitable approach for understanding the brain-behavior, or brain-mind relationship. In the brain-mind paradigm, we presume that the mind has emerged from the brain.

Identification and Assessment of Impairment of Psychological Functions

Psychological examination of patients with disorders of the brain is used for detecting: (1) impairment in neurocognitive processing of the brain, (2) the effects of impairment on personal, social, and occupational, functioning of the individual. This is carried out by identifying signs of specific deficits in psychological tests and behavioral tests, and eliciting the presence of focal deficits associated with focal lesions of the brain. Deficits may be specific based on the system impaired by the lesion, whether it is a focal, extended, or diffused lesion. The most important aim of the examination is to identify presence of characteristic signs, which would indicate the presence of involvement of specific functional systems, precipitated by the lesion interrupting the participation of specific brain areas processing. On the other hand, it may also be necessary to determine the impairment of cognitive abilities in terms of premorbid functional level. Estimating the degree of impairment of cognitive abilities is considered most difficult and often inaccurate as a true estimation can be derived only with respect to the premorbid level of functioning of the patient, which may not have been quantified earlier and hence not available. On the one hand, (1) one may want to assess the performance pattern of a patient for detecting presence of specific deficit features in performance because of which the patient is not able to perform the test satisfactorily. On the other hand, (2) one may want to assess the ability level of a patient in comparison with that of normal control for deciding if the patient has impairment in the ability tested and the magnitude of the disability. First, it has to be understood clearly that a clinical neuropsychological assessment is not used for assessing the intellectual and cognitive potentialities of a patient. Its purpose is to detect various deficits or dysfunctions that may be manifested by the presence of a lesion or disorder in the brain. The lesion would indeed impair intellectual abilities and the level of current functioning can be understood from psychometric assessments. This is indeed useful for settling the medico-legal liabilities of a case. On the other hand, the routine neuropsychological assessment of a patient is to understand and evaluate the varying effects of the brain disorder, which are responsible for the performance decrement in psychometric test outcome. The neuropsychological assessment evaluates the multiple subcomponents of neurocognitive processes, which contribute to a wholesome cognitive ability or functional system in a person. This is based on the assumptions and findings that different cortical areas in the brain contribute to different components of a functional system, and understanding of the deficits in the different subcomponents produces a dysfunction profile of the brain. Lesion in a specific neural substrate disables its specific functional contribution in the sensory-motor or cognitive processing of the brain. This would leave a specific dysfunctional feature impairing the total functional system, which is identified in the clinical neuropsychological assessment of the patient. There are multiples of such functional subcomponents, which together contribute to each functional system in the brain. This requires very subtle examination procedures so that such dysfunction features can be identified, if present in a patient. Neuropsychology is the science of understanding such multiples of subcomponents involved in processing in the different functional domains of the brain. Several of these features, especially some of the functions of the sensory-motor systems are normally elicited in the neurological examination of a patient and the remaining and the neurocognitive features are picked up in a neuropsychological examination of a patient. Such examination of a normal person will not elicit any deficit and there cannot be a normal distribution of the deficits. Some of the normal functional attributes can indeed be tested by using neuroimaging techniques and their spatial localization can be determined. The functional deficits can be elicited only by careful clinical examination of the patient. However, understanding and accepting neuroplasticity of the brain indicate that a lost functional capability can be developed by adjacent and other areas in the brain if the brain is retrained. Examining and estimating the functional profiles are also important part of neuropsychological assessment from the point of various treatment programs. The improvements shown by treatment programs have to be supported by improved functional efficiency in the patient. The emphasis is not only on looking out for reduced dysfunctions, but also on improvement in functional capabilities compared to pre-intervention levels and normalization of functions if present. The procedures may indeed extend from clinical assessments to neurocognitive experimental methods for demonstrating the recovery pattern in the patients.

Neurorehabilitation of a patient is equally challenging and important when total restoration of impaired functions is not possible to achieve. The patient needs to be rehabilitated at a different level, commensurate with the capabilities remaining intact and the level to which the patient can be retrained. It involves the use of new technologies as well as retraining of the patients. Cognitive rehabilitation is the challenge for neuropsychologists as well as other professionals involved in the psychosocial, emotional, cognitive, and occupational rehabilitation of patients. Contributions from other professionals, social institutions are indeed important. Medicolegal liabilities, especially compensations in accident victims can be decided only by assessing the current levels of abilities, and by estimating what the victim has lost in the accident. Estimation of cognitive deficits has to be often made in comparison with comparable normative data, though a comparison with the premorbid levels of efficiency is the most accurate. The difficulty may be partly overcome by comparing performance to those skills, like language skills, which do not easily deteriorate or show impairment during the early stages of the illness, unless the lesion has specifically impaired these abilities. These are vocabulary and general information repertoire of a person. From these as well as educational and occupational levels attained by the subject a reference point for premorbid level of functioning may be arrived at.

Neuropsychological Assessment

The primary aim of clinical neuropsychological assessment is to identify and estimate the nature of impairment of psychological functions and behavior due to damage to the brain as an outcome of neurological diseases, trauma, and other pathophysiological conditions. The psychological and behavioral domain consists of functions of reception of information in the brain, attending to the stimulus inputs, their encoding and transcoding, perception and recognition, working memory operations, storage of information and its retrieval, thinking, psychomotor execution, complex motor programming, responding to various external conditions, verbal awareness, emotions and motivation (drive). Arousal of emotions, emotional experience, and expressions are closely attached to all forms of cognitive processes that the two are inseparable interactive processes in the brain. The cognitive and emotional impairments may easily have deleterious effects on daily activities of life, occupational, and social functioning of the patient. Neuropsychological tests help in many ways to help the patient. Some of them are: (a) for understanding the nature and magnitude of deficits and consequent disabilities; (b) the diagnostic implications of such deficits; (c) estimation of the progressiveness of the deficits and the possibilities of restoration of the functions through retraining program; (d) implementation of cognitive retraining, conceptual and behavioral enrichment programs; and (d) subsequent rehabilitation of the patient whenever needed. The nature and extensiveness of the lesion is investigated separately using neuroimaging techniques and the correlational inferences between site and extensiveness of the lesion and psychological deficits could be ascertained. Such validation of the psychological tests gives them clinically useful predictive powers. The technique underscores that there are typical deficits, which could be identified and evaluated, associated with specific lesion condition or disorder of the brain.

Deficits are abnormalities of normal psychological functions and skills of an individual and therefore, a comprehensive understanding of the normal function is extremely important. Identification and evaluation of deficits may be carried out by both qualitative observation, as well as their quantification, in whatever form possible. There are several deficits, which cannot be quantified as they are related to a loss of normal functions. Identifying the inability to do simple normal functions are therefore, sure ways of identifying these deficits. Examination of a patient is carried out with various psychomotor tests, tests of attention, visuospatial performance tests, tests of perception in different sensory modalities, working memory tests, tests of verbal and visual learning memory functions, etc. The deficits need to be accurately described in terms of their expression in patients and the manner in which they are elicited by tests.

Neuropsychological deficits are elicited by simple clinical examination procedures using tests and procedures. The purpose of the tests is never to estimate the potentiality level that one may reach, but to understand if the patient can carry out simple processes in the normal manner, or fails to perform even if given extra time. The tests must show how simple and basic functional components are impaired or absent in the cognitive and emotional processes and expressive behavior of the patient. Standardized testing/examination procedure may be used and in addition, improvisation of procedure is possible as long as the deficit could be elicited. However, there are areas in which such inferences are difficult to make as in the case of intelligence and memory testing. There may be actual impairment seen as decrements in the IQ and MQ scores, though the total performance of a patient may still be within normal range and hence it may escape to be noticed. The patient, on the other hand, may report changes and concern in his cognitive processing ability compared to what he used to perform. Therefore, all complains and personal estimates of personal performance of a patient must be taken seriously and recorded.

An important requirement of the clinical examination model called the "idiometric" approach is that it must be possible to demonstrate the deficit in repeat examination of the patient. The deficit may be demonstrated by using more than one test procedure. The emphasis is on accurate description of the deficits, how they are expressed by the patient and observed by the examiner. A group of such deficits may be elicited in a patient and the analysis and interpretation of the deficits has been called Neuropsychological Syndrome Analysis. Deficit in one area may have deleterious effect on many other functions, and therefore, it is very important to identify those basic deficits, which influence adversely other functions. For example, deficit in the application of the central executive of working memory can affect several other functions such as verbal and visual encoding, spatial planning, visuospatial perception, verbal and abstract reasoning, etc. Presence of dyscalculia can impair performance on working memory test using mental arithmetic. Deficit in visuospatial perception in the form of distortions can impair performance on visual memory and encoding. Different functions are interrelated as the same structures mediate different functions in the brain. The commonality in the mediation of different functional systems is still to be understood adequately.

A deficit and its association with a lesion in a specific site in the brain do not necessarily indicate that the associated normal function is controlled exclusively by that area. Lesion in more than one area in any part of a functional circuit has the propensity to produce the same or more or less the same type of deficit. This is discussed in detail elsewhere in the book. The wealth of clinical findings of neuropsychological deficits amply support that there is no exclusive one to one relationship between a site and a deficit. Therefore, a profile of deficits does not strongly indicate a lesion in a particular area. On the other hand, it is considered indicative of the involvement of a functional system subserved by the neural circuit that is affected by the lesion.

Identification and evaluation of dysfunction has paramount clinical importance and clinical neuropsychology is essentially a study of profile of such dysfunction in the different domains of psychological functioning of a patient. As there is a close one to one relationship between various primary sensory-motor functions and the brain, diagnosis of lesion from sensory-motor deficits is a reliable clinical approach. Focal deficits of perception, memory, and motor programming are also seen in relation to focal lesions of the brain and their identification and evaluation help to localize the structures of the brain producing such deficits. However, a one to one relationship between a deficit and the site of a lesion reduces, as the function affected is complex and abstract. Therefore, focal deficits of perception, memory, etc. may not necessarily have a one to one relationship with exclusive sites of lesion. Larger areas involving network of structures contribute to subserving such complex functional systems and therefore, the deficits result because of lesion in any of the part of the network that supports the function.

The veracity of the concept of normal deterioration of brain functions in the absence of a disease process of the brain has been questioned. Clinically significant deficits are typically produced by the pathology in the brain. During old age, there is a natural decline of skeleto-muscular abilities and therefore, in functions used by these system. The decline found in skeleto-muscular functions during the old age is considered normal decline. Therefore, speed of response, especially the psychomotor type could show decrement as age advances. A one standard deviation decline on tests that involves both cognitive processing and speed of response has been indicated from 20 years to 70 years. However, there is no evidence to show that either thinking or reasoning processes shows such natural decline in individuals who maintain cognitive activity throughout. It is also not presumed that there is a normal distribution of brain damage due to neurological disorders and hence there may be normal distribution of associated deficits. There may be exception to this with regard to certain disorders in childhood and old age. Scholastic backwardness and specific learning disabilities are not considered associated with a disease or damage of the brain. Specific learning disability is widely considered a problem related to the programming of the brain contributed by inadequate or disordered network circuits.

The clinical neuropsychological assessment procedures described here are based on the procedures learnt and made use of by the author and his team during the years 1975-1990 at the All India Institute of Mental Health, which later became the National Institute of Mental Health & Neuro Science, Bengaluru, as part of the attempts to develop clinical neuropsychological services.

Clinical Neuropsychological Assessment

The first step in a neuropsychological assessment is to get to know as much details as possible about the case. This includes information about the present complains, history of present illness in detail from the patient as well as informants, and finally reports of other investigations, especially findings of neuroradiological and MRI investigations, and clinical diagnosis including differential diagnosis if any. This will help to make a neuropsychological formulation and decide on the various functions that need to be examined thoroughly. The case could have been referred for one of the following reasons: (1) Presence of neurocognitive deficits in the patient, which will offer further diagnostic confirmation, (2) monitoring the prognosis of the patient during the ongoing therapeutic regime, (3) as part of pre-post assessments during neurosurgery, (4) for neurocognitive evaluation in epilepsy, epilepsy surgery, head injury, vascular conditions, etc., (5) for dementia evaluation by determining the nature and degree of neurocognitive deficits, and (6) for neurocognitive retraining as part of neurological rehabilitation. The strategy of neuropsychological assessment and the tests used are likely to be different for different conditions.

Observation of the Patient

Keen observation of a patient's behavior is the primary step in neuropsychological examination. Observation includes how the patient is kempt, the pattern of walking, moving around, using limbs, posture, gestures if any, the manner in which he scans the environment, looks at the examiner and others, attends to speech, manner of speaking, facial expressions, etc.

1. Appearance of the Patient

While meeting a patient for the first time, it may not be possible to know if the patient had dressed himself or he has been helped by relatives or attendants. However, if the patient does not appear adequately dressed or appearing reasonably clean and tidy, it is necessary to note down the same. Only if the patient has been deteriorating as in the case of dementia or is having an episode of depression or psychosis, it is generally possible that the patient is ill kempt.

2. Locomotion and Use of Limbs

The ease and freedom with which the patient may walk in will be different based on gait, muscular conditions of the lower limbs, etc. Difficulty in walking and using limbs may be because of impairment of associated muscle control functions or indicate presence of apraxia, which will require careful evaluation.

3. Arousal of Attention

Presence of spontaneous arousal of attention in the patient can be easily observed. Its absence, make it necessary to arouse the attention of the patient by repeated commands and instructions. On the other hand, hyper arousal of attention will cause distractibility and the patient will find it difficult to focus attention while speaking to the examiner and performing the tasks presented. Inability to attend to the examiner may also be because of loss of drive and motivation in the patient. It may also be the result of preoccupation and associated emotional state of a person, as in the case of depression. A checklist for observing the state of attention is given in the Neuropsychological battery.

4. Speech

The manner of speaking requires careful evaluation and needs special attention from the examiner. Appropriateness of the loudness and flow of speech, ability to articulate are to be evaluated as soon as the patient starts speaking. As speech may require careful evaluation for identifying the presence of different types of deficits, it is to be done as part of speech assessment separately.

5. Emotions

The general behavior and task specific performance reveal important clues about the emotional state of a patient. Patient's response as he enters the testing room, the anticipation that may be seen on his face and the readiness to answer questions, are important aspects to be noted. The patient may be seen as preoccupied, without any concern or distressed. The patient may sit in front of the examiner without any concern and the examiner will have to repeatedly ask or coax the patient to respond to questions. Non-cooperativeness on the part of the patient to respond to the examiner itself is a significant condition to be observed.

It is equally important that the patient be closely observed during test performance. Several of the test findings are drawn from observation of patient's performance. Such observation is important to make note of the strategies used by the patient and his specific difficulties in performance. These are important observations, which help to formulate the nature of the deficits the patient may have. For example, in Block Design test, if a patient arranges the four blocks in a line or one on the top of the other, this needs to be recorded as it has significant diagnostic implication. A patient may be found to leave the task in between and instructions have to be repeated or the patient may resume the task on his own on prompting. The subtle difference between the two approaches has important differential implication, and therefore, they must be recorded accurately.

The clinical methods of patient examination and interpretations used by the author were based on the clinical and research findings of contemporary neuropsychologists especially that of A.R. Luria (1996a, b) in the years 1975-1992, along with a few additional original tests, for developing clinical neuropsychological practice at the National Institute of Mental Health & Neuro Sciences, Bengaluru. The normative data described for the Neuropsychological battery of tests were collected by the team during the years 1980-1998.

Neuropsychological tests constitute items, most of which adapted or used in the originally described form for the local patient population and some developed based on the knowledge available on cerebral localization and lateralization of higher mental functions. This is a loosely packed battery of tests, from which appropriate tests can be chosen according to diagnostic and other test needs. The main feature of the battery is its emphasis on eliciting dysfunction or impairment of brain function using rather simple testing methods. Therefore, there is considerable stress on identifying various basic functional components and employing appropriate tests for eliciting their impairment. The examiner must have a good knowledge of what is expected of a normal subject, if he or she is presented with a certain question, problem, or task. This will help the examiner to detect the deviations of performance and then make judgment of impairment. It is the difference or the inability to perform that attracts the attention of the examiner who must readily make note of it.

A. Tests for Eliciting Frontal Lobe Dysfunctions

Attention, visual search, mental set, psychomotor performance, ideational fluency, abstraction, working memory, spatial planning and personality changes are the major areas examined for drawing a Frontal dysfunction profile in a patient.

1. Attention

(a) Spontaneous arousal of attention is absent.

(b) Attention has to be aroused by repeated commands.

(c) Attention is easily distracted.

(d) Instructions have to be repeatedly given.

(e) Excessive broadening or narrowing of attention is present.

Interpretation of attentional processes can be made only after careful observation of the patient during the interview and testing. Spontaneous arousal of attention is the first component that may be considered for evaluation. Spontaneous attention may be considered adequate when the patient looks up in anticipation at the examiner. Absence of spontaneous arousal of attention and the need to arouse attention by repeated instructions are commonly associated with lesions of the mediobasal areas of the frontal cortex. On the other hand, the opposite profile may be found in lesions of the orbitofrontal cortex. In this case, attention is easily aroused and the patient responds to even irrelevant stimuli around him, which interferes with sustained attention related performance. An impairment of ability to broaden or expand attentional span may result in increased narrowing of attention and the patient will be unable to attend simultaneously to several aspects of an object or stimulus field. A right orbitofrontal lesion thus may easily result in distractibility. Therefore, there are three major aspects of attention to be judged, viz., spontaneous arousal of attention, responding to irrelevant stimuli or distractibility, and ability for focused and sustained attention. Impaired attention will have a significant adverse effect on all other performance tests. An accurate understanding of attentional process in the patient is essential before commenting on performance on other tests.

2. Visual Search [visual exploration]

(a) Visual scanning of numbers.

(b) Visual scanning of picture.

(c) Visual Exploration test. (Weintraub-Messulam 1987)

Serial scanning of numbers printed at random on a paper allows the examiner to observe the smoothness and rapidity with which the individual systematically searches a given visual space. Firstly, a slow shifting of the gaze leads to slow scanning. Secondly, tardy exploration of the visual space because of absence of a spatial plan and difficulty in serially looking for numbers can affect the speed and accuracy of visual search. The first item is a relatively simple one and has numbers from 1 to 20 printed in a space of 4 cm × 15 cm. The second item has numbers from 1 to 60 and printed in a larger space of 12 cm ×

15 cm. The third item has 12 numbers out of 36 repeating twice or more and the subject is expected to score out all the repeated numbers one by one. The total time taken to scan each number series and the errors are recorded. If the patient is illiterate and cannot read numbers, visual scanning of a picture was used. A picture with 5-6 distinctly visible items was used for this. The test was administered to normal adult subjects for determining the time taken by them to perform this simple task. These scores were used to compare the score of a patient. The picture scanning is not as sensitive as the former one. But, if a patient has difficulty to identify the items in the picture, it could be an indication of a visual scanning difficulty or at times visual agnosia. The third test is the visual exploration test described by Weintraub and Mesulam (1987, 1988) in which subject has to choose targets from non-targets and cancel them in the right and left spatial halves on a paper placed in front. Their studies have shown a normal preference of the left half of the visual field over the right, and significantly greater deficit or visual neglect of contralateral visual field by right frontal lesion patients on scanning both the halves compared to left lesion patients.

Instructions for visual scanning tests 1 & 2: "Numbers 1 to 20 are arranged at random on this sheet of paper. Please strike of the numbers in serial order, for example, 1,2,3, up to 20" (or 1-50 for item 2). For item 3 the instruction may be as follows: "Here is list of numbers starting from 1 to 40. Some of the numbers are repeated once or more. You have to search out those numbers, which are repeated, and strike them out. You have to cancel as many as possible within 2 minutes."

Interpretation

When there is difficulty for visual search, the patient may not be able to search more than a few numbers (3-5) in serial order. Failure to search out the number in sequence is the main difficulty that the examiner looks for. If the patient has difficulty to hold on to the numbers serially, the examiner can help the patient with the number that he has to look out. The real difficulty that is considered is the impairment in searching the visual space for the numbers. Serial counting can be affected by working memory difficulty and hence the examiner may help the patient in that respect. Speed of search may also be affected by general state of the patient. Difficulty to move visual search to different spatial locations is what is tested. This is different from ability to shift visual gaze fixation, which is important for reading, though impairment in shifting gaze fixation too can impair visual search. The left visual dominance seen in studies is because of a right visual dominance in the brain. Such lateralized visual dominance improves the chances of detection and responding to stimuli in the left visual field. The patient will be stuck after searching out the first few numbers with the help of the examiner and would find it hard to search out the numbers further. The patient would make mistakes and call out wrong numbers. The impairment in visual search is normally apparent and can be identified without referring to normative data. Even when the patient makes a wrong choice, he would not be aware that he has called out a wrong number. Patients with present slowness in search may be because of lethargy or inadequate drive to perform. Impairment in visual search functions seen as reduced speed or impaired performance indicate a right frontal involvement. Patients with visual search difficulty would find difficulty to locate objects routinely used in everyday life. Visual search is a function of visual attention and hence it has to be evaluated along with attention.

3. Mental Set: Psychomotor Perseveration

Psychomotor perseveration can be detected in (a) motor alternation tests and (b) continuous drawing tests. The motor alteration test as described by Luria has been used. One method of this test involves asking the patient to stretch out first his right hand or preferred hand, and showing a fist, and then put the hand down and to stretch out again showing a ring with the thumb and the index finger. The patient has to continue to alternating this act several times until the examiner is satisfied that the patient can carry out the task smoothly and the alternation is correctly maintained. The examiner may demonstrate the movement of hand and even train the patient to carry out. Impairment is seen as inability to continuously alternate when patient will throw fist or the ring alone.

Continuous Drawing test: The patient is first asked to draw small circle, triangle and a cross on a sheet of paper one by one. Once the examiner is satisfied that the subject can draw these with ease, the patient is told that he has to draw the figures as the examiner calls out their names. The examiner then calls out the names at random order from a prepared list. Keep the pace convenient for the subject to draw the figure fully. Impairment will be inability of the patient to change the figures as and when they are changed by the examiner. The patient will be seen drawing the same figure repeatedly. This is recorded as perseveration.

Interpretation: Perseveration of the above type is seen generally when there is extensive lesion of the frontal lobes especially the orbitofrontal areas. In less extensive lesions perseveration may be seen in other performance tests such as the visuospatial tests viz., Bender Gestalt test or Benton's Visual Retention test, etc.

4. Psychomotor Deficits

Kinetic Melody Disturbances (tapping test)

To test kinetic melody, first instruct/demonstrate the patient how to rhythmically tap the table with the fingers of the two hands—tap twice with the right hand and once with the left hand fingers, and maintain the rhythm for about a minute. Very seldom, a patient may be seen who does not understand the instructions for finger tapping. If the patient can spontaneously tap after the examiner has demonstrated, there will be no further need to test the patient. Sometimes it may be necessary to increase the complexity of tapping especially if the patient is a musician who has a special ear to music or plays percussion instruments. The number of tapping can be then changed, for example, tap thrice with right hand and twice with left or changing the timings, which the examiner must demonstrate first. As impairment is a significant indicator of a frontal lobe involvement, a hasty decision about it is unwarranted. It is also extremely important to know that tapping ability can be impaired in cerebellar lesions. In this case, the tapping may become rigid and devoid of smoothness and at times the patient may be unable to tap at all. Therefore, it is essential to know if the patient also has a cerebellar involvement before arriving at an inference about a frontal lobe involvement. Luria (1985) has described impairment in kinetic melody because of premotor area lesions.

5. Deficits in Working Memory

Delayed Response Ability Test: Tests for Mental Control

Working memory refers to an online memory configuration in which a certain block of information is held in awareness or span of attention for use in an ongoing information processing. It is a partitioned awareness achieved through division of attention for holding on to important piece of information needed, while individual is engaged in processing another. A simple example is the serial subtraction test in which 1 has to be serially subtracted from 20. For calling out 19, the subject has to remember the previous number 20. In the next step, the subject holds on to number 19 so that he can call out the number 18 and so on. Once a number has been called out, the previous number need not be further held on. Thus working memory is a buffer memory from where information can be transferred for use in an ongoing processing. It is obvious that if the subject is not able to hold on to number 19, he will not be able to say the next number 18. Yet another similar test is the digits forward and backward tests, which are often used in the mental state examination of psychiatric patients. Frontal lobe patients have sever difficulty in both and would give up the test generally after two digits presentations. Another formal Working Memory test is by using mental arithmetic calculations, which was devised and used first in the 1975-1976, and became a stable part of the battery of neuropsychological tests because of its high efficiency to indicate presence of frontal lobe dysfunction, if present, in various types of lesion cases (Mukundan et al. 1979a, b, 1991; Mukundan 1996). In this, the subject is presented with a problem to "add 2 and 3 and subtract the total from the sum of 5 and 6", presented only once in total. The test has thus three parts to execute. Subject has to first mentally hold on to the whole problem and then work on the first part of finding '2 + 3' and then on hold on 5 and then work on 5 + 6 which was held on. Once the answer to the second addition is available as 11, then he must do the third stage of subtracting 5 from 11.

The typical difficulty seen on this test is the inability to hold on to the part while processing the second. The patient may often ask for the repetition of the first part, as he does not remember it as he says. The test contains 20 items. It is essential to find out at the outset itself if the subject can carry out simple single digit arithmetical operations before the test is administered by asking him to add or subtract single digit numbers both mentally.

If the patient asks for repetition of the test, this may be recorded. The test is not to be presented in parts even if the patient asks for it.

Interpretation: The test is very sensitive to detect frontal lobe involvement provided the patient can carry out simple arithmetic spontaneously. The inability to either carry out arithmetic of the first part or hold on to the solution of the first part will be clearly seen in these patients. The test is exceptionally sensitive in both unilateral and bilateral frontal lobe lesions indication bilateral representation of the function that is involved. The results of the test have been discussed in detail elsewhere in the book. When the patient does not have difficulty in this area, it is easily evident as the responses are made spontaneously. Even minimal deficits shown by a patient with good premorbid arithmetical ability, is indicative of a frontal lobe involvement, unless the difficulty can be explained in terms of stress reaction.

6. Deficits of Ideational Function

Name objects made of [a] wood, [b] round objects, each for 2 minutes.

Ideational Fluency test: Spontaneity and ideation are the key factors that affect the performance in the tests. The test measures sematic fluency by instructing the subject to name objects, which are "round" and objects, which are made of "wood". It is suitable for all patients. Subject has to name "round things" and "wooden things" for two minutes each and the number of names so described constitutes the scores on each.

7. Deficits in Visuospatial Analysis—Synthesis and Visual Integration

Ability for visuospatial analysis and synthesis and visual integration are considered important right hemisphere functions and involves engagément of right frontal, temporal, and parietal cortical areas. Impairment in visuospatial analysis and synthesis, and visual integration are to be observed from the performances on various drawing and construction tests. Absence of ability in these areas manifest as specific difficulties during visuosptial performance and the features representing such difficulty can be observed when the patient is engaged is different visuoperceptual and construction tasks. These tasks could be part of various intelligence or perceptual tests. For example, tests used for eliciting such dysfunctions were Bender Gestalt Test, Minnesota Percepto-diagnostic (MPD) Test, Koh's Block Design Test, Object Assembly Test, and Alexander's Passalong Test, and Maze Test. However, as a neuropsychological procedure these tests were not used for measuring a potential functional capability, but for identifying the presence of specific features of dysfunction in visuospatial perception. Therefore, the performance of the patient needs to be closely observed and recorded. If there is no indication of such deficits, the testing was not continued. The presence of such deficits cannot be obtained from normative data, as normal subjects do not have such difficulties. For example, despite informing the patient that he has to accommodate all the figures of the Bender Gestalt test on a single sheet of paper, the patient would find it difficult to draw more than 3 or 4 figures as the drawings are macrographic and spatially ill arranged on the sheet. In the Bender Gestalt test, a patient may start drawing the first figure from the middle of the page and would find it difficult to complete all the figures on the same page. Some of them still would draw all the figures in the top half or quarter of the paper and find it difficult to maintain a proper spatial separation and size representation of the original figures. Performance on the Block Design test, the Object Assembly test and the Passalong test are also used for interpreting visual perceptual anomalies. As these tests are used as tests of visual integration they are discussed in the next section. The role of spatial planning in the Maze test is well known. Spatial planning is associated with right frontal areas than with left frontal lobes, and the deficits of this type are more frequent in right frontal lesions. However, this cannot be generalized to planning in general. It is also often difficult to differentiate between spatial planning and spatial construction (including drawing), even though the two are contributed by the right frontal and parietal lobes respectively. The two needs to be applied in a combined manner and the features of difficulty cannot be easily differentiated in the performance. However, when the patient has difficulty in performance, its presence is seen as specific features of functional deficits that can be detected straightaway. Despite giving unlimited time for performance, the patient struggles to progress in the task and would be stuck with one difficulty or the other. Instructing the patient and giving clues do not help him to overcome difficulty. These impairment features could also be elicited by other similar tests, where the patient has to complete a task by visually organizing the constituent parts. In object assembly, the first task is to examine the parts and guess that the object or the picture would be when the parts are assembled. If one cannot guess that the parts represent the fingers, he cannot assemble the palm from them. Similarly, if he cannot guess that another set of parts represent the nose, mouth, ears, and eyes he would not be able to assemble a face with those parts.

Gestalt perception is an important aspect of visual perception, as discussed earlier, and the failure of the strategies needed for effective visual perception and reproduction of the perceived figure produces several independent deficits in the performance or the drawing accomplished by a patient. The typical features indicating deficits in visuospatial perception are the following (also discussed elsewhere):

1. Size estimation (Micrographia and Macrographia).
2. Impairment in Verticality and Horizontality and diagonal representations.

3. Fragmentation while drawing as the patient misses parts.
4. Distorted figures, unable to maintain original profile.
5. Impairment in perpendicularity, angularity, curviness, etc.
6. Visual extinction.
7. Unilateral neglect in perception, Hemi-inattention.
8. Constructional Apraxia: Cannot draw any aspect of figure through, there is no drawing difficulty.
9. Perseveration of components and figures.
10. Impairment in visual integration—parts are not joined.

The examiner has to examine carefully the performance of the patient to decide the presence of the above features and make note of the presence of each and any descriptive detail, if possible are necessary.

8. Expressive Speech Disturbances (Not included)

9. Changes in Voluntary Activity, Personality, and Affect

Frontal lesions may result in changes in voluntary movements and activities of a person. On the one hand, this may be related to reduced purposefulness and goal directedness and on the other hand, it may be related to deficits of regulation of motor behavior. In clinical terms, purposefulness in a person can be measured in terms of explanations and justifications of the activities that he is engaged in and the goals of life could be understood from the ambitions and aspirations. The lifestyle and activities one develops will be geared for achieving these goals. Therefore, a diminished view and concern of these can drastically alter the life pattern of the affected person. A significant result will be reduction in the familial, social, and occupational activities of the patient. The patient loses interest in spending time with the immediate family members and withdraws from family and social engagements. Lack of initiative could also affect several daily chores, which were voluntarily carried out by a person. In acute condition produced by extensive frontal lobe lesion the patient becomes apathetic, akinetic and abulic (Luria 1981). On the other hand, personality changes resulting from disinhibition indicated a different neuropsychological deficit profile. The specific personality changes that the examiner must look for are mentioned below.

Personality, Emotional, Cognitive and Behavioral Changes in Lesions of the Frontal Lobes.

I. Features of ACC Dysfunction

1. Akinetic mutism (patient is unable to speak though does not have expressive aphasia) in bilateral lesions.
2. Transient akinetic mutism in unilateral lesions.
3. Absence of spontaneous speech.
4. Speaks in monosyllables if made to speak.
5. Apathy—absence of emotion.
6. Absence of emotion even when hurt and in pain.
7. Absence of interest in self and surroundings.
8. Absence of initiative in the patient and the patient becomes indifferent.
9. Does not ask for food, eat and drink only if fed.

The above changes are indicative of involvement of the Anterior Cingulate Cortex and the subcortical system connected to this area.

II. Features of Orbitofrontal Dysfunction

1. Change in the tolerance levels: Patient has become intolerant, impatient, and aggressive.
2. Change in affective state: Patient who was shy and inhibited becomes outspoken and less inhibited in comments and behavior with others.
3. Change in affective state: Person with an earlier serious disposition has become frivolous.
4. Change in occupational attitudes: Person who was actively involved in his professional life/occupation becomes less or not concerned about the same.
5. Change in purposiveness in life: Patient shows reduced or total absence of interest in the welfare of self, the family, and the cause for which he has been striving.

III. Features of Dorsolateral Prefrontal Dysfunction

1. Executive Functions and Working Memory impaired.
2. Sequential Motor Programming impaired.
3. Ability to change Mental (Response set) set for doing different tasks is impaired.
4. Verbal and Design Fluency impaired.
5. Capacity to organize various semantic materials for Learning is impaired.
6. Constructional Strategy (planning and execution) for copying—constructing Complex Designs impaired.

10. Frontal Amnesia (Source Memory Deficits)

Frontal amnesia is not considered a true memory disturbance. It is the inability to recall spontaneously names, information, or events, when one attempts to recall them. The affected person will be able to recall the same at a later stage without effort. The amnesia may be considered as an inability to evoke the tempero-spatial coordinates of the information as and when required leading to a non-recall. Frontal amnesia is often found in heavy social drinkers and alcohol dependent subjects.

Affective changes are also seen in the form of labile affect, depression, and euphoria. Emotional labiality occurs when a patient is unable to associate right affective responses to ongoing psychomotor activity or thinking process. The inappropriateness of the affect may also be accompanied by swings of unwarranted changes. Extremes of happiness and sadness may switch in the patient.

Recent history of impulsiveness and need for immediate gratification, decline in personal care, disinhibition, irritability or aggressiveness, poor social judgment, anhedonia, and lack of interest in personal life and occupation are some of the personality changes seen in frontal lobe lesion patients. Impairment in ability to plan and delay activities lead to need for immediate gratification and impulsiveness. It is apparent that these changes can be ascertained and confirmed only by detailed interview of the patient and the informant. The changes may be insidious, but of shorter durations than seen in psychotic patients, or acute with a definite period of onset. Personality changes may be early signals of deterioration of brain functions as it may precede even cognitive changes. In the absence of cognitive changes, the patient may present a psychiatric profile and seek psychiatric help first.

B. Tests for Eliciting Temporal Lobe Dysfunction

1. Deficits of Visual Integration

(a) Block Design Test

(b) Object Assembly Test

(a) Block Design Test: The purpose of giving this test is primarily to see if the patient can assemble or put together four or nine blocks of cubes. The accuracy of the pattern is the second aspect that is tested. After giving a demonstration of the task, the patient is instructed to carry on his own, giving as much time as needed, unless the examiner wants to terminate the tests, as patient is desperate as he is not able to carry out the task. It is observed that one may use an explicit or implicit method to construct the pattern. If the patient resorts to an explicit method, he would compare the design already made with that of the pattern. If he uses an implicit method, he would build the pattern systematically from a corner or side.

Interpretation: Spontaneous performance is of great significance and greater the time taken by the patient more is the possibility of impairment. It may also be noted that the patient's ability to assemble the blocks can be impaired by a basic visuospatial impairment due to a Parietal Lobe lesion and hence it may not be possible to comment on the integration ability of the patient. This dysfunction can be seen in various drawing tests. In the absence of such dysfunction an inability to put together the blocks is an indication of integrative difficulty and can be considered as an indication of right temporal-frontal lobe involvement. An implicit method will require a primary visuospatial analysis of the pattern and only then, it can be reconstructed using the blocks. This spatial analysis may be largely absent in the explicit approach and the patient often notices the discrepancies in the pattern that he has built only when he is made to take note of by the examiner. The patient will otherwise sit back with a notion that he has correctly designed the blocks. Visuospatial analysis involves careful study of the pattern and analysis of the different components of the patterns and their shades. One has to look for fragmented models, closing-in phenomenon, and rotation of the completed models, all of which may indicate a parietal lobe involvement. Constructional apraxia can render performance on this test impaired. In the absence of constructional apraxia of an executive type, the impairment seen on the Block Design Test can be attributed to either a right parietal or a right temporal lesion.

(b) Object Assembly Test: The patient is first asked to examine the parts and identify the object that he has to assemble. He may be allowed to take the parts in the hand and examine them one by one. If the patient has difficulty to report what the assembled object is, he may be assisted in gradually identifying the object from the various parts and this information recorded. There is no time limit for the test, but the time taken on each may be recorded. It is essential to allow the patient first to perform on his own, and express that he has or not completed the task. The examiner can give cues or ask for comments after this stage. If the patient promptly assembles two of the tasks, there may be no need to proceed further.

Interpretation: Object Assembly Test is a more complex and adequate test of visual integration than the Block Design Test. This test involve certain degree of abstraction which is absent in the Block Design test and in which the pattern to be constructed is kept in front of the subject. Right frontal lesion patients may also have difficulty in making the inference about the object they are assembling from the parts. The right temporal and parietal lesion patients have greater difficulty in visually arranging or integrating the parts into a whole. Further, the subject also has to make use of visual imagery and an understanding of the position of parts is essential. Even if they may know what the object they are assembling, they will struggle to decide the positions of the parts. There is also spatial planning involved, as the subject has to decide from which part he has to proceed and which parts have to be assembled in sequential manner. As the tests are administered without time limits, the true difficulty would be seen in the greater amount of time taken by the patients. If the test is administered with time limits, the failure rate would be very high. However, false positivity would be also high as several normal subjects also have difficulty in completing all the items within short time limits.

There are different difficulties encountered by a patient on this test. Firstly, it may be difficult for the patient to guess what the object is. Examination of the parts may not give any clue about what it belongs. This difficulty to identify the total from components indicates primarily a Parietal lobe involvement. These patients may also show impairment on other visuospatial tests used for eliciting Parietal dysfunction. However, in the absence of a definite visuospatial difficulty, the impairment may be considered due to an inability to anticipate the object and hence may be associated with a frontal lobe lesion. The whole process of putting the parts together in a meaningful way is the integrative part, which is generally affected in right Temporal lobe lesions. Therefore, impairment on this test may reflect a Fronto-Parietal or Fronto-Temporal involvement or both. The difference between the Object Assembly Test and the Block Design Test is the Frontal involvement in the former and its absence in the latter. Presence of Constructional Apraxia can again confound the performance on this test and therefore interpretation has to be made with caution if the patient has constructional apraxia.

2. Testing Verbal Comprehension

Comprehension is an integral component of communication skills. It is the ability to understand in a meaningful way what another person speaks or understand the meaning of a situation, which will enable to make an adequate response, if needed. Generally, it refers to both verbal and nonverbal comprehension. Hence, it may be considered global in nature. Diffused lesions of the brain as in degenerative disorder affect comprehension in a global way whereas a unilateral lesion can produce a material specific comprehension difficulty. Thus, in a left lateralized lesion involving the posterior speech centres, verbal comprehension alone can be affected. If expressive speech is intact or partly affected, the patient will communicate through speech and gestures. There will be no difficulty to verify that he makes contact with reality, though he does not understand spoken or written speech. The impairment of comprehension that is tested in this section is not this material specific difficulty, but loss of grasp of the external world communicated through symbols and language. The test starts with simple question viz. "What is your name?" to complex and abstract questions. As the aim of the test is to evaluate comprehension ability, the appropriateness of the answer has to be judged with caution. For example, if the patient responds to the former question by "I have no name", it is acceptable as the patient has understood the question. A patient may not respond to many more questions. The answers will be easily affected by the distress due to illness and other affective state of the patient. It is often noticed a dementia patient has less expressive difficulty compared to comprehension difficulty. Though the patient may not adequately understand the question, he may have a lot to speak in answer.

Speech evaluation: Speech evaluation has to be carried out carefully with standard tools. Speech evaluation is not part of this neuropsychological examination protocol. However basic deficits of speech such reception, expression and conduction are to be tested through standard clinical procedures. It starts with recording of the answers to simple direct questions, followed by recording of writing skills of the patient to dictation and copying. Once speech reception and expression abilities are ascertained and found to be satisfactory for examining other cognitive processing, the examiner may start with neuropsychological examination of the patient. This speech examination may also include procedures for detecting Nominal Aphasia, Conduction Aphasia, and Agraphia, if any present.

3. Sentence Repetition Test

This test contains 20 sentences of increasing length. Ask the subject to carefully listen and reproduce each sentence after they are spoken out. It is very important that the sentences be reproduced verbatim. Read out the sentence at a steady pace so that there is no difficulty for the subject to listen to the sentences. There is no bar regarding the language to be used.

Interpretation: The purpose of the test is to determine a patient can hear a sentence being read out and reproduce it without any change. This involves not only hearing, but also reception of speech and its verbatim reproduction. This function can be affected if there is a deficit in reception, conduction of speech from receptive areas to the expressive areas in the left half of the brain and its expression. If verbal comprehension is adequate and the subject has the capacity to express freely himself, an inability to reproduce the sentences in a verbatim manner is due to conduction of speech.

4. Learning and Memory Impairment

Neuroanatomically memory impairment can be classified as axial or Korsakoff amnesia produced by lesions of the hippocampus, focal amnesia—a material specific amnesia produced by unilateral lesions in the right or left cerebral hemispheres, global amnesia—combination of both axial and focal types of Amnesia, associated with diffused cerebral lesions, and Transient Global Amnesia—loss of selected events or information seen in recovering head injury and temporal lobe epilepsy patients. Axial amnesia represents the primary type of memory disturbance in which there is a progressive loss of newly learnt information. The rate of loss could be acute and rapid or gradual depending on the severity of the lesion. Simple tests can often be used to confirm axial amnesia. For example, asking the patient what he had for his breakfast or lunch or asking him to repeat a simple postal address after allowing him to learn it. In more pronounced conditions, the patient is likely to forget even after a few minutes and at times it can be so severe that the amnesia leads to disorientation in new place. The patient generally has normal memory for events that took place before the onset of the lesion. The patient will perform well on other tests of higher mental functions as long as it does not involve memory for newly learnt information.

Other cortical lesions can affect learning mechanism and the channel capacity of the nervous system. Therefore, a poor learning can lead to poor memory. Learning impairment could be material or mode specific disorders. For example, a left cerebral hemisphere lesion may affect verbal learning and consequently verbal memory and a similar right lesion may affect visuospatial learning and visual memory. Hence it is essential to assess the learning functions of a subject before an accurate evaluation of memory can be made. A method of repeated performance was developed for testing rate of learning with verbal and visual materials in the years 1975-1979 (Mukundan et al, 1979a, b, 1991). The verbal passage was read out three times, whereas the visual design was exposed for limited time in three consecutive trials, with each presentation followed by immediate recall from the patient.

4.1 The Verbal Learning & Memory Functions Test (VBLMF Test)

Test description: The verbal form uses four passages, which are read out to the patient one at time and the patient has to recall the contents of the passage immediately or after a delay. Passage A and B are considered equivalent passages in terms of the number of words, and passage C is lengthier than A and B and passage D is a child version. The test is administered in two parts. In the first part, there are three consecutive trials, and each time the passage is read out, the subject has to immediate recall the passage and the recall is recorded and quantified. In the second part, which comes after the third trial recall, the subject is told that he will be asked to recall the same passage ten minutes later from memory. During the interval, the subject is engaged in any non-stressful task such as drawing or copying test. The delayed recall is also recorded and quantified.

Interpretation: Interpretation of the scores is done in a stepwise manner. A low first trial score alone is not to be given too much significance, especially when the II and III trial scores show significant improvement. If the improvement is below the levels shown above it is indicative of a learning deficit. A verbal learning deficit is strongly suggestive of a left temporal and frontal involvement. Memory impairment may be confirmed if the delayed recall performance falls below the levels shown above. As can be seen the delayed recall is compared with the third trial recall. Even though the delayed recall is low, if the patient is able to recall most of his third trial recall, the performance is considered within normal limits. Therefore performance on I through III trials indicate the learning curve of the subject the IV trial performance as function of the III trial is indicative of memory impairment. The performance on this test has to be further interpreted in terms of performance on other tests especially Ideational Fluency test and Sentence Repetition test. It is interesting to consider the often seen discrepancy between Sentence Repetition test and VBLMF test which reveals the complexity of information processing in the VBLMF test. The patient would have immediately recalled even long sentences containing 10-15 words, while his performance on the three trials would be extremely poor. The passages for recall in the VBLMF test contain complex logical associations in a sequential manner while the Sentence Repetition test has just one central meaning. Patients may find it difficult to recall the passage even if he has to reproduce the units of information in his own words, it may be more difficult than reproducing a long sentence verbatim. The VBLMF test requires longer focused attention than the Sentence Repetition test and this may also contribute to increased difficulty seen on this test.

The three passages used for determining Verbal Learning and Memory are the following:

Passage 1: Asha Kumari/ of South Kanara/ employed/ as a work woman/ in an office building/ reported/ at the City Police/ Station/ that she has been robbed/ of fifteen rupees/. She had four/ little children/, the rent/ was due/ and they had not eaten/ for 2 days/. The officers/ touched by the woman's story/ gave some money/ for her/.

Passage 2: The Indian/ship/Jaldeep/struck a rock/ near Cape Comorin/Monday/evening/. Inspite of a blinding/snow storm/ and darkness/the sixty/passengers including 18/ women/ were all rescued/though the boats/ were tossed about/ like corks in the heavy sea/. They were brought to land/ the next day/ by an Indian/ Steamer.

Passage 3: Ram/ Mohan/ Rao/ a 40-year old/ carpenter/ from the rural district/ of Andhra Pradesh,/ was engaged/ by a rich/ businessman/ to design and make/ the furniture/ for an estate/ house on a coffee/ plantation/ in Coorg/. He commenced/

his work/ with enthusiasm/ drawing upon the ideas/ of the famous/ 19th century craftsmen/. At the conclusion/ of the contract,/ he had executed/ with brilliance/ in rose wood and teak/ the job/ detailed in the contract/. While he was acclaimed/ by all/ for the excellent work/ he was criticized/ by his boss/ for having overshot/ the budget.

4.2 Visual Learning and Memory Functions Test (VSLMF Test)

Test description: The stimulus is a complex pattern presented on a 6″ × 4″ card. Twenty-three components are identified in the pattern and scored individually. The stimulus card is shown to subject for 15 sec and he is asked to draw the pattern from memory on a sheet of paper of the same dimension. The copy is taken away a fresh paper is provided to the subject and he is shown the pattern again for the same duration. After immediate recall, the test is repeated for a third time. After the third trial recall the subject is told that he would be asked to draw the pattern from memory after an interval of 10 minutes. After the IV trial delayed recall, the subject is shown the stimulus card and asked to copy it on a sheet of paper.

Instruction: "I will show you a complex visual pattern printed on a card for a short time and take it away. You must try to study the pattern as intently as possible. I would require you to draw the design from memory immediately after I take it away. I will show the design two more times and every time you are required to draw the design from your memory."

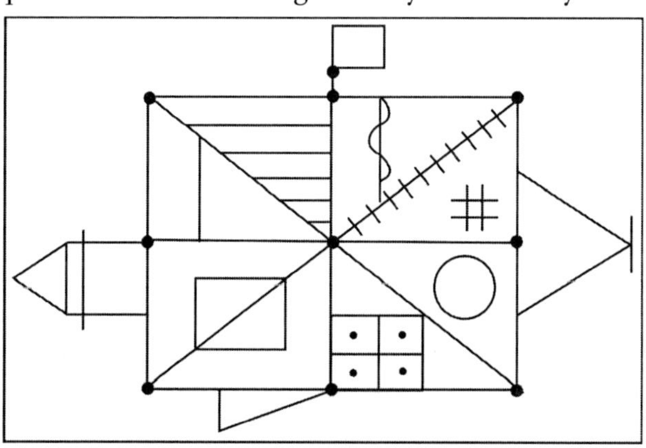

Complex Figure for VSLMF Test

The Scoring Scheme:

Item	Score
1. Large Rectangle	1
2. Diagonals	2
3. Perpendicular lines	2
4. Flag on Top	1
5. Horizontal Rectangle with vertical line	2
6. Triangle downward at bottom	1
7. Rectangle with triangle on left side with vertical line	2
8. Vertical line in the first quadrant	1
9. Horizontal lines in first quadrant	2
10. Lines on the diagonal cut in the second quadrant	1
11. Vertical line with curve in the second quadrant	2
12. Double cross marks in the second quadrant	2
13. Smaller rectangle perpendicular lines and dots in the third quadrant	2
14. Circle in the third quadrant	1
15. Smaller rectangle in the fourth quadrant	1
TOTAL SCORE	23

Interpretations: The tests were originally designed in 1975-76 for assessing verbal and visual learning deficits in the left and right temporal lobe lesions respectively. The increment in the recall from Trial I to III was considered to reflect the rate of learning in a person. Our early data showed that both verbal and visual learning was impaired not only in the left temporal lobe lesion patients but also in the left frontal lobe lesion patients. A frontal and left temporal lesion may result in confabulation on the VBLMF test. A right cortical lesion will seldom cause impairment on the VBLMF test, except hippocampal lesions or lesions in the axial structures or lesions that affect the functioning of these structures produce delayed recall deficits in both verbal and visual modes. Loss of information seen on the IV trial gives vital clues and confirms primary memory impairment. The lesion effects on the two tests have been discussed in detail in the earlier sections.

A low initial score (trial 1 score) is often found to be associated with a functional overlay or involvement. It occurs when the patient is not attentive enough while listening or visually observing the test material. Though the trial I score is low, they catch up in the subsequent trials and show significant improvement. It is also often noticed that many of these patients may have a greater IV trial score compared to their III trial score. This could be the effect of reminiscence and rehearsal effect during the interval between the III and the IV trials often reported in patients with anxiety.

The VSLMF test is a complex and sensitive test as performance on it may be affected by impairment of focused attention, visual scanning, transcoding difficulties, and difficulty to form visual imagery. The design is too complex for a total search within 15 sec of exposure. Normally one improves the recall of the design by trials. One has to hold on to several items of the design. Sequential association is possible with respect to any few of the items. One can visualize or verbalize and hold on to the details for the immediate recall performance. For example, one may visualize or transcode the rectangle divided by two straight lines vertically and horizontally and two diagonals running through the centre. Remaining components are there without any particular rationale and subject has to consciously take note of them as well as visually recall them for reproduction. Visuospatial processing significantly depends on parallel processing, a major functional attribute of the right brain. Impairment of this mode of processing interferes with the visual learning process. This may explain the absence of association between the VSLMF recalls in the first three trials and the BVRT delayed recall.

5. Benton's Visual Retention Test (BVRT)

There are several modes of administration of this test. Administration Mode C is often used as it has a limited stimulus exposure and a delay before recall. Method of administration and interpretation are as given in the manual of the test.

6. Recent History of Acute Emotional Change and Memory Disturbance

7. Examination of the Patient for Identifying the Presence of Progressive Amnesia, Recent and Remote Memory Loss, Loss of Memory for Autobiographical Episodes

C. Tests for Eliciting Parietal Lobe Dysfunction Profile

The tests for Parietal lobe dysfunctions consist of tests for visuospatial perception, visual memory, spatial organization of numbers and testing for presence of focal signs of Prosopagnosia, Gerstmann's syndrome, Visual agnosia, agnosia for body parts, body schema disturbances, root finding difficulty and constructional apraxia.

1. Tests for visuospatial perception: Three major spatial aspects evaluated are perception of form, size, and depth. The deficits in these areas looked for are distortions, micrographia, macrographia, spatial disorientation, visual neglect, closing-in-phenomenon, mirror drawing, exploded copying, fragmentation, and simplification.

(a) Bender Gestalt test.

(b) Block Design test.

(c) Spatial Comparison tests.

(d) Spatial Comparison using verbal report of differences.

The above tests have been already discussed.

Interpretation: Performance on the Bender Gestalt test, the Block Design test and the Spatial Comparison tests are compared with one another for interpretation. Though several features of dysfunction may be present, a definite identification of a single deficit is enough to presume a Parietal lobe involvement. Distortion is the most convincing impairment of form. Macrographia and micrographia indicate deficits of size estimation. Rotation is a sign of impairment of spatial orientation of verticality and horizontality. Impairment of three-dimensional viewing and depth perception are other features of Parietal dysfunction. Visual neglect is the result of a unilateral parietal lesion in which parts of a figure in the contralateral visual half is ignored and therefore not drawn by the patient. A lesion on the right side will produce a left sided neglect. This neglect may be more severe in magnitude than produced by a left lesion. A left parietal lesion may result in contralateral neglect of lesser magnitude. A right parietal lobe lesion will produce more prominent features of visuo-perceptual impairment than a left lesion. In left lesion the patient may resort to simplification of the figure with only a few large details of the figure are drawn leaving out most of the details. If the left lesion produces constructional apraxia, the patients' performance will be severely affected in terms of ability to draw or construct objects in two or three dimensions. It may be necessary to identify if the deficits are a result of constructional apraxia or visuospatial perceptual difficulty. A test for spatial comparison using verbal reporting of spatial differences can be used for this. The test is described below.

2. Test for spatial comparison using verbal report of difference: This test contains 6 items. In each item there is a target figure presented in the centre of 4′ × 5′ card. The comparison figures for each item are printed on eight cards of similar size. One card has the stimulus figure identical to the target and presented in the centre. The other five cards have the exact target figure presented on the (1) top, at the (2) bottom, near the (3) right edge, near the (4) left edge, (5) bigger in size and in the centre, (6) smaller in size and in the centre, (7) slightly different in form. Each comparison card is presented side by side of the target card and the subject is asked to report verbally the difference between the figures in the two cards.

3. Presence of ideational and ideomotor apraxia, finger agnosia, visual agnosia, prosopagnosia, hemisomatognosia, anasognosia, simultanagnosia, disturbance of topographic memory and body schema disturbances are to be elicited using appropriate clinical methods.

a. Apraxia:

   Test patient for the presence of constructional apraxia, ideational and ideomotor apraxia, dressing apraxia.

b. Presence of Acalculia, Alexia and Agraphia.

c. Presence of left-right disorientation.

d. Impaired spatial organization of numbers.

D. Tests for Eliciting Occipital Lobe Dysfunction Profile

1. Presence of visual memory and imagery deficits.
2. Presence of visual agnosia, simultanagnosia.
3. Visual inattention, visual neglect.
4. Color recognition and naming difficulty.
5. Deficits in visuospatial perception.
6. Topographic memory disturbances.

ANNEXURE 2

NEUROPSYCHOLOGICAL ASSESSMENT GUIDELINES LOBE-SYSTEM-WISE DYSFUNCTION PROFILE

I. Examination of Frontal Cortex Dysfunctions

Prefrontal Lesions

1. Motor sequencing: Cannot perform motor sequencing—Frontal apraxia—disturbance of preliminary synthesis (cannot light and smoke a cigarette).
2. Absence of distress at mistakes or attempts at correction of mistakes.
3. Presence of motor perseveration.
4. Difficulty to perform serial tasks and commands.
5. Difficulty to understand complicated pictures, thematic pictures and comprehension of written text.
6. Difficulty in visual scanning, tracking.
7. Difficulty to reproduce drawings from memory.
8. Difficulty to make planned movements.
9. Responds to irrelevant stimuli—distractibility present.
10. Impairment in working memory abilities—verbal and visual.
11. Impairment in other executive functions—Trail making, digit-symbol substitution test, etc.
12. Difficulty in ideational fluency.
13. Presencee of confabulation.
14. Difficulty in design fluency.
15. Difficulty in abstract thinking ability.
16. Difficulty to delay, impulsiveness.
17. Difficulty for shifting mental set.
18. Difficulty for visual planning.
19. Difficulty in temporal sequencing—Subtraction of serial 3 from 40 and 7 from 100; holding information for sequencing of themes during recall.
20. Impairment in encoding.

21. Difficulty in spontaneous speech, and lack of self-correction and absence of distress during mistakes.
22. Difficulty in understanding new ideas, creative ideas.
23. Difficulty in comprehension of propositional instructions (e.g. "place a cross beneath the circle").
24. Difficulty to perform consecutive acts with one time verbal instructions.
25. Difficulty to shift set if instructions are varied—difficulty on 'go-no go' test.
26. If instructed to squeeze a rubber bulb, the patient will:
    - make verbal statement but not squeeze the ball or squeezes without stopping.
    - can give verbal statements but can't make proper response.
    - difficulty in alternating mental set in responses, for example: press left button to red light, right button to green light.
27. Difficulty to recall an already learnt response, and if he is aware of it, even after the patient has learnt to perform a response.
28. Difficulty in altering response sequence.
29. Impairment in the detection of signal value of a stimulus.
30. Impairment in active visual scanning.
31. Difficulty in moving objects.
32. Difficulty for detecting hidden figures (Embedded figures).
33. Difficulty to make quick generalizations using isolated or part facts.
34. Tends to respond to temporally proximal instructions.
35. Reproduces only the last part of a sentence or instruction while sentence recall.
36. Elation, hyperactivity or apathy.

II. Analysis of Motor Functions

Prerequisite for Psychomotor Examination

1. Test Muscle strength.
2. Test Muscle tone.
3. Stand/sit facing patient.
4. Examiner raise right hand—instruct patient to repeat the same.
5. Examiner position hand frontally, sagittally, horizontally—instruct patient to repeat the same.
6. Examiner touch eye and ear—instruct patient to repeat.
7. Examiner show two hands position—instruct patient to repeat.
8. Examiner repeat with spoken commands—instruct patient to perform to command.

III. Pre-motor Cortex

Testing Kinetic Organization

1. Touch fingers with thumb as fast as possible (AFAP) (reveals paresis, lack of precision, pathological dystonia, ataxia).
2. Separate and close fingers AFAP.
3. Clinch and relax fingers (both hands) AFAP (reveals fatigue).
4. Place hands in front (tap twice with right, once with left)—Reverse Test for kinetic melody—Pre-motor patients carries out indiscreet steps rather than a series—Frontal patients—tap haphazardly without correction.
5. Fist—ring test—cannot do them in series.
6. Reverse sequence produces problems.
7. Fist—edge-palm test—non automatic performance.
8. Keyboard playing test (first forward then reverse) frontal patients can't reverse; pre-motor may improve with spoken commands or feedback; frontals—may repeat correctly but still can't make proper movement.

IV. Investigation of Oral Praxis

1. Test smile.
2. Test tongue extension and movement.
3. Test automatism and fluency of speech.
4. Test order of words.
5. Test if patient could speak complete sentence or speaks in telegraphic style.

V. Dysfunctions Associated with Post Central Gyrus Lesions

Kinesthetic Sensation and Movement

1. Eyes closed—patient is to position hand to match position of other as set by examiner.
2. Passive finger detection.
3. Test kinesthetic sensation—Two-point threshold.
4. Test kinesthetic sensation—Vibration sense.
5. With lesion—most severe changes seen in distal parts of limbs; pain returns first pressure and touch next; temperature next; position sense and passive movement.
6. Fasten a button.
7. Tie a shoelace.
8. Thread beads.
9. Test pin—point vs. head.
10. Touch area on skin and have patient point to area on contralateral side.

VI. Dysfunctions Associated with Supramarginal Gyrus Lesions

1. Test astereognosis.
2. Test fingertip number writing ability.
3. Right-Left disorientation—confusion.
4. Test for finger agnosia.
5. Test for Gerstmann's syndrome—left inferior parietal lesion R-L confusion, finger agnosia, agraphia, and acalculia.

VII. Dysfunctions Associated with Angular Gyrus Lesions

1. Test for Pure word blindness (cannot read aloud or comprehend written words).
2. Can copy words but not write from dictation.
3. Dyslexia, dysgraphia.
4. Test for spelling loss.
5. Test for loss of ability to name objects.
6. Test for loss of color naming and color matching ability.

VIII. Examination of Temporal Cortex Dysfunctions

Right Temporal Lobe

1. Test patients to reproduce patterns presented acoustically.
2. Test to reproduce verbal instructions.
3. Test discreet taps—poor rhythm.
4. Test verbal rehearsal—temporal lesion patients improve, frontals do not.
5. Present minimal visual information—confused by sketchy drawings.
6. Test ability to quickly visually search for a paragraph previously observed.
7. Problems on recurrent nonsense figures.
8. Test stylus maze learning.
9. Test recognition using repeated presentation of nonsense figures and photographs, which cannot be named.
10. Test recognition of auditory tonal patterns.
11. Test on timbre (Seashore M of M Talents).

Left Temporal Lobe

1. Test ability to locate sound.
2. May see HH (upper homonymous quadranopoia).
3. Wernicke's area—word deafness.
4. Tinnitus—reception to pathway disease.
5. Impairment on dichotic listening test.
6. Greatest impairment on retest after one hour unannounced.

7. Test learning of words, nonsense syllables.
8. Test ability to decipher the phonemic code.
9. Test writing from dictation and copying.
10. Test for anomia.
11. Test for word memory.
12. Test for musical hearing—may not be disturbed.
13. Test patient extensively for learning and memory loss—impairment on both auditory and visual (those requiring transcoding) tasks.

Anterior Temporal

1. Test presence of Deja vu.
2. Test if the patient has feelings of remoteness.
3. Test the presence of hallucinations (auditory and/or visual).
4. Disinhibition syndromes.

Middle-Posterior Temporal

1. Test if the patient has sudden arrest of speech.
2. Test if the patient has difficulty to remember words presented orally.
3. Test if phonemic reproduction is intact but defect in audio verbal memory.
4. Test for receptive and conduction aphasia.
5. Test for conduction aphasia—sentence repetition test.
6. Test for modality specific memory loss—verbal vs. visual.

IX. Parietal Lobes

Right Parietal Lobe

1. Test for ability to perceive Gestalt.
2. Test for ability to copy figures.
3. Test for ability for spatial comparisons.
4. Test for ability for size and distance estimation.
5. Test for ability to recognize horizontality and verticality.
6. Test for ability for spatial positioning.
7. Test for ability to recognize hidden figures.

8. Test for visual agnosia.
9. Test for prosopagnosia.
10 Test for visuomotor coordination.
11. Test for ability draw a clock.
12. Test for ability for drawing three-dimensional figures.
13. Test for immediate visual memory.

Left Parietal Lobe

1. Test for Right-Left confusion.
2. Test for difficulty in dressing.
3. Test for ability to locate places on a map.
4. Test for presence of constructional apraxia.
5. Test for ability to draw letters.
6. Test for ability for organization of positions of numbers.
7. Test for dysgraphia.
8. Test for dyscalculia.

Parieto-occipital Cortex

1. Right-left homonymous heminopsia.
2. Paragnosia—difficulty with visual recognition of objects.
3. Prosopagnosia—recognition of faces.
4. Spatial loss.
5. Spatial agnosia.
6. Lack of awareness of own defects.

Parieto-temporal-occipital cortex

1. Understands meaning of individual words but cannot comprehend meaning of the whole sentence.
2. Ability to evoke visual images in response to a given word is impaired.
3. Gross inability to draw the picture of an object named.

X. Examination of Occipital Cortex Dysfunctions

Area 17

1. Unilateral ablation of area 17 produces complete homonymous hemianopsia of the contralateral field.
2. Bilateral ablation of 17 produces in bilateral homonymous hemianopsia.
3. Test for cortical blindness (sometimes called Anton's syndrome).
4. Test if the individual denies blindness and confabulates.
5. Test for macular sparing. Ablation of the optic radiations can be differentiated from lesions of area 17 as damage to area 17 is more often characterized by macular sparing.

Areas 18 and 19

1. Deficits may occur in visual recognition and reading.
2. If the lesion does not extend beyond 18 and 19 but involves both hemispheres or its connections then a visual agnosia results.
3. Rare to find this type of deficit without involvement of parieto-occipital and/or inferior parietal regions.
4. Unilateral lesion may produce deficits in visual following:
   - Unilateral lesion extending past 17, 18, and 19 may produce 'unilateral spatial agnosia'.
   - Severe lesion may produce impairment of recognition of even simple objects. If the lesion is less severe, simple objects may be recognized.
   - Recognition of object by part recognition will be impaired.

ANNEXURE 3

NEUROPSYCHOLOGICAL TESTS FOR ASSESSING BRAIN DYSFUNCTION

ASSESSMENT FORMAT—PART I

I. Frontal Lobes Dysfunction Test

1. Attention

(a) Spontaneous arousal of attention is absent.

(b) Attention has to be aroused by repeated commands.

(c) Attention is easily distracted.

(d) Instructions have to be repeatedly given.

(e) Fatigability of attention.

(f) Excessive broadening/narrowing of attention present.

(g) Sensory Inattention.

2. Visual Search [visual exploration]

(a) Visual scanning of numbers.

(b) Visual scanning of picture.

3. Mental Set—Perseveration

(a) Psychomotor perseveration.

(b) Continuous drawing test.

4. Psychomotor Deficits

(a) Kinetic Melody disturbances [tapping test].

5. Deficits in Working Memory

(a) Test of mental control—Serial Subtraction Tests

(b) Delayed Response Ability Test.

(c) Trail Making Test—Form A and Form B.

6. Deficits of Ideational and Design Fluency Tests

(a) Name objects made of—

[i] wood,

[ii] round objects, each for 2 minutes.

(b) Design Fluency test.

7. Deficits in Visuospatial Perception Tasks

(a) Bender Gestalt Test.

(b) Alexander's Passalong test.

(c) Object Assembly test.

(e) Maze tests.

8. Abstract Reasoning

(a) Raven's Progressive Matrices.

9. Expressive Speech Disturbances (not included here)

II. Tests for Eliciting Temporal and Fronto-temporal Dysfunction Profile

1. Deficits of Visual Integration

(a) Block Design Test.

(b) Object Assembly Test.

3. Visual Memory Tests—Benton-Visual Retention Test

(a) Immediate Recall.

(b) Delayed Recall.

4. Verbal and Visual Learning and Memory Functions Test (Fronto-Temporal Dysfunction)—Encoding and Transcoding Deficits

(a) Verbal Form—Passage Learning Test—Passage A, B, C —Trial I, Trial II, Trial III.

(b) Visual Form—Complex Figure Test—Trial I, Trial II, Trial III.

5. Progressive Amnesia, Recent-Remote, Autobiographic Memory Impairment

III. Tests for Eliciting Parietal Lobe Dysfunction Profile

1. Tests for Visuospatial Perception

(a) Bender Gestalt test.

(b) Block Design test.

(c) Spatial comparison tests.

(d) Spatial comparison using verbal report of differences.

(e) Root finding difficulty.

(f) Object Assembly Test.

2. Focal Tests

Tests for

(a) Apraxia,

(b) Acalculia,

(c) Agraphia,

(d) Alexia,

(e) Visual Agnosias,

(f) Finger Agnosia,

(g) Left-Right disorientation.

IV. Tests for Eliciting Occipital Lobe Dysfunction Profile

1. Presence of visual memory and imagery deficits.
2. Presence of visual agnosia, simultanagnosia.
3. Visual inattention, visual neglect.
4. Color recognition and naming difficulty.
5. Deficits in visuospatial perception.

ANNEXURE 4

CLINICAL NEUROPSYCHOLOGICAL PROFILE—PART II

Name:	No:
Sex:	Education:
Age:	Handedness:
Date of Examination:	Present - P :: Absent - A

Dysfunction	P/A
1. Disorientation to time	
2. Disorientation to place	
3. Disorientation to person	
4. Absence of arousal of attention, spontaneous arousal is absent—Attention must be aroused by command	
5. Distractibility—Response to irrelevant stimuli	
6. Confusion, perplexity, impaired judgments (any P1, P2, P3, all—P)	
7. Apathy—Absence of emotions, Emotionally withdrawn, impassive	
8. Akinesia—akinetic mutism—constant or transient, absence of speech, reduced or nil movements	
9. Emotional liability—inappropriate emotions and moods	
10. Personality Change—elevation in mood/ depression	
11. Imitation behavior	
12. Utilization behavior	
13. Lack of initiative	
14. Eat and drink only if fed	
15. Disinhibition in expressive speech (more outspoken)	
16. Sensory disinhibition—hallucinations, delusions	
17. Psychomotor disinhibition	

(*Contd...*)

Dysfunction	P/A
18. Emotional disinhibition	
19. Sexual disinhibition	
20. Indifferent—lack of concern for family and friends, events and things	
21. Impulsiveness and need for immediate gratification, inability to delay responses	
22. Irritability	
23. Violence	
24. Perseveration in speech and psychomotor behavior	
25. Perseveration in psychomotor behavior	
26. Incontinence	
27. Amnesia—Semantic Amnesia	
28. Episodic Amnesia	
29. Post Traumatic Amnesia	
30. Retrograde Amnesia	
31. Anterograde Amnesia	
32. Axial amnesia: progressive forgetting of newly learnt information	
33. Apraxia: ideational	
34. Apraxia: ideomotor	
35. Apraxia: other type	
36. Constructional Apraxia: seen in copying and constructional tasks	
37. Aphasia—expressive speech disturbance, impaired language function	
38. Aphasia—receptive speech disturbance, impaired language function	
39. Conduction aphasia—sentence repetition	
40. Nominal aphasia—naming difficulty (knows functions)	

(Contd...)

Dysfunction	P/A
41. Visual agnosia—inability to identify real objects or objects in pictures 42. Finger agnosia—inability to identify one's own fingers 43. Astereognosis—inability to identify objects by touch 44. Discalculia—inability to carry out simple arithmetic (on paper) 45. Prosopagnosia—inability to visually identify persons, faces 46. Finger agnosia—inability to identify one's own fingers 47. Astereognosis—inability to identify objects by touch 48. Left-right disorientation—inability to identify one's own left/right 49. Discalculia—inability to carry out simple arithmetic (on paper) 50. Route finding difficulty 51. Dysgraphia—difficulty in writing, changes in handwriting 52. Semantic speech impaired—inability to spontaneously speak 53. Body schema disturbance—difficulty to localize sensations on the body 54. Neglect of half—neglect of one full or part half (left or right) of the body 55. Reasoning, judgment, critical abilities, General Intelligence	
Examiner: **Comments:**	

References

Abrams, D.A., Nicol, T., Zecker, S., Kraus, N. (2008). Right-hemisphere auditory cortex is dominant for coding syllable patterns in speech. *The journal of neuroscience*, 28(15): 3958-65.

Adler, A.C., Warum, D., Sapire, J.M. (2012). Transient global amnesia caused by hippocampal infarct: case report and review of literature. *Clinical Imaging,* 36(5): 584-86.

Aggleton, J.P., Brown, M.W. (1999). Episodic memory, amnesia, and the hippocampal-anterior thalamic axis. *Behavior Brain Science,* 22: 425-44.

Alario, F.X., Chainay, H., Lehericy, S., Cohen, L. (2006). The role of the supplementary motor area (SMA) in word production. *Brain Research,* 3: 1076(1): 129-43.

Alcock, K. (2006). The development of oral motor control and language. *Down Syndrome Research and Practice,* 11(1): 1-8.

Alexander, G.E., Crutcher, M.D., Delong, M.R. (1990). Basal ganglia-thalamocortical circuits: parallel substrates for motor, oculomotor, 'prefrontal' and 'limbic' functions. *Progress in Brain Research,* 85: 119-46.

Alexander, G.E., Delong, M.R., Strick, P.L. (1986). Parallel organization of functionally segregated circuits linking basal ganglia and cortex. *Annual review of Neurosciences*, 9: 351-82.

Alexander, M.P., Schmitt, M.A. (1980). The aphasia syndrome of stroke in the left anterior cerebral artery territory. *Archives of Neurology*, 37: 97-100.

Alvarez, J.A., Emory, E. (2006). Executive function and the frontal lobes: A meta-analyticreview. *Neuropsychology Review,* 16(1): 17-42.

American Psychiatric Association (1994). *Diagnostic and Statistical Manual of Mental Disorders: DSM-IV*. Washington, DC: American Psychiatric Association.

Amick, M.M., Schendan, H.E., Ganis, G., Cronin-Golomb, A. (2006). Frontostriatal circuits are necessary for visuomotor transformation: mental rotation in Parkinson's disease. *Neuropsychologia,* 44: 339-49.

Andermann, L.F., Savard, G., Meencke, H.J., McLachhan, R., Moshé, S., Andermann, F. (1999). Psychosis after resection of ganglioglioma or DNET: evidence for an association. *Epilepsia,* 40: 83-87.

Anderson, J.M., Gilmore, R., Roper, S., Crosson, B., Bauer, R.M., Nadeau, S., Beversdorf, D.Q., Cibula, J., Rogish, M. 3rd, Kortencamp, S., Hughes, J.D., Gonzalez, Rothi, L.J., Heilman, K.M. (1999). Conduction aphasia and the arcuate fasciculus: A reexamination of the Wernicke-Geschwind model. *Brain Language,* 70(1): 1-12.

Anderson, A.K., Phelps, E.A. (1998). Intact recognition of vocal expressions of fear following bilateral lesions of the human amygdala. *Neuroreport*, 9(16): 3607-13.

Anderson, T., Heitger, M., Macleod, A.D. (2006). Concussion and mild head injury. *Practical Neurology*, 6(6): 342-57.

Andrea, S., Christian, L., John, A.R. (2010). Conditional Routing of Information to the Cortex: A Model of the Basal Ganglia's Role in Cognitive Coordination. *Psychological Review,* 117(2): 541-74.

Andreasen, N.C., O'Leary, D.S., Arndt, S., Cizadlo, T., Hurtig, R., Rezai, K., Watkins, G.L., Ponto, L.L., Hichwa, R.D. (1995). Short-term and long-term working memory: a positron emission tomography study. *Proceedings of National Academy of Science, U.S.A.,* 92: 5111-15.

Annet, C., Mukundan, C.R. (1996a). Social drinking—part I: Neuropsychological changes in social drinkers, *NIMHANS Journal*, 14(1): 15-21.

Annet, C., Mukundan, C.R. (1996b). Social drinking—part-II: Auditory evoked potentials, P300 responses and contingent negative variation in social drinkers, *NIMHANS Journal*, 14(1): 22-30.

Angel, R.W. (1976). Efference copy in the control of movement. *Neurology*, 26(12): 1164-68.

Arch, J.J., Craske, M.G. (2006). Mechanisms of mindfulness: Emotion regulation following a focused breathing induction. *Behaviour Research and Therapy*, 44(12): 1849-58.

Arnold, S.E., Hyman, B.T., Flory, J., Damasio, A.R., Van Hoesen, G.W. (1991). The Topographical and Neuroanatomical Distribution of Neurofibrillary Tangles and Neuritic Plaques in the Cerebral Cortex of Patients with Alzheimer's Disease. *Cortex*, 1(1): 103-16.

Aron, A.R., Shahakian, B.J., Robbins, T.W. (2003). Distractibility during selection-for-action: differential deficits in Huntington's disease and following frontal lobe damage. *Neuropsychologia*, 41: 1137-47.

Arseneault, L., Tremblay, R.E., Boulerice, B., Séguin, J.R., Saucier, J-F (2000). Minor physical anomalies and family adversity as risk factors for violent delinquency in adolescence. *American Journal of Psychiatry*, 157: 917-23.

Astor-Jack, T., Haggard, P. (2005). Intention and reactivity. In G.W. Humphreys, M.J. Riddoch (Eds.), *Attention in Action* (109-29). Hove: Psychology Press.

Atkinson, R.C., Shiffrin, R.M. (1968). Human memory: A proposed system and its control processes. In K.W. Spence, J.T. Spence (Eds.), *The psychology of learning and motivation* (Vol. 2: 89-195). New York: Academic Press.

Aumann, R.J. (2008). Game Theory: Introduction, *The New Palgrave Dictionary of Economics*, 2nd Edition.

Azari, N.P., Nickel, J., Wunderlich, G., Niedeggen, M., Hefter, H., Tellmann, L., Herzog, H., Stoerig, P., Birnbacher, D., Seitz, R.J. (2001). Neural correlates of religious experience. *European Journal of Neuroscience*, 13: 1649-52.

Azevedo, F.A., Carvalho, L.R., Grinberg, L.T., Farfel, J.M., Ferretti, R.E., Leite, R.E., Jacob Filho, W., Lent, R., Herculano-Houzel, S. (2009). Equal numbers of neuronal and nonneuronal cells make the human brain an isometrically scaled-up primate brain. *J. Comparative Neurology,* 513(5): 532-41.

Aziz-Zadeh, L., Damasio, A. (2008). Embodied semantics for actions: findings from brain functional imaging. *J. Physiology-Paris*, 102(1-3): 35-39.

Babiloni, C., Babiloni, F., Carducci, F., Cincotti, F., Vecchio, F., Cola, B., Rossi, S., Miniussi, C., Rossini, P.M. (2004a). Functional frontoparietal connectivity during short-term memory as revealed by high-resolution EEG coherence analysis. *Behavioral Neuroscience,* 118(4): 687-97.

Babiloni, C., Babiloni, F., Carducci, F., Cappa, S., Cincotti, F., Del Percio, C., Miniussi, C., Moretti, D.V., Pasqualetti, P., Rossi, S., Sosta, K., Rossini, P.M. (2004b). Human cortical EEG rhythms during long-term episodic memory task: A high-resolution EEG study of the HERA model. *NeuroImage*, 21: 1576-84.

Babiloni, C., Vecchio, F., Cappa, S., Pasqualetti, P., Rossi, S., Miniussi, C., Rossini, P.M. (2006). Functional frontoparietal connectivity during encoding and retrieval processes follows HERA model: A high-resolution study. *Brain Research Bulletin*, 68: 203-12.

Backhaus, J., Junghanns, K., Born, J., Hohaus, K., Faasch, F., and Hohagen, F. (2006). Impaired declarative memory consolidation during sleep in patients with primary insomnia: Influence of sleep architecture and nocturnal cortisol release. *Biological Psychiatry*, 60: 1324-30.

Baddeley, A. (2000). The episodic buffer: a new component of working memory? *Trends in Cognitive Science,* 4, 417-23.

Baddeley, A. (1998). Recent developments in working memory. *Curr. Opin. Neurobiol. 8*(2): 234-38.

Baddeley, A. (1992). Working Memory: The Interface between Memory and Cognition. *Journal of Cognitive Neuroscience,* 4(3): 281-88.

Baddeley, Alan D. (1986). *Working memory*. Oxford: Clarendon Press.

Baddley, A., Hitch, G. (1974). Working memory. In: G. Bower (ed.), *Recent Advances in Learning and Motivation*. Academic Press, New York, vol. 8: 47-90.

Baerentsen, K.B. (2001). Onset of meditation explored with fMRI. *NeuroImage, 13*: S297.

Balkin, T.J., Braun, A.R., Wesensten, N.J., Jeffries, K., Varga, M., Baldwin, P., Belenky, G., Herscovitch, P. (2002). The process of awakening: A PET study of regional brain activity patterns mediating the re-establishment of alertness and consciousness. *Brain, 125*: 2308-19.

Balota, D.A., Faust, M.E. (2001). Attention in dementia of the Alzheimer type. In F. Boller & S.F. Cappa (Eds.), Handbook of neuropsychology (2nd ed., Vol. 6: 51-80). Amsterdam: Elsevier Science.

Ball, H., Berch, D.B., Helmers, K.F., Jobe, J.B., Leveck, M.D., Marsike, M., Morris, J., Rebok, G.W., Smith, D.M., Tennstedt, S.L., Unverzagt, F.W., Willis, S.L. (2002). Effects of cognitive training interventions with older adults: a randomized controlled trial. *Journal of American Medical Association,* 288: 2271-81.

Baird, A., Dewar, B.K., Critchley, H., Dolan, R., Shallice, T., Cipolotti, L. (2006). Social and emotional functions in three patients with medial frontal lobe damage including the anterior cingulate cortex. *Cognitive Neuropsychiatry*. 11(4): 369-88.

Baker, S.C., Frith, C.D., Frackowiak, R.S.J., Dolan, R.J. (1996). Active representation of shape and spatial location in man. *Cerebral Cortex*, 6: 612-19.

Banich, M.T. (2009). Executive function: The search for an integrated account. *Current Directions in Psychological Science,* 18(2): 89-94.

Barbas, H. (1993). Organization of cortical afferent input to orbitofrontal areas in the rhesus monkey. *Neuroscience*, 56(4): 841-64.

Barbas, H. (1995). Anatomic basis of cognitive-emotional interactions in the primate prefrontal cortex. *Neuroscience Biobehavioral Review,* 19(3): 499-510.

Barbizet, J. (1971). Human Memory and its Pathology. Translated by A.K. Jardines. W.H. Freeman & Co. Ltd.

Barker-Collo S. (2000). Initial evaluation of a structured group format memory rehabilitation program. *Journal of Cognitive Rehabilitation,* 18(2): 16-21.

Barker-Collo, S., Feigin, V.L. (2008). Memory deficit after traumatic brain injury: how big is the problem in New Zealand and what management strategies are available? *Journal of the New Zealand Medical Association,* 121: 1268.

Bartsch, T., Deuschl, G. (2010). Transient global amnesia: functional anatomy and clinical implications. *Lancet Neurology*, 9(2): 205-14.

Bates, E., Benigni, L., Bretherton, I., Carnaioni, L., Volterra, V. (1979). *The Emergence of Symbols: Cognition and Communication in Infancy*. New York: Academic Press.

Batty, M.J., Cave, K.R., Pauli, P. (2005). Abstract stimuli associated with threat through conditioning cannot be detected preattentively. *Emotion*, 4: 418-430.

Baum, W.B. (1994). *Understanding behaviorism: Science, behavior, and culture*. New York: HarperCollins.

Baumgaertner, A., Weiller, C., Buchel, C. (2002). Event-related fMRI reveals cortical sites involved in contextual sentence integration. *NeuroImage,* 16: 736-45.

Baxter, L.R. Jr., Phelps, M.E., Mazziotta, J.C., Schwartz, J.M., Gerner, R.H., Selin, C.E., Sumida, R.M. (1985). Cerebral metabolic rates for glucose in mood disorders. Studies with positron emission tomography and fluorodeoxyglucose. *Archives of General Psychiatry,* 42(5): 441-47.

Bechara, A., Damasio, H., Damasio, A.R. (2000). Emotion, decision-making, and the orbitofrontal cortex. *Cerebral Cortex,* 10: 295-307.

Beck, A.T., Rush, A.J., Shaw, B.F. & Emery, G. (1979). *Cognitive therapy of depression.* New York: Guilford Press.

Beck, A.T. (1975). *Cognitive Therapy and the Emotional Disorders.* International Universities Press, New York, 1976.

Beck, A.T., Freeman, A., Davis, D.D. (2003). *Cognitive Therapy of Personality Disorders.* The Guilford Press.

Bedford, (2012). A perception theory in mind-body medicine: guided visual imagery and mindful meditation as cross-modal adaptation. *Psychomomic Bulletin and Review,* 19(1): 24-45.

Beek, P.J., Peper, C.E., Daffertshofer, A. (2002). Modeling rhythmic interlimb coordination: beyond the Haken-Kelso-Bunz model. *Brain Cognition,* 48: 149-65.

Beck, D.M., Rees, G., Christopher, D., Frith, C.D., Lavie, N. (2001). Neural correlates of change detection and change blindness. *Nature Neuroscience*, 4: 645-50.

Belleville, S., Gilbert, B., Fontaine, F., Gagnon, L., Ménard, E., Gauthier, S. (2006). Improvement of Episodic Memory in Persons with Mild Cognitive Impairment and Healthy Older Adults: Evidence from a Cognitive Intervention Program. *Dementia Geriatric Cognitive Disorders,* 22(5-6): 486-99.

Belin, P., Zilbovicius, M., Crozier, S., Thivard, L., Fontaine, A., Masure, M.C., Samson, Y. (1998). Lateralization of speech and auditory temporal processing. *Journal of Cognitive Neuroscience*, 10: 536-40.

Berli, R., Hutter, A., Waespe, W., Bachli, E.B. (2009). Transient global amnesia—not so rare after all. *Swiss Medical Weekly*, 16, 139 (19-20): 288-92.

Bertalanffy, L. von (1962). General System Theory—A critical review, *General Systems*, 7: 1-20.

Bertalanffy, L. von (1974). *Perspectives on General System Theory* Edited by Edgar Taschdjian. George Braziller, New York.

Besnard, J., Allain, P., Aubin, G., Chauviré, V., Etcharry-Bouyx, F., Le Gall, D. (2011). A contribution to the study of environmental dependency phenomena: the social hypothesis. *Neuropsychologia*, 49(12): 3279-94.

Beynon-Davies, P. (2010). Dances with bees: exploring the relevance of the study of animal communication to informatics. *International Journal of Information Management,* 30 (1): 185-98.

Biederman, I. (1987). Recognition-by-components: A theory of human image understanding. *Psychological Review, 94*, 115-47.

Biederman, I. (2001). Recognizing Depth-Rotated Objects: A Review of Recent Research and Theory. *Spatial Vision*, 13: 241-53.

Binder, L.M. (1986). Persisting Symptoms after Mild Head Injury: A Review of the Postconcussive Syndrome. *Journal of Clinical and Experimental Neuropsychology,* 8 (4): 323-46.

Birbaumer, N., Veit, R., Lotze, M., Erb, M., Hermann, C., Grodd, W., Flor, H. (2005). Deficient fear conditioning in psychopathy: a functional magnetic resonance imaging study. *Archives of General Psychiatry*, 62(7): 799-805.

Bishop, D.V.M. (2002). Motor immaturity and specific speech and language impairment: Evidence for a common genetic basis. *American Journal of Medical Genetics*, 114(1): 56-63.

Blair, R.J.R. (2007). The amygdala and ventromedial prefrontal cortex in morality and psychopaths. *Trends In Cognitive Sciences,* 11: 387-92.

Blair, R.J.R., Budhani, S., Colledge, E., Scott, S. (2005). Deafness to fear in boys with psychopathic tendencies. *Journal Child Psychology and Psychiatry,* 46: 327-36.

Blair, R.J.R., Cipolotti, L. (2000). Impaired social response reversal: a case of acquired sociopathy. *Brain*, 123: 1122-41.

Bledowski, C., Rahm, B., Rowe, J.B. (2009). What 'works' in working memory? Separate systems for selection and updating of critical information. *The Journal of Neuroscience,* 29(43): 13735-41.

Boemio, A., Fromm, S., Braun, A., Poeppel, D. (2005). Hierarchical and asymmetric temporal sensitivity in human auditory cortices. *Nature Neuroscience*, 8: 389-95.

Bogen, J.E. (1979). The Callosal syndrome. In K.L. Heilman & E. Valenstein (ed), *Clinical Neuropsychology*. Oxford University Press.

Booth, J.R., Burman, D.D., Meyer, J.R., Gitelman, D.R., Parrish, T.B., Mesulam, M.M. (2002). Modality independence of word comprehension. *Human Brain Mapping*, 16: 251-61.

Bor, D., Cumming, N., Scott, C.E., Owen, A.M. (2004). Prefrontal cortical involvement in verbal encoding strategies. *European Journal of Neuroscience, 19*(12): 3365-70.

Bor, D., Duncan, J., Wiseman, R.J., Owen, A.M. (2003). Encoding strategies dissociate prefrontal activity from working memory demand. *Neuron, 37*(2): 361-67.

Bowker, R.M., Coulter, J.D. (1981). Intracortical connectivities of somatic sensory and motor areas: Multiple cortical pathways in monkeys. In C.N. Woolsey (ed), *Cortical Sensory Organization*, vol. 1: Multiple Somatic Areas. Humana Press.

Bogousslavsky, J., Van Melle, G., Regli, F. (1988). The Lausanne Stroke Registry: analysis of 1,000 consecutive_patients with first stroke. *Stroke,* 19(9): 1083-92.

Braitenberg, V., Schüz, A (1991). *Anatomy of the Cortex: Statistics and Geometry*. NY: Springer-Verlag.

Braun, C.M., Dumont, M., Duval, J., Hamel-Hébert, I., Godbout, L. (2003). Brain modules of hallucination: an analysis of multiple patients with brain lesions. *Journal of Psychiatry Neuroscience,* 28(6): 432-49.

Braver, T.S., Barch, D.M., Gray, J.R., Molfese, D.L., Snyder, A. (2001). Anterior Cingulate Cortex and Response Conflict: Effects of Frequency, Inhibition and Errors. *Cerebral Cortex*, Vol. 11, No. 9: 825-36.

Braver, T.S., Cohen, J.D. (2000). On the control of control: The role of dopamine in regulating prefrontal function and working memory. In S. Monsell & J. Driver (Eds.), *Attention and Performance XVIII*; Control of cognitive processes, 713-37.

Braver, T.S., Cohen, J.D., Nystrom, L.E., Jonides, J., Smith, E.E., Noll, D.C. (1997). A parametric study of prefrontal cortex involvement in human working memory. *NeuroImage,* 5: 49-62.

Bressler, S.L., Kelso, J.A. (2001). Cortical coordination dynamics and cognition. *Trends in Cognitive Sciences,* 5: 26-36.

Broadbent, D.E. (1958). Perception and Communication. Pergamum Press, New York.

Brown, J.W. (1977). *Mind, Brain and Consciousness: The Neurophysiology of Cognition.* Academic Press.

Brown, K.W., Ryan, R.M. (2003). The benefits of being present: Mindfulness and its role in psychological well-being. *Journal of Personality and Social Psychology,* 84(4): 822-48.

Brooks, N., Campsie, L., Symongton, C., Beattie, A., McKinlay, W. (1986). The five-year outcome of severe blunt head injury: a relative's view. *Journal of Neurology, Neurosurgery & Psychiatry*, 49: 764-70.

Bruce, D. (2001). Fifty years since Lashley's In search of the Engram: refutations and conjectures. *Journal of the History of the Neurosciences*, 10(3): 308-18.

Bruce, V., Green, P., Georgeson, M. (1996). Visual Perception: Physiology, psychology and ecology. (3rd Ed.): 110.

Buchanan, T.W., Lutz, K., Mirzazade, S., Specht, K., Shah, N.J., Zilles, K. Jancke, L. (2000). Recognition of emotional prosody and verbal components of spoken language: an fMRI study. *Brain Research Cognitive Brain Research*, 9: 227-38.

Buchsbaum, M.S., Cappelletti, J., Ball, R., Hazlett, E., King, A.C., Johnson, J., Wu, J., DeLisi, L.E. (1984). Positron emission tomographic image measurement in schizophrenia and affective disorders. *Annals of Neurology,* 15: S157-65.

Buckner, R.L., Kelly, W.M., Petersen, S.E. (1999). Frontal cortex contributes to human memory formation. *Nature Neurosciences,* 4: 311-14.

Burgess, N., Maguire, E.A., O'Keefe, J. (2002). The human hippocampus and spatial and episodic memory. *Neuron,* 35: 625-41.

Burgess, P.W., Quayle, A., Frith, C.D. (2001). Brain regions involved in prospective memory as determined by positron emission tomography. *Neuropsychologia,* 39(6): 545-55.

Burgess, P., Shallice, T. (1997). The relationship between prospective and retrospective memory: Neuropsychological evidence. In: M.A. Conway **(Ed.)** *Cognitive Models of Memory.* Psychology Press, 249-56.

Burke, J.G., Dursun, S.M., Reveley, M.A. (1999). Refractory schizophrenia resulting from frontal lobe lesion: response to clozapine. *Journal of Psychiatry and Neuroscience,* 24: 456-61.

Butters, N., Salmon, D., Heindel, W.C. (1994). Specificity of the memory deficits associated with basal ganglia dysfunction. *Review of Neurology,* 150: 580-87.

Cabeza. R., Prince, S.E., Daselaar, S.M., Greenberg, D.L., Budde, M., Dolcos,, F., LaBar, K.S., Rubin, D.C. (2004). Brain activity during episodic retrieval of autobiographical and laboratory events: an fMRI study using a novel photo paradigm. *Journal of Cognitive Neuroscience,* 16(9): 1583-94.

Cabeza, R., Grady, C.L., Nyberg, L., McIntosh, A.R., Tulving, E., Kapur, S., Jennings, J.M., Houle, S., Craik, F.I. (1997). Age related differences in neural activity during memory encoding and retrieval: A positron emission tomography study. *The Journal of Neuroscience,* 17: 391-400.

Cahn, B.R., Polich, J. (2006). Meditation States and Traits: EEG, ERP, and Neuroimaging Studies. *Psychological Bulletin,* 132, No. 2: 180-211.

Carlson, N.R., Donald, H.C. (2010). Psychology the Science of Behaviour Ontario, CA: Pearson Education Canada 20-22.

Capek, C.M., Bavelier, D., Corina, D., Newman, A.J., Jezzard, P., Neville, H.J. (2004). The cortical organization of audio-visual sentence comprehension: an fMRI study at 4 Tesla. *Brain Research Cognitive Brain Research*, 20: 111-19.

Caplan, D. (2006). Why is Broca's Area Involved in Syntax? *Cortex,* 42(4): 469-71.

Cannon, W.B. (1929). Organization for Physiological Homeostasis. *Physiological Review,* 9(3): 399-421.

Cannon, W.B. (1927). The James-Lange theory of emotion: A critical examination and an alternative theory. *The American Journal of Psychology,* 39: 106-24.

Cantu, R.C. (2001). Posttraumatic Retrograde and Anterograde Amnesia: Pathophysiology and Implications in Grading and Safe Return to Play. *Journal of Athletic Training,* 36(3): 244-48.

Carmichael, S.T., Price, J.L. (1995). Sensory and premotor connections of the orbital and medial prefrontal cortex of macaque monkeys. *Journal of Comparative Neurology,* 25; 363(4): 642-64.

Cassidy, J.D., Carroll, L.J., Peloso, P.M., Borg, J., von Holst, H., Holm, L., Kraus, J., Coronado, V.G. (2004). Incidence, risk factors and prevention of mild traumatic brain injury: Results of the WHO Collaborating Centre Task Force on Mild Traumatic Brain Injury. *Journal of Rehabilitation Medicine,* 36(Supplement 43): 28-60.

Cassileth, B. (1998). The Alternative Medicine Handbook: *The Complete Reference Guide to Alternative and Complementary Therapies*. New York, NY: W.W. Norton.

Castaneda, C. (2003). Diabetes control with physical activity and exercise. *Nutrition in Clinical Care,* 6: 89-96.

Catani, M., Jones, D.K., ffytche, D.H. (2005). Perisylvian language networks of the human brain. *Annals of Neurology,* 57(1): 8-16.

Catani, M., ffytche, D.H. (2005). The rises and falls of disconnection syndromes. *Brain,* 128(10): 2224-39.

Cattaert, D., Semjen, A., Summers, J.J. (1999). Simulating a neural cross-talk model for between-hand interference during bimanual circle drawing. *Biological Cybernetics,* 81: 343-58.

Castelli, F., Happé, F., Frith, U., Frith, C. (2000). Movement and mind: a functional imaging study of perception and interpretation of complex intentional movement patterns. *Neuroimage,* 12(3): 314-25.

Cavada, C., Schultz, W. (2000). The Mysterious Orbitofrontal Cortex. Foreword. *Cerebral Cortex,* 10(3): 205.

Celone, K.A., Calhoun, V.D., Dickerson, B.C., Atri, A., Chua, E.F., Miller, S.L., DePeau, K., Rentz, D.M., Selkoe, D.J., Blacker, D., Albert, M.S., Sperling, R.A. (2006). Alternations in memory networks in mild cognitive impairment and Alzheimer's disease: An independent component analysis. *Journal of Neuroscience*, 26: 10222-31.

Cervone, Barbara Tucker; Duren, Bill; Kohn, J.J.; Snell, J. Laurie; Stein, Marjorie L. (1995). A.W. Tucker: some reminiscences, *Notices of the American Mathematical Society,* 42(10): 1143-47.

Chan, R.C.K., Shum, D., Toulopoulou, T., Chen, E.Y.H. R., Shum, D., Toulopoulou, T., Chen, E. (2008). Assessment of executive functions: Review of instruments and identification of critical issues. *Archives of Clinical Neuropsychology,* 223(2): 201-16.

Chan, J.L, Ross, E.D. (1997). Alien hand syndrome: influence of neglect on the clinical presentation of frontal and callosal variants. *Cortex,* 33(2): 287-99.

Chakravarthy, V.S., Denny, J., Raju, B.S. (2010). What do the basal ganglia do? A modeling perspective. *Biological Cybernetics,* 103(3): 237-53.

Chee, M.W., O'Craven, K.M., Bergida, R., Rosen, B.R, Savoy, R.L. (1999). Auditory and visual word processing studied with fMRI. *Human Brain Mapping*, 7: 15-28.

Chen, Z., Cowan, N. (2005). Chunk limits and length limits in immediate recall: a reconciliation. *Journal of Experimental Psychology, Learning, Memory, and Cognition,* 31(6): 1235-49.

Chen, S.S., Tu, P.C., Su, T.P., Hsieh, J.C., Lin, Y.C., Chen, L.F. (2008). Impaired frontal synchronization of spontaneous magnetoencephalographic activity in patients with bipolar disorder. *Neuroscience Letters,* 14; 445(2): 174-78.

Chiesa, A., Serretti, A. (2011). Mindfulness based cognitive therapy for psychiatric disorders: A systematic review and meta-analysis. *Psychiatry Review*, 187: 441-53.

Chiron, C., Jambaque, I., Nabbout, R., Lounes, R., Syrota, A., Dulac, O. (1997). The right brain hemisphere is dominant in human infants. *Brain,* 120, 1057-65.

Chiu, P., Ambady, N., Deldin, P. (2004). Contingent Negative Variation to Emotional In- and Out-Group Stimuli Differentiates High- and Low-Prejudiced Individuals. *Journal of Cognitive Neuroscience,* 16; 10: 1830-39.

Chu, B.C., Millis, S.R., Arango-Lasprilla, J.C., Hanks, R., Novack, T., Hart, T. (2007). Measuring recovery in new learning and memory following traumatic brain injury: a mixed-effects modeling approach. *Journal of Clinical and Experimental Neuropsychology,* 29: 617-25.

Christina, S., Anita, R., Mukundan, C.R. (2009). Technology in Rehabilitation: A Computer Based Cognitive Retraining Programme for Patients with Head Injury. *Indian Journal of Clinical Psychology*, 1. 1: 11-22.

Cinel, C., Humphreys, G., Poli, R. (2002). Cross-modal illusory conjunctions between vision and touch. *Journal of Experimental Psychology: Human Perception and Performance*, 28(5): 1243-66.

Clark, L., Bechara, A., Damasio, H., Aitken, M.R.F., Sahakian, B.J., Robbins, T.W.L., Bechara, A., Damasio, H., Aitken, M.R.F., Sahakian, B.J., Robbins, T.W. (2008). Differential effects of insular and ventromedial prefrontal cortex lesions on risky decision making. *Brain,* 131(5): 1311-22.

Clarke, S., Assal, G., Bogousslavsky, J., Regli, F., Townsend, D.W., Leenders, K.L., Blecic, S. (1994). Pure amnesia after unilateral left polarthalamic infarct: topographic and sequential neuropsychological and metabolic (PET) correlations. *Journal of Neurology, Neurosurgery and Psychiatry,* 57: 27-34.

Clayton, N.S., Dickinson, A. (1998). Episodic-like memory during cache recovery by scrub jays. *Nature,* 395(6699): 272-74.

Cleghorn, J.M., Franco, S., Szechtman, B., Kaplan, R.D., Szechtman, H., Brown, G.M., Nahmias, C., Garnett, E.S. (1992). Toward a brain map of auditory hallucinations. *American Journal of Psychiatry,* 149(8): 1062-69.

Clemo, H.R., Allman, B.L., Donlan, M.A., Meredith, M.A. (2007). Sensory and multisensory representations within the cat rostral suprasylvian cortex. *Journal of Comparative Neurology,* 503: 110-27.

Clemo, H.R., Sharma, G.K., Allman, B.L., Meredith, M.A. (2008). Auditory projections to extrastriate visual cortex: Connectional basis for multisensory processing in 'unimodal' visual neurons. *Experimental Brain Research,* 191: 37-47.

Cogan, D.G. (1973). Visual hallucinations as release phenomena. *Graefe's Archives for Clinical and Experimental Ophthalmology,* 188: 139-50.

Cohen, J.D., Perlstein, W.M., Braver, T.S., Nystrom, L.E., Noll, D.C., Jonides, J., Smith, E.E. (1997). Temporal dynamics of brain activation during a working memory task. *Nature,* 386: 604-08.

Cohen, S.O., Walco, G.A. (1999). Dance/movement therapy for children and adolescents with cancer. *Cancer Practice,* 7: 34-42.

Colavita, F.B. (1974). Human sensory dominance. *Perception & Psychophysics,* 16(2): 409-12.

Colebatch, J.G. (2007). Bereitschaftspotential and movement-related potentials: origin, significance, and application in disorders of human movement. *Movement Disorders,* 15; 22(5): 601-10.

Collette, F., Hogge, M., Salmon, E., Van der Linden, M. (2005). Exploration of the neural substrates of executive functioning by functional neuroimaging. *Neuroscience,* 28; 139(1): 209-21.

Constable, R.T., Pugh, K.R., Berroya, E., Mencl, W.E., Westerveld, M., Ni, W., Shankweiler, D. (2004). Sentence complexity and input modality effects in sentence comprehension: an fMRI study. *NeuroImage*, 22: 11-21.

Conway, M.A., Pleydell-Pearce, C.W., Whitecross, S.E., Sharpe, H. (2003). Neurophysiological correlates of memory for experienced and imagined events. *Neuropsychologia*, 41(3): 334-40.

Cooke, A., DeVita, C., Gee, J., Alsop, D., Detre, J., Chen, W., Grossman, M. (2003). Neural basis for sentence comprehension deficits in frontotemporal dementia. *Brain Language*, 85: 211-21.

Cooke, A., Grossman, M., Devita, C., Gonzalez-Atavales, J., Moore, P., Chen, W., Gee, J., Detre, J. (2006). Large-scale neural network for sentence processing. *Brain Language*, 96: 14-36.

Corbetta, M., Miezin, F.M., Dobmeyer, S., Shulman, G.L. Petersen, S.E. (1991). Selective and divided attention during visual discriminations of shape, color and speed: functional anatomy by Positron Emission Tomography. *Journal of Neuroscience,* 11: 2383-2402.

Corbetta, M., Miezin, F.M., Shulman, G.L., Petersen, S.E. (1993). A PET study of visuospatial attention. *Journal of Neuroscience,* 13(3): 1202-26.

Corbetta, M., Shulman, G.L., Miezin, F.M., Petersen, S.E. (1995). Superior parietal cortex activation during spatial attention shifts and visual feature conjunction. *Science,* 270: 802-05.

Corbetta, M., Gordon L. Shulman, G.L. (2002). Control of goal-directed and stimulus-driven attention in the brain. *Nature Reviews Neuroscience*, 3, 201-15.

Coull, I.T., Frackowiak, R.S., Frith, C.D. (1998a). Monitoring for target objects: activation of right frontal and parietal cortices with increasing time on task. *Neuropsychologia*, 36(12): 1325-1334.

Coull, I.T., Frith, C.D., Frackowiak, R.S.J., Grasby, P.M. (1996). A fronto-parietal network for rapid visual information processing: a PET study of sustained attention and working memory. *Neuropsychologia,* 34: 1085-95.

Coull, I.T., Frith, C.D., Nobre, A.C. (1997). fMRI reveals distinct neuronal netwroks for attention to time or space. *Society for Neuroscience Abstract*, 23: 620.11.

Coull, J.T. (1998b). Neural correlates of attention and arousal: insights from electrophysiology, functional neuroimaging and psychopharmacology. *Progress in Neurobiology*, 55: 343-61.

Courtney, S.M., Petit, L., Maisog, J.M., Ungerleider, L.G., Haxby, J.V. (1998). An area specialized for spatial working memory in human frontal cortex. *Science,* 279: 1347-51.

Courtney, S.M., Ungerleider, L.G., Keil, K., Haxby, J.V. (1996). Object and spatial visual working memory activate separate neural systems in human cortex. *Cerebral Cortex*, 6: 39-49.

Courtney, S.M., Ungerleider, L.G., Keil, K., Haxby, J.V. (1997). Transient and sustained activity in a distributed system for human working memory. *Nature*, 386: 608-11.

Cowan, N. (2001). The magical number 4 in short-term memory: A reconsideration of mental storage capacity. *Behavioral and Brain Sciences,* (1): 87-114.

Craighero, L., Metta, G., Sandini, G., Fadiga, L. (2007). The mirror-neurons system: data and models. *Progress in Brain Research*, 164: 39-59.

Crinion, J., Price, C.J. (2005). Right anterior superior temporal activation predicts auditory sentence comprehension following aphasic stroke. *Brain*, 128: 2858-71.

Cummings, J.L. (1995). Anatomic and behavioral aspects of frontal-subcortical circuits. *Annals of New York Academy of Sciences,* 769: 1-13.

Cummings, J.L. (1993). Frontal-Subcortical circuits and human behavior. *Archives of Neurology*, 50: 873-80.

Cummings, J.L., Cunningham, K. (1992). Obsessive-compulsive disorder in Huntington's disease. *Biological Psychiatry,* 31: 263-70.

Cunnington, R., Windischberger, C., Moser, E. (2005). Premovement activity of the pre-supplementary motor area and the readiness for action: studies of time-resolved event-related functional MRI. *Human Movement Science,* 24(5-6): 644-56.

Cutting, L.E., Clements, A.M., Courtney, S., Rimrodt, S.L., Schafer, J.G., Bisesi, J., Pekar, J.J., Pugh, K.R. (2005). Differential components of sentence comprehension: Beyond single word reading and memory. *Neuroimage*, 29: 429-38.

Curtis, C.E., D'Esposito, M. (2003). Persistent activity in the prefrontal cortex during working memory. *Trends in Cognitive Sciences,* 7(9): 415-23.

Curran, T., DeBuse, C., Woroch, B., Hirshman, E. (2006). Combined Pharmacological and Electrophysiological Dissociation of Familiarity and Recollection. *The Journal of Neuroscience*, 26: 1979-85.

Cycowicz, Y.M., Friedman, D., Rothstein, M., Snodgrass, J.G. (1997). Picture naming by young children: norms for name agreement, familiarity, and visual complexity. *Journal of Experimental Child Psychology*, 65: 171-237.

Cycowicz, Y.M., Friedman, D., Snodgrass, J.G., Duff, M. (2001). Recognition and source memory for pictures in children and adults. *Neuropsychologia,* 39(3): 255-67.

Daffner, K.R., Mesulam, M.M., Scinto, L.F., Acar, D., Calvo, V., Faust, R., Chabrerie, A., Kennedy, B., Holcomb, P. (2000a). The central role of the prefrontal cortex in directing attention to novel events. *Brain,* 123(5): 927-39.

Daffner, K.R., Mesulam, M.M., Holcomb, P.J., Calvo, V., Acar, D., Chabrerie, A., Kikinis, R., Jolesz, F.A., Rentz, D.M., Scinto, L.F. (2000b). Disruption of attention to novel events after frontal lobe injury in humans. *J. Neurol. Neurosurg. Psychiatry,* 68(1): 18-24.

Dalla Barba, G., Parlato, V., Jobert, A., Samson, Y., Pappata, S. (1998). Cortical networks implicated in semantic and episodic memory: common or unique? *Cortex,* 34: 547-61.

Damasio, A.R. (1979). The frontal lobes. In K.M. Heilman and E. Valenstein (Eds.), *Clinical Neuropsychology.* New York, Oxford Univrsity Press. 360-412.

Damasio, A.R. (1990). Synchronous activation in multiple cortical regions: a mechanism for recall. *Seminars in Neuroscience,* 2: 287-96.

Damasio, A.R., Van Hosoesen, G.W. (1980). Structure and the function of supplementary motor area. *Neurology,* 30: 359.

Damasio, H. (2000). The lesion method in cognitive neuroscience. In F. Boller, J. Grafman, G. Rizzolati (Eds.), *Handbook of Neuropsychology* (2nd ed.). Amsterdam: Elsevier. 1: 77-102.

Damasio, H. (2001). Neural basis of language disorders. In R. Chapey (Ed.), *Language Intervention Strategies in Aphasia and Related Neurogenic Communication Disorders*, Philadelphia, PA: Lippincott William & Wilkins (4th ed.): 18-36.

Damasio, H., Grabowski, T.J., Tranel, D., Hichwa, R.D., Damasio, A.R. (1996). A neural basis for lexical retrieval. *Nature*, 380: 499-505.

Damasio, H., Tranela, D., Grabowskia, T., Adolphsa, R., Damasio, A. (2004). Neural systems behind word and concept retrieval. *Cognition*, 92(1-2): 179-229.

Darwin, C., Paul, E., Phillip, P. (1998). *The Expression of the Emotions in Man and Animals*, 3rd edn. London: Harper Collins.

Daum, I., Ackermann, H. (1994a). Frontal-type memory impairment associated with thalamic damage. *International Journal of Neuroscience*, 77(3-4): 187-98.

Daum, I., Ackermann, H. (1994b). Dissociation of declarative and nondeclarative memory after bilateral thalamic lesions: a case report. *International Journal of Neuroscience*, 75(3-4): 153-65.

David, L.S., Kabat-Zinn, J. (2008). Mindfulness in Medicine. *Journal of the American Medical Association,* 300.11: 1350-52.

Debaere, F., Wenderoth, N., Sunaert, S., Van-Hecke, P., Swinnen, S.P. (2003). Internal vs external generation of movements: differential neural pathways involved in bimanual coordination performed in the presence or absence of augmented visual feedback. *NeuroImage,* 19(3): 764-76.

Decety, J., Jackson, P.L. (2004). The functional architecture of human empathy. *Behavioral and Cognitive Neuroscience Reviews*, 3: 71-100.

Decety, J., Sommerville, J.A. (2003). Shared representations between self and other: a social cognitive neuroscience view. *Trends in Cognitive Science,* 7(12): 527-33.

Deecke, L. (1985). Cerebral potentials related to voluntary actions: Parkinsonian and normal subjects. *Clinical Neurophysiology in Parkinsonism*. P.J. Delwaide and A. Agnoli (Eds.), Amsterdam and Oxford: Elsevier. 91-105.

Deecke, L. (1987). Bereitschaftspotential as an indicator of movement preparation in supplementary motor area and motor cortex. *Ciba Foundation Symposium*, 132: 231-50.

Deecke, L. (1990). Electrophysiological correlates of movement initiation. *Review of Neurology*, 10: 612-19.

Deecke, L. (2000). The Bereitschaftspotential as an electrophysiological tool for studying the cortical organization of human voluntary action. *Supplements in Clinical Neurophysiology*, 53: 199-206.

Deecke, L. Kornhuber, H.H. (1978). An electrical sign of participation of the mesial supplementary motor cortex in human voluntary finger movement. *Brain Research*, 159: 473-76.

Deecke, L., Eisinger, H., Kornhuber, H.H. (1980). Comparison of Bereitschaftspotential, promotion positivity and motor potential preceding voluntary flexion and extension movements in man. *Progress in Brain Research*, 54: 171-76.

Deecke, L., Heise, B., Kornhuber, H.H., Lang, M., Lang, W. (1984). Brain potentials associated with voluntary manual tracking: Bereitschaftspotential, conditioned premotion positivity, directed attention potential, and relaxation potential. Anticipatory activity of the limbic and frontal cortex. *Annals of New York Academy of Sciences*, 425: 450-64.

Deecke, L., Lang, W. (1996). Generation of movement-related potentials and fields in the supplementary sensorimotor area and the primary motor area. *Advances in Neurology,* 70: 127-46.

de Gelder, B., Morris, J.S., Dolan, R.J. (2005). Unconscious fear influences emotional awareness of faces and voices. *Proceedings of National Academy of Sciences, U.S.A.* 20; 102(51): 18682-87.

de Gelder, B., Rouw, R. (2000). Paradoxical configuration effects for faces and objects in prosopagnosia. *Neuropsychologia*, 38: 1271-79.

de Gelder, B., Vroomen, J., Pourtois, G., Weiskrantz, L. (1999). Non-conscious recognition of affect in the absence of striate cortex. *Neuroreport*, 10: 3759-63.

de Fiorio, M., Tinazzi, M., Aglioti, S.M. (2006). Selective impairment of hand mental rotation in patients with focal hand dystonia. *Brain,* 129: 47-54.

de Lange, F.P., Hagoort, P., Toni, I. (2005). Neural topography and content of movement representations. *Journal of Cognitive Neuroscience*, 17: 97-12.

DeLuca, J., Schultheis, M.T., Madigan, N.K., Christodoulou, C., Averill, A. (2000). Acquisition versus retrieval deficits in traumatic brain injury: implications for memory rehabilitation. *Archives of Physical Medicine and Rehabilitation,* 81(10): 1327-33.

Demonet, J.F., Chollet, F., Ramsay, S., Cardebat, D., Nespoulous, J.L., Wise, R., Rascol, A., Frackowiak, R. (1992). The anatomy of phonological and semantic processing in normal subjects. *Brain,* 115: 1753-68.

Denes, G., Semenza, C., Stoppa, E., Lis, A. (1982). Unilateral spatial neglect and recovery from hemiplegia: a follow-up study. *Brain,* 105 (Pt 3): 543-52.

Depue, R.A., Collins, P.F. (1999). Neurobiology of the structure of personality: Dopamine, facilitation of incentive motivation, and extraversion. *Behavioral and Brain Sciences,* 22(3): 491-517.

D'Esposito, M., Detre, J.A., Alsop, D.C., Shin, R.K., Atlas, S., Grossman, M. (1995). The neural basis of the central executive system of working memory. *Nature,* 378: 279-81.

Deutsch, J.A., Deutsch, D. (1963). Attention: some theoretical consdierations. *Psychological Review*, 70: 80-90.

Dikmen, S.S., Machamer, J.E., Powell, J.M., Temkin, N.R. (2003). Outcome 3 to 5 years after moderate to severe traumatic brain injury. *Archives of Physical Medicine and Rehabilitation,* 84: 1449-57.

Dierks, T., Linden, D.E., Jandl, M., Formisano, E., Goebel, R., Lanfermann, H., Singer, W. (1999). Activation of Heschl's gyrus during auditory hallucinations. *Neuron,* 22(3): 615-21.

Dirnberger, G., Lang, W., Lindinger, G. (2008). A new method to determine temporal variability in the period of pre-movement electroencephalographic activity. *International Journal of Psychophysiology,* 70(3): 165-70.

Dietz, N.A., Jones, K.M., Gareau, L., Zeffiro, T.A., Eden, G.F. (2005). Phonological decoding involves left posterior fusiform gyrus. *Human Brain Mapping*, 26: 81-93.

Doody, R.S., Jankovic, J. (1992). The alien hand and related signs. *Journal of Neurology, Neurosurgery, and Psychiatry*, 55(9): 806-10.

Douglas, J.J., Wilkinson, D.A. (1993). Evidence of normal emotional responsiveness in alcoholic Korsakoff's syndrome in the presence of profound memory impairment. *Addiction*, 88(12): 1637-45.

Dringenberg, C. 1998. The basal forebrain cholinergic system: direct cortical activator and mediator of activation induced by excitation of secondary brain systems. *INABIS98 SYMPOSIUM.*

Dronkers, N.F., Plaisant, O., Iba-Zizen, M.T., Cabanis, E.A. (2007). Paul Broca's historic cases: high resolution MR imaging of the brains of Leborgne and Lelong. *Brain,* 130 (5): 1432-41.

Duchek, J.M., Balota, D.A., Storandt, M., Larsen, R. (2007). The power of personality in discriminating between healthy aging and early-stage Alzheimer's disease. *Journals of Gerontology: Series B,* 62(6): 353-61.

Dudai, Y. (2004). The neurobiology of consolidations, or, how stable is the engram? *Annual Review of Psychology*, 55: 51-86.

Duncan, J., Owen, A.M. (2000). Common regions of the human frontal lobe recruited by diverse cognitive demands. *Trends in Neuroscience,* 23: 475-83.

Dutta, P.K. (1999). Strategies and Games: Theory and Practice, MIT Press.

Dwivedi, P., Mukundan, C.R. (1993). Lateralization visual attention and distractibility. *NIMHANS Journal*, 1993. 11(1): 27-34.

Eichenbaum, H. (2001). The Hippocampus and Declarative Memory: Cognitive Mechanisms and Neural Codes. *Behavioural Brain Research*, 127: 199-207.

Eichenbaum, H., Otto, T., Cohen, N.J. (1994). Two functional components of the hippocampal memory system. *Behavioral and Brain Science*, 17: 449-518.

Eisenberg, N., Fabes, R.A., Karbon, M., Murphy, B.C., Wosinski, M., Polazzi, L., Carlo, G., Juhnke, C. (1996). The relations of children's dispositional prosocial behavior to emotionality, regulation, and social functioning. *Child Development, 67:* 974-92.

Eliassen, J.C., Baynes, K., Gazzaniga, M.S. (2000). Anterior and posterior callosal contributions to simultaneous bimanual movements of the hands and fingers. *Brain,* 123(12): 2501-11.

Elizabeth, A.F., Rowse, A., Ballantine, B. (2002). Does handedness determine which hand leads in a bimanual task? *Journal of Motor Behavior*, 34(4): 402-12.

Ellis, A. (2004). *Rational Emotive Behavior Therapy: It Works for Me—It Can Work for You by Albert Ellis*. Prometheus Books.

Ellis, A., Grieger, R. (1977). Handbook of rational emotive therapy. New York: Springer.

Ellis, R. (1994). *Rational Emotive Therapy*. Allein & Bacon, New Jersey.

Elliott, R. (2003). Executive functions and their disorders. *British Medical Bulletin,* (65): 49-59.

Engel, A.K., Singer, W. (2001). Temporal binding and the neural correlates of sensory awareness. *Trends in Cognitive Neurosciences*, 5: 16-25.

Epstein, C.M., Sekino, M., Yamaguchi, K., Kamiya, S., Ueno, S. (2002), Asymmetries of prefrontal cortex in human episodic memory: effects of transcranial magnetic stimulation on learning abstract patterns. *Neuroscience Letters*, 320: 5-8.

Erdler, M., Beisteiner, R., Mayer, D., Kaindl, T., Edward, V., Windischberger, C., Lindinger, G., Deecke, L. (2000). Supplementary motor area activation preceding voluntary movement is detectable with a whole-scalp magnetoencephalography system. *NeuroImage,* 11(6 Pt 1): 697-707.

Ericsson, K.A., Kintsch, W. (1995). Long-term working memory. *Psychological Review*, 102(2): 211-45.

Evans, J.J., Heggs, A.J., Antoun, N., Hodges, J.R. (1995). Progressive prosopagnosia associated with selective right temporal lobe atrophy. A new syndrome? *Brain,* 118: 1-13.

Eysenck, H.J. (1967). *The biological basis of personality*. Springfield, IL: Thomas Publishing.

Faber, P.L., Lehmann, D., Gianotti, L.R.R., Kaelin, M., Pascual-Marqui, R.D. (2004). *Scalp and intracerebral (LORETA) theta and gamma EEG coherence in meditation.* Paper presented at the meeting of the International Society for Neuronal Regulation, Winterthur, Switzerland.

Fadiga, L., Craighero, L., Fabbri Destro, M., Livio Finos, Cotilon-Williams, N., Smith, A.T., Castiello, U. (2006). Language in Shadow. *Social Neuroscience,* 1(2): 77-89.

Faw, B. (2006). Latest Findings in the Mechanisms of Cortical 'Arousal': 'Enabling' Neural Correlates for All Consciousness. *Electroneurobiología,* 14(2): 199-210.

Fernandez, T., Harmony, T., Silva-Pereyra, J., Fernandez-Bouzas, A., Gersenowies, J., Galan, L., Carbonell, F., Marosi, E., Otero, G., Sergio, I., Valdes, S.I. (2000). Specific EEG frequencies at specific brain areas and performance. *Neuroreport,* 11: 2663-68.

Filley, C.M., Kleinschmidt, B.K. (1995). Neurobehavioral presentations of brain neoplasms. *Western Journal of Medicine,* 163: 19-25.

Fisk, A.D., Schneider, W. (1984). Memory as a function of attention, level of processing, and automatization, *Journal of Experimental Psychology: Learning, Memory and Cognition,* 10(2): 181-97.

Fletcher, P.C., Henson, R.N. (2001). Frontal lobes and human memory: insights from functional neuroimaging. *Brain,* 124: 849-81.

Fletcher, P.C., Frith, C.D., Grasby, P.M. (1995). Brain systems for encoding and retrieval of auditory-verbal memory. *Brain*, 118: 401-16.

Fletcher, P.C., Shallice, T., Dolan, R.J. (1998a). The functional roles of prefrontal cortex in episodic memory: I Encoding. *Brain*, 121: 1239-48.

Fletcher, P.C., Shallice, T., Frith, C.D., Frackowiak, R.S., Dolan, R.J. (1998b). The functional role of prefrontal cortex in episodic memory: II Retrieval. *Brain*, 121: 1249-56.

Fletcher, P.C., Frith, C.D., Rugg, M.D. (1997). The functional neuroanatomy of episodic memory. *Trends in Neuroscience*, 20: 213-18.

Fletcher, P.C., Frith, C.D., Grasby, P.M. (1995). Brain systems for encoding and retrieval of auditory-verbal memory. *Brain,* 118: 401-16.

Foley, E., Baillie, A., Huxter, M., Price, M., Sinclair, E. (2010). Mindfulness-based cognitive therapy for individuals whose lives have been affected by cancer: A randomized controlled trial. *Journal of Consulting and Clinical Psychology, 78*(1): 72-79.

Forman, W.B. (2012). Transient global amnesia: a case report and literature review. *American Journal of Hospice and Palliative Care,* 29(7): 563-65.

Francis, D.J., Fletcher, J.M., Stuebing, K.K., Davidson, K.C., Thompson, N.M. (1991). Analysis of change: modeling individual growth. *Journal of Consulting and Clinical Psychology,* 59: 27-37.

Franz, V.H., Gegenfurtner, K.R., Bülthoff, H.H., Fahle, M. (2000). Grasping visual illusions: no evidence for a dissociation between perception and action. *Psychology Science*, 11(1): 20-25.

Friederici, A.D. (2001). Syntactic, prosodic, and semantic processes in the brain: evidence from event-related neuroimaging. *Journal of Psycholinguistic Research,* 30: 237-50.

Friederici, A.D. (2002). Towards a neural basis of auditory sentence processing, *Trends in Cognitive Science*, 6: 78-84.

Friederici, A.D., Ruschemeyer, S.A., Hahne, A., Fiebach, C.J. (2003). The role of left inferior frontal and superior temporal cortex in sentence comprehension: localizing syntactic and semantic processes. *Cerebral Cortex*, 13: 170-77.

Frith, C. (2005). The self in action: lessons from delusions of control. *Conscious Cognition*, 14(4): 752-70.

Frojan-Parga, M.X., Calero-Elvira, A., Montano-Fidalgo, M. (2009). Analysis of the therapist's verbal behavior during cognitive restructuring debates: a case study. *Psychotherapy Research*, 19: 30-41.

Fullerton, C.S., Ursano, Wang (2004). Acute Stress Disorder, Posttraumatic Stress Disorder, and Depression in Disaster or Rescue Workers. *American Journal of Psychiatry,* 161(8): 1370-76.

Fuster, J.M. (1980). The Prefrontal Cortex. Anatomy, Physiology, and Neuropsychology of the Frontal Lobe. New York: Raven Press.

Fuster, J.M., Alexander, G.E. (1971). Neuron activity related to short-term memory. *Science,* 13; 173(3997): 652-54.

Gabrieli, J., Kao, Y. (2007). Development of the Declarative Memory System in the Human Brain. *Nature Neuroscience*, 10: 1198-05.

Gardiner, J.M., Java, R.I. (1990). Recollective experience in word and nonword recognition. *Memory & Cognition*, 18: 23-30.

Gais, S., Molle, M., Helms, K., Born, J. (2002). Learning-dependent increases in sleep spindle density. *Journal of Neuroscience*, 22: 6830-34.

Galaburda, A.M., Pandya, D.N. (1982). Role of architectonic and connections in the study of primate brain evolution. In E. Armstrong and D. Falk (eds), *Primate Brain Evolution: Methods and Concepts*.

Gallopin, T., Fort, P., Eggermann, E., Cauli, B., Luppi, P.H., Rossier, J., Audinat, E., Mühlethaler, M., Serafin, M. (2000). Identification of sleep-promoting neurons *in vitro*. *Nature*, 404: 992-95.

Gallagher, S. (2000). Philosophical conceptions of the self: Implications for cognitive neuroscience. *Trends in Cognitive Neuroscience,* 4: 14-21.

Galvin, J.E., Powlishta, K.K., Wilkins, K., McKeel, Jr., D.W., Xiong, C., Grant, E.A., Storandt, M., Morris, J.C. (2005). Predictors of preclinical Alzheimer disease and dementia: A clinicopathologic study. *Archives of Neurology*, 62: 758-65.

Ganis, G., Thompson, W.L., Kosslyn, S.M. (2004). Brain areas underlying visual mental imagery and visual perception: an fMRI study. *Brain Research Cognitive Brain Research*, 20(2): 226-41.

Garland, E., Gaylord, S., Park, J. (2009). The role of mindfulness in positive reappraisal. *Explore—The Journal of Science and Healing,* 5(1): 37-44.

Gazzaniga, M.S. (1970). *The Bisected Brain.* New York: Appleton-Century-Crofts.

Gershberg, F.B., Shimamura, A.P. (1995). Impaired use of organizational strategies in free recall following frontal lobe damage. *Neuropsychologia*, 13: 1305-33.

Gilbertson, M.W., Orr, S.P., Rauch, S.L., Pitman, R.K. (2008). Trauma and posttraumatic stress disorder. In: T.A. Stern, J.F. Rosenbaum, M. Fava, J. Biederman, S.L. Rauch (Eds.), *Massachusetts General Hospital Comprehensive Clinical Psychiatry,* 1st ed. Philadelphia, Pa: Mosby Elsevier; chap. 34.

Giloba, A., Winocur, G., Grady, C.L., Hevenor, S.J., Moscovitch, M. (2004). Remembering our past: functional neuroanatomy of recollection of recent and very remote personal events. *Cerebral Cortex,* 14(11): 1214-25.

Glover, S. (2004). Separate visual representations in the planning and control of action. *Behavioral Brain Sciences*, 27(1): 3-24.

Godschalk, M., Lemon, R.N., Kuypers, H.G., Ronday, H.K. (1984). Cortical afferents and efferents of monkey postarcuate area: An anatomical and electrophysiological study. *Experimental Brain Research,* 56: 410-24.

Goldar, J.C., Rojas, D., Outes, M. (1993). A neurobiological model of mind. *Acta Psiquiatrica Psicologica Americana Latina,* 39(1): 33-44.

Goldberg, G. (1985). Supplementary motor area structure and function: Review and hypotheses. *The Behavior and Brain Sciences*. 567-615.

Goldberg, B., Goldberg, M.A. (2002). *Alternative Medicine: The Definitive Guide, Celestial Arts.*

Goldberg, G., Bloom, K.K. (1990). The alien hand sign. Localization, lateralization and recovery. *American Journal of Physical Medicine and Rehabilitation*, 69(5): 228-38.

Goldberg, G., Mayer, N.H., Toglia, J.U. (1981). Medial frontal cortex infarction and alien hand sign. *Archives of Neurology,* 38: 663-68.

Goldstein, R.Z., Alia-Klein, N., Tomasi, D., Carrillo, J.H., Maloney, T., Woicik, P.A., Wang, R., Telang, F., Volkow, N.D. (2009). Anterior cingulate cortex hypoactivations to an emotionally salient task in cocaine addiction. *Proceedings of National Academy of Sciences, U.S.A.* 9; 106(23): 9453-58.

Gillihan, S.J., Farah, M.J. (2005). Is Self Special? A Critical Review of Evidence From Experimental Psychology and Cognitive Neuroscience. *Psychological Bulletin,* 131(1): 76-97.

Graham, K.S., Lee, A.C., Brett, M., Patterson, K. (2003). The neural basis of autobiographical and semantic memory: new evidence from three PET studies. *Cognitive, Affective & Behavioral Neuroscience*, 3: 234-54.

Gray, C.M. (1999). The temporal correlation hypothesis of visual feature integration: Still alive and well. *Neuron,* 24: 31-47.

Griffiths, K., Camic, P.M., Hutton, J.M. (2009). Participant experiences of a mindfulness-based cognitive therapy group for cardiac rehabilitation. *Journal of Health Psychology*, 14: 675-81.

Groenewegen, H.I., Berendse, H.W., Wolters, J.G., Lohman, A.H. (1990). The anatomical relationship of the prefrontal cortex with the striatopallidal system, the thalamus, and the amygdala: evidence of a parallel organization. *Progress in Brain Research*, 85: 95-116.

Grossman, P., Niemann, L., Schmidt, S., Walach, H. (2004). Mindfulness-based stress reduction and health benefits. A meta-analysis. *Journal of Psychosomatic Research*, 57(1): 35-43.

Gruzelier, J.H. (2006). Frontal functions, connectivity and Neural Efficiency Underpinning Hypnosis and Hypnotic Susceptibility. *Contemporary Hypnosis, 23*(1): 15-32.

Gusnard, D.A., Akbudak, E., Shulman, G.L., Marcus, E. Raichle, M.E. (2007). Medial prefrontal cortex and self-referential mental activity: Relation to a default mode of brain function. *National Academy of Sciences, USA*. 98(7): 4259-64.

Gusnard, D.A., Akbudak, E., Shulman, G.L., Raichle, M.E. (2001). Medial prefrontal cortex and self referential mental activity: relation to a default mode of brainfunction. *Proceedings of National Academy of Sciences, U.S.A.*, 27; 98(7): 4259-64.

Gyung, H.O., Chunga, G.H.C., Hana, Y.M., Jeonga, S.H., Jack Jr., C.R. (2005). Functional Heterogeneity of the Supplementary Motor Area. *American Journal of Neuroradiology*, 26: 1819-23.

Habib, R., Nyberg, L., Tulving, E. (2003). Hemispheric asymmetries of memory: the HERA model revisited. *Trends in Cognitive Sciences*, 7(6): 241-45.

Huckabee, M.L., Deecke, L., Cannito, M.P., Gould, H.J., Mayr, W. (2003). Cortical control mechanisms in volitional swallowing: the Bereitschaftspotential. *Brain Topography*, 16(1): 3-17.

Haggard, P. (2005). Conscious intention and motor cognition. *Trends in Cognitive Sciences*, 9: 290-95.

Haggard, P., Clark, S. (2003). Intentional action: Conscious experience and neural prediction. *Consciousness and Cognition*, 12: 659-707.

Haggard, P., Aschersleben, G., Gehrke, J., Prinz, W. (2002a). Action, binding, and awareness. In W. Prinz, B. Hommel (Eds.), *Common mechanisms in perception and action: Attention & Performance, XIX*. Oxford: Oxford University Press.

Haggard, P., Clark, S., Kalogeras, J. (2002). Voluntary action and conscious awareness. *Nature Neuroscience*, 5: 382-85.

Haist, F., Bowden Gore, J., Mao, H. (2001). Consolidation of human memory over decades revealed by functional magnetic resonance imaging. *Nature Neuroscience,* 4: 1139-45.

Hallanger, A.H., Levey, A.I., Lee, H.G., Rye, D.B., Warner, B.H. (1987). The origins of cholinergic and other subcortical afferents to the thalamus in the rat. *Journal of Comparative Neurology,* 262: 104-24.

Hamann, S. (2001). Cognitive and neural mechanisms of emotional memory. *Trends in Cognitive Science,* 5: 394-400.

Hamano, T., Lüders, H.O., Ikeda, A., Collura, T., Comair, Y.G., Shibasaki, H. (1997). The cortical generators of the contingent negative variation in humans: A study with subdural electrodes. *Electroencephalography Clinical Neurophysiology*, 104: 257-68.

Hanna, J.L. (1995). The power of dance: health and healing. *J. Altern. Complement. Med.,* 1: 323-31.

Harmony, T., FemGndez, T., Silva, J., Bemal, J., Diaz-Comas, L., Reyes, A., Marosi, E., Rodriguez, M. (1996). EEG delta activity: an indicator of attention to internal processing during performance of mental tasks. *International Journal of Psychophysiology*, 24: 161-71.

Harris, D.M., Kay, J. (1995). I recognize your face but I can't remember your name: is it because names are unique? *British Journal of Psychology,* 86: 345-58.

Hartcher-O'Brien, J., Levitan, C., Spence, C. (2010). Extending visual dominance over touch for input off the body, *Brain Research,* 1362: 48-55.

Haxby, J.V., Ungerleider, L.G., Horwitz, B., Maisog, J.M., Rapoport, S.I., Grady, C.L. (1996). Face encoding and recognition in the human brain. *Proceedings of the National Academy of Sciences, U.S.A.,* 93: 922-27.

Hayden, B.Y., Platt, M.L. (2010). Neurons in Anterior Cingulate Cortex Multiplex Information about Reward and Action. *Journal of Neuroscience,* 30 (9): 3339-46.

Hebb, D.O. (1949). The organization of behavior. New York: Wiley.

Hebb, D.O. (1961). "Distinctive features of learning in the higher animal" in J.F. Delafresnaye (Ed.), *Brain Mechanisms and Learning.* London: Oxford University Press.

Haber, S.N., Kunishio, K., Mizobuchi, M., Lynd-Balta, E. (1995). The orbital and medial prefrontal circuit through the primate basal ganglia. *Journal of Neuroscience*, 15(7 Pt 1): 4851-67.

Heilman, K.M., Valenstein, E. (1972a). Frontal lobe neglect in man. *Neurology,* 22(6): 660-64.

Heilman, K.M., Valenstein, E. (1972b). Auditory neglect in man. *Archives of Neurology*, 26(1): 32-35.

Heim, S., Opitz, B., Muller, K., Friederici, A.D. (2003). Phonological processing during language production: fMRI evidence for a shared production-comprehension network. *Brain Research Cognitive Brain Research*, 16: 285-96.

Himanen, L., Portin, R., Tenovuo, O., Taiminen, T., Koponen, S., Hiekkanen, H., Helenius, H. (2009). Attention and depressive symptoms in chronic phase after traumatic brain injury. *Brain Injury*, 23(3): 220-27.

Himanen, L., Portin, R., Isoniemi, H., Helenius, H., Kurki, T., Tenovuo, O. (2006). Longitudinal cognitive changes in traumatic brain injury: a 30-year follow-up study. *Neurology*, 66: 187-92.

Heidenreich, T., Tuin, I., Pflug, B., Michal, M., Michalak, J. (2006). Mindfulness-based cognitive therapy for persistent insomnia: A pilot study. *Psychotherapy and Psychosomatics*, 75: 188-89.

Henson, R.N., Hornberger, M., Rugg, M.D. (2005). Further dissociating the processes involved in recognition memory: An fMRI study. *Journal of Cognitive Neuroscience*, 17: 1058-73.

Henson, R.N., Rugg, M.D., Shallice, T., Dolan, R.J. (2000). Confidence in recognition memory for words: Dissociating right prefrontal roles in episodic retrieval. *Journal of Cognitive Neuroscience*, 12: 913-23.

Henson, R.N., Shallice, T., Dolan, R.J. (1999). Right prefrontal cortex and episodic memory retrieval: A functional MRI test of the monitoring hypothesis. *Brain*, 122: 1367-81.

Herzog, H., Lele, V.R., Kuwert, T., Langen, K.J., Kops, E.R., Feinendegen, L.E. (1990). Changed pattern of regional glucose metabolism during yoga meditative relaxation. *Neuropsychobiology*, 23: 182-87.

Hicks, J.L., Marsh, R.L. (2001). False recognition occurs more frequently during source recognition than during old-new recognition. *Journal of Experimental Psychology: Learning, Memory and Cognition*, 27: 375-83.

Hill, E.L. (2001). Non-specific nature of specific language impairment: a review of the literature with regard to concomitant motor impairments. *International Journal of Language & Communication Disorders*, 36(2): 149-71.

Hillier, S.L., Sharpe, M.H., Metzer, J. (1997). Outcomes 5 years post-traumatic brain injury (with further reference to neurophysical impairment and disability). *Brain Injury*, 11(9): 661-75.

Hilton, G. (1994). Behavioral and cognitive sequelae of head trauma. *Orthop Nurs.*, 13(4): 25-32.

Hobson, J.A. (2005). Sleep is of the brain, by the brain and for the brain. *Nature,* 27; 437(7063): 1254-56.

Hobson, J.A., Pace-Schott, E.F., Stickgold, R. (2000). Consciousness: Its Svicissitudes in waking and sleep. In Gazzaniga, M.S. (Ed.), *New Cognitive, Neurosciences: Second Edition.* MIT Press. 1341-54.

Hobson, R.P., Lee, A. (1999). Imitation and identification in autism. *Journal of Child Psychology and Psychiatry,* 40(4): 649-59.

Hodges, J.R., Warlow, C.P. (1990a). The aetiology of transient global amnesia. A case-control study of 114 cases with prospective follow-up. *Brain*, 13(3): 639-57.

Hodges, J.R., Warlow, C.P. (1990b). Syndromes of transient amnesia: towards a classification. A study of 153 cases. *Journal of neurology, neurosurgery, and psychiatry,* 53(10): 834-43.

Hodges, J.R., Patterson, K., Ward, R., Garrard, P., Bak, T., Perry, R., Gregory, C. (1999). The differentiation of semantic dementia and frontal lobe dementia (temporal and frontal variants of frontotemporal dementia) from early Alzheimer's disease: a comparative neuropsychological study. *Neuropsychology*, 13(1): 31-40.

Hoeks, J.C.J., Stowe, L.A., Doedens, G. (2004). Seeing words in context: the interaction of lexical and sentence level information during reading, *Cognitive Brain Research,* 19: 59-73.

Hothersall, D. (2004). *History of Psychology* (4th ed.). New York, NY: McGraw-Hill.

Hölzel, B.K., Carmody, J., Vangel, M., Congleton, C., Yerramsetti, S.M., Gard, T., Lazar, S.W. (2011). Mindfulness practice leads to increases in regional brain gray matter density. *Psychiatry Research*, 30; 191(1): 36-43.

Homae, F., Hashimoto, R., Nakajima, K., Miyashita, Y., Sakai, K.L. (2002). From perception to sentence comprehension:

the convergence of auditory and visual information of language in the left inferior frontal cortex. *NeuroImage,* 16: 883-900.

Hope, D.A., Burns, J.A., Hyes, S.A., Herbert, J.D., Warner, M.D. (2010). Automatic thoughts and cognitive restructuring in cognitive behavioral group therapy for social anxiety disorder. *Cognitive Therapy Research*, 34: 1-12.

Horiike, A., Kuroki, T., Sato, K., Terada K., Li-qun, W., Nakane, H., Nishimura, C. (2004). An fMRI study on autobiographical memory retrieval. *International Congress Series,* 1270: 306-10.

Hubl, D., Koenig, T., Strik, W., Federspiel, A., Kreis, R., Boesch, C., Maier, S.E., Schroth, G., Huckabee, M.L., Deecke, L., Cannito, M.P., Gould, H.J., Mayr, W. (2003). Cortical control mechanisms in volitional swallowing: the Bereitschaftspotential. *Brain Topography,* 16(1): 3-17.

Hugenholtz, H., Stuss, D.T., Stethem, L.L., Richard, M.T. (1988). How long does it take to recover from a mild concussion? *Neurosurgery,* 22(5): 853-58.

Hummel, J.E., Biederman, I. (1992). Dynamic binding in a neural network for shape recognition. *Psychological Review,* 99: 480-517.

Humphries, C., Love, T., Swinney, D., Hickok, G. (2005). Response of anterior temporal cortex to syntactic and prosodic manipulations during sentence processing. *Human Brain Mapping,* 26: 128-38.

Humphrey, G. (1924). The psychology of the gestalt. *Journal of Educational Psychology,* 15(7): 401-12.

Iber, C., Ancoli-Israel, S., Chesson, A., Quan, S.F. (2007). The AASM Manual for the Scoring of Sleep and Associated Events: Rules, Terminology and Technical Specifications. Westchester: American Academy of Sleep Medicine.

Iidaka, T., Sadato, N., Yamada, H., Yonekura, Y. (2000). Functional asymmetry of human prefrontal cortex in verbal and non-verbal episodic memory as revealed by fMRI. *Brain Research Cognitive Brain Research,* 9(1): 73-83.

Ikeda, A., Lüders, H.O., Collura, T.F., Burgess, R.C., Morris, H.H., Hamano, T., Kimura, J., Luders, H.O., Shibasaki, H. (1996). Subdural potentials at orbitofrontal and mesial prefrontal areas accompanying anticipation and decision-making in humans: A comparison with Bereitschaftspotential. *Electroencephalography Clinical Neurophysiology*, 98: 206-12.

Ikeda, A., Lüders, H.O., Burgess, R.C., Shibasaki, H. (1992). Movement-related potentials recorded from supplementary motor area and primary motor area: Role of supplementary motor area in voluntary movements. *Brain*, 115: 1017-43.

Ikeda, A., Lüders, H.O., Burgess, R.C., Shibasaki, H. (1993). Movement-related potentials associated with single and repetitive movements recorded from human supplementary motor area. *Electroencephalography Clinical Neurophysiology*, 89: 269-77.

Ikeda, A., Lüders, H.O., Shibasaki, H., Collura, T.F., Burgess, R.C., Morris, H.H. 3rd, Hamano, T. (1995). Movement-related potentials associated with bilateral simultaneous and unilateral movement recorded from human supplementary motor area. *Electroencephalography Clinical Neurophysiology*, 95: 323-34.

Ikeda, A., Shibasaki, H., Nagamine, T., Terada, K., Kaji, R., Fukuyama, H., Kimura, J. (1994). Dissociation between contingent negative variation and Bereitschaftspotential in a patient with cerebellar efferent lesion. *Electroencephalography Clinical Neurophysiology*, 90: 359-64.

Ikeda, A., Taki, W., Kunieda, T., Terada, K., Mikuni, N., Nagamine, T., Yazawa, S., Ohara, S., Hori, T., Kaji, R., Kimura, J., Shibasaki, H. (1999). Focal ictal direct current shifts in human epilepsy as studied by subdural and scalp recording. *Brain*, 122: 827-38.

Ingvar, D.H. (1985). "Memory of the future": an essay on the temporal organization of conscious awareness, *Human Neurobiology*, 4: 127-36.

Ingvar, D.H. (1979). "Hyperfrontal" distribution of the cerebral grey matter flow in resting wakefulness; on the functional anatomy of the conscious state, *Acta Neurologica Scandinavica,* 60: 12-25.

Jackson, P.L., Brunet, E., Meltzoff, A.N., Decety, J. (2006). Empathy examined through the neural mechanisms involved in imagining how I feel versus how you feel pain: An event-related fMRI study. *Neuropsychologia,* 44: 752-61.

Jain, S., Shapiro, S.L., Swanick, S., Roesch, S.C., Mills, P.J., Bell, I., Schwartz, G.E. (2007). A randomised controlled trial of mindfulness meditation versus relaxation training: Effects on distress, positive states of mind, rumination, and distraction. *Annals of Behavioral Medicine,* 33(1): 11-21.

James, W. (2005). Dilemma of Determinism. Kessinger Publishing, USA.

James, F.D. (2008). Basal Ganglia and the Striatal Motor System. *Neuroanatomy (Board Review Series)* (4th ed.). Baltimore: Wulters Kluwer and Lippincott Wiliams & Wilkins. 274-81.

Janowsky, J.S., Shimamura, A.P., Kritchevsky, M., Squire, L.R. (1989). Cognitive impairment following frontal lobe damage and its relevance to human amnesia. Cognitive impairment following frontal lobe damage and its relevance to human amnesia. *Behavioral Neuroscience*, 103(3): 548-60.

Jevning, R., Anand, R., Biedebach, M., Fernando, G. (1996). Effects on regional cerebral blood flow of transcendental meditation. *Physiology and Behavior, 59:* 399-402.

Jha, A.P., Stanley, E.A., Kiyonaga, A., Wong, L., Gelfand, L. (2010). Examining the protective effects of mindfulness training on working memory capacity and affective experience. *Emotion,* 10(1): 54-64.

Jobard, G., Crivello, F., Tzourio-Mazoyer, N. (2003). Evaluation of the dual route theory of reading: a metanalysis of 35 neuroimaging studies. *Neuroimage*, 20: 693-712.

Jolicoeur, P. (1998). Modulation of the attentional blink by on-line response selection: evidence from speeded and unspeeded Task—sub-1 decisions. *Memory and Cognition,* 26: 1014-32.

Jolicoeur, P. (1999). Concurrent response-selection demands modulate the attentional blink. *J. Exp. Psychol. Hum. Percept. Perform. Mem. Cogn.*, 25: 979-92.

Joliot, M., Ribary, U., Llinas, R. (1994). Human oscillatory brain activity near 40 Hz coexists with cognitive temporal binding. *Proceedings of the National Academy of Science, USA*, 91: 11748-51.

Jonas, S. (1981). The supplementary motor region and speech emission. *Journal of Communication Disorders,* 14: 349-73.

Jones-Gotman, M., Milner, B. (1977). Design Fluency: The invention of nonsense drawings after focal cortical lesions. *Neuropsychologia*, 15(1): 653-74.

Jonathan, R.L., Roth, T. (2008). Neurophysiology of Sleep and Wakefulness: Basic Science and Clinical Implications. *Current Neuropharmacology*, 6(4): 367-78.

Jones, B.E. (2003). Arousal systems. *Frontiers in Bioscience*, 8: 438-51.

Jones, B.E. (1998). Why and how is the basal forebrain important for modulating cortical activity across the sleep-waking cycle? *INABIS98 SYMPOSIUM.*

Jones, T.C., Jacoby, L.L., Gellis, L. (2001). Cross-modal feature and conjunction errors in recognition memory. *Journal of Memory and Language,* 44: 131-52.

Jones, E.G., Coulter, J.D., Hendry, S.H.C. (1978). Intracortical connectivity of architectonic fields in the somatic sensory, motor, and parietal cortex of monkeys. *Journal of Comparative Neurology,* 181: 291-348.

John, J., Wu, M.F., Boehmer, L.N., Siegel, J.M. (2004). Cataplexy-active neurons in the hypothalamus: implications for the role of histamine in sleep and waking behavior. *Neuron*, 42: 619-34.

Johnson, D.L., Wiebe, J.S., Gold, S.M., Andreasen, N.C. (1999). Cerebral blood flow and personality: A positron emission tomography study. *American Journal of Psychiatry,* 156(2): 252-57.

Jonides, J., Schumacher, E.H., Smith, E.E., Koeppe, R.A., Awh, E., Reuter-Lorenz, P.A., Marshuetz, C., Willis, C.R. (1998). The role of parietal cortex in verbal working memory. *The Journal of Neuroscience,* 18(13): 5026-34.

Jonides, J., Smith, E., Koeppe, R.A., Awh, E., Minoshima, S., Mintun, M.A. (1993). Spatial working memory in humans as revealed by PET. *Nature*, 363: 623-25.

Joyce, E.M., Robbins, T.W. (1991). Frontal lobe function in Korsakoff and non Korsakoff alcoholics: planning and spatial working memory. *Neuropsychologia*, 29(8): 703-23.

Jung, C. (1921). *Psychologischen Typen.* Rascher Verlag, Zurich—translation H.G. Baynes, 1923.

Jung, C. (1995). *Memories, Dreams, Reflections.* London: Fontana Press. 414-15.

Kandel Eric, R., Schwartz James, H., Jessell Thomas, M. (2000). *Principles of Neural Science. Fourth Edition.* United State of America: McGraw-Hill. 324.

Kanter, J.W., Schildcrout, J.S., Kohlenberg, R.J. (2005). In vivo processes in cognitive therapy for depression: Frequency and benefits. *Psychotherapy Research*, 15: 366-73.

Kapur, S., Craik, F.I., Jones, C., Brown, G.M., Houle, S., Tulving, E. (1995). Functional role of the prefrontal cortex in retrieval of memory: a PET study. *Neuroreport,* 6: 1880-84.

Kapur, S., Rose, R., Liddle, P.F., Zipursky, R.B., Brown, G.M., Stuss, D. Houle, S., Tulving, E. (1994a). The role of the prefrontal cortex in verbal processing: semantic processing or willed action? *Neuroreport,* 5: 2193-96.

Kapur, S., Craik, F.I.M., Tulving, E., Wilson, A.A., Houle, S., Brown, G.M. (1994b). Neuroanatomical correlates of encoding in episodic memory: levels of processing effect. *Proceedings of the National Academy of Sciences, U.S.A.*, 91: 2008-11.

Kapur, N. (1990). Korsakoff's psychosis. *Journal of Neurology, Neurosurgery, and Psychiatry*, 53(3): 270.

Keeton, W.T., Gould, J.L. (1986). *Biological Science* (4th Edition). W.W. Norton & Co. Ltd., New York.

Keller, T.A., Carpenter, P.A., Just, M.A. (2001). The neural bases of sentence comprehension: a fMRI examination of syntactic and lexical processing. *Cerebral Cortex,* 11: 223-37.

Kelley, W.M., Miezin, F.M., McDermott, K.B., Buckner, R.L., Raichle, M.E., Cohen, N.J., Ollinger, J.M., Akbudak, E., Conturo, T.E., Snyder, A.Z., Petersen, S.E. (1998). Hemispheric specialization in human dorsal frontal cortex and medial temporal lobe for verbal and nonverbal memory encoding. *Neuron*, 20: 927-36.

Kelso, J.A.S. (1995). Dynamic Patterns: The Self-Organization of Brain and Behavior, MIT Press, Cambridge, MA.

Kelso, J.A., Southard, D.L., Goodman, D. (1979). On the coordination of two-handed movements. *Journal Experimental Psychology: Human Perception and Performance*, 5: 229-38.

Kelso, J.A., Fink, P.W., DeLaplain, C.R., Carson, R.G. (2001). Haptic information stabilizes and destabilizes coordination dynamics. *Proceedings of Royal Society London Series B: Biological Sciences,* 268: 1207-13.

Kessler, H.R., Cohen, R.A., Lauer, K., Kausch, D.F. (1992). The relationship between disability and memory dysfunction in multiple sclerosis. *International Journal of Neuroscience,* 62(1-2): 17-34.

Kessels, R.P., Hensken, L.M. (2009). Effects of errorless skill learning in people with mild-to-moderate or severe dementia: a randomized controlled pilot study. Neuro Rehabilitation, 5(4): 307-12.

Kessels, R.P., Kortrijk, H.E., Wester, A.J., Nys, G.M. (2008). Confabulation behavior and false memories in Korsakoff's syndrome: role of source memory and executive functioning. *Psychiatry Clinical Neuroscience*, 62(2): 220-25.

Khanna, S., Mukundan, C.R., Channabasavanna, S.M. (1989). Bereitschaftspotential in melancholic depression. *Biological Psychiatry*, 26: 526-29.

Khushu, S., Telles, S., Kumaran, S., Naveen, K.V., Tripathi, R.P. (2000). Frontal activation during meditation based on functional magnetic resonance imaging (fMRI). *Indian Journal of Physiology and Pharmacology, 44:* 34.

Kitamura, J., Shibasaki, H., Takagi, A., Nabeshima, H., Yamaguchi, A. (1993). Enhanced negative slope of cortical potentials before sequential as compared with simultaneous extensions of two fingers. *Electroencephalography Clinical Neurophysiology,* 86(3): 176-82.

Kochanska, G., Murray, K.T., Harlan, E.T. (2000). Effortful control in early childhood: Continuity and change, antecedents, and implications for social development. *Developmental Psychology,* 36: 220-32.

Koenig, P., Smith, E.E., Moore, P., Glosser, G., Grossman, M. (2007). Categorization of novel animals by patients with Alzheimer's disease and corticobasal degeneration. *Neuropsychology*, 21(2): 193-206.

Kondo, H., Osaka, N., Osaka, M. (2004). Cooperation of the anterior cingulate cortex and dorsolateral prefrontal cortex for attention shifting. *NeuroImage,* 23(2): 670-79.

Konishi, S., Nakajima, K., Uchida, I., Kikyo, H., Kameyama, M., Miyashita, Y. (1999). Common inhibitory mechanism in human inferior prefrontal cortex revealed by event-related functional MRI. *Brain*, 122: 981-91.

Koppen, C., Spence, C. (2007a). Seeing the light: exploring the Colavita visual dominance effect. *Experimental Brain Research,* 180: 737-54.

Koppen, C., Alsius, A., Spence, C. (2008). Semantic congruency and the Colavita visual dominance effect. *Experimental Brain Research,* 184: 533-46.

Koppen, C., Spence, C. (2007b). Audiovisual asynchrony modulates the Colavita visual dominance effect. *Brain Research,* 224-32.

Kopelman, M.D., Thomson, A.D., Guerrini, I., Marshall, E.J. (2009). "The Korsakoff syndrome: clinical aspects, psychology, and treatment". *Alcohol and Alcoholism,* 44(2): 148-54.

Kornhuber, H.H., Deecke, L. (1965). Hirnpotentialänderungen bei Willkürbewegungen und passiven Bewegungen des Menschen: Bereitschaftspotential und reafferente Potentiale. *Pflüger. Archives Ges. Physiol.*, 284: 1-17.

Kosslyn, S.M., Thompson, W.L., Sukel, K.E., Alpert, N.M. (2005). Two types of image generation: evidence from PET. *Cognitive, Affective, & Behavioral Neuroscience,* 5(1): 41-53.

Kosslyn, S.M., Pascual-Leone, A., Felician, O., Camposano, S., Keenan, J.P., Thompson, W.L., Ganis, G., Sukel, K.E., Alpert, N.M. (1999). The role of area 17 in visual imagery: convergent evidence from PET and rTMS. *Science,* 284(5411): 167-70.

Kosslyn, S.M., Thompson, W.L., Alpert, N.M. (1997). Neural systems shared by visual imagery and visual perception: a positron emission tomography study. *NeuroImage,* 6(4): 320-34.

Klimesch, W., Doppelmayr, M., Rohm, D., Pollhuber, D., Stadler, W. (2000). Simultaneous desynchronization and synchronization of different alpha responses in the human electroencephalograph: a neglected paradox? *Neuroscience Letters,* 284: 97-100.

Klimesch, W., Schimke, H., Schwaiger, J. (1994). Episodic and semantic memory: an analysis in the EEG theta and alpha band. *Electroencephalography Clinical Neurophysiology,* 91: 428-41.

Kramer, J.H., Jurik, J., Sha, S.J., Rankin, K.P., Rosen, H.J., Johnson, J.K., Miller, B.L. (2003). Distinctive neuropsychological patterns in frontotemporal dementia, semantic dementia, and Alzheimer disease. *Cognitive Behavioral Neurology,* 16(4): 211-18.

Kringelbach, M.L. (2005). The orbitofrontal cortex: linking reward to hedonic experience. *Nature Reviews Neuroscience,* 6: 691-702.

Kruggel, F., Brückner, M.K., Arendt, T., Wiggins, C.W., Yves von Cramon, D. (2003). Analysing the neocortical fine-structure. *Medical Image Analysis,* 7(3): 251-64.

Kirshner, H.S. (2011). Transient global amnesia: a brief review and update. *Current Neurology and Neuroscience Report,* (6): 578-82.

LaBar, K.S., Cabeza, R. (2006). Cognitive neuroscience of emotional memory. www.nature.com/reviews/neuro, Nature Publishing Group, 7: 54-64.

LaBar, K.S., Gatenby, J.C., Gore, J.C., LeDoux, J.E., Phelps, E.A. (1998). Human amygdala activation during conditioned fear acquisition and extinction: a mixed-trial fMRI study. *Neuron,* 20(5): 937-45.

LaBar, K.S., Phelps, E.A. (1998). Arousal-mediated memory consolidation: role of the medial temporal lobe in humans. *Psychol. Science,* 9: 527-40.

Ladd, D.R. (1996). *Intonational Phonology.* Cambridge: Cambridge University Press.

Lane, R.D., Fink, G.R., Chau, P.M., Dolan, R.J. (1997). Neural activation during selective attention to subjective emotional responses. *Neuroreport,* 22; 8(18): 3969-72.

Lawrie, S., McIntosh, A., Nadeem, Z. (2002). Schizophrenia. *Clinical Evidence,* (8): 1019-49.

Lazar, S.W., Bush, G., Gollub, R. L., Fricchione, G. L., Khalsa, G., Benson, H. (2000). Functional brain mapping of the relaxation response and meditation. *Neuroreport, 11:* 1581-85.

Lazarus, R. (1991). *Emotion and adaptation.* New York: Oxford University Press.

Laberge, M., Fournier, S., Freeston, M.H., Ladouceur, R., Provencher, M.D. (2000). Structured and free-recall measures of worry themes: effect of order of presentation on worry report. *Journal of Anxiety Disorders,* 14(4): 429-36.

Laplane, D., Degos, J.D., Baulac, M., Gray, F. (1981). Bilateral infarction of the anterior cingulate gyri and of the fornices. Report of a case. *Journal of Neurological Science,* 51(2): 289-300.

LeDoux, J. (1996). Emotional networks and motor control: A fearful view. *Progress in Brain Research*, 107: 437-46.

LeDoux, J. (1998). Fear and the brain: Where have we been, and where are we going? *Biological Psychiatry*, 44: 1229-38.

LeDoux, J. (2003). The emotional brain, fear, and the amygdala. *Cellular and Molecular Neurobiology*, 23: 727-38.

Le Moal, M., Galey, D., Cardo, B. (1975). Behavioral effects of local injection of 6-hydroxydopamine in the medial ventral tegmentum in the rat. Possible role of the mesolimbic dopamingergic system. *Brain Research,* 25; 88(1): 190-94.

Lee, C.C., Winer, J.A. (2008). Connections of cat auditory cortex: III. Corticocortical system. *Journal of Comparative Neurology,* 507: 1920-43.

Lee, A.C., Robbins, T.W., Pickard, J.D., Owen, A.M. (2000). Asymmetric frontal activation during episodic memory: the effects of stimulus type on encoding and retrieval. *Neuropsychologia*, 38: 677-92.

Lee, L.K. (2007). Controversies in the sequelae of pediatric mild traumatic brain injury. *Pediatric Emergency Care,* 23(8): 580-83.

Lehmann, D., Faber, P.L., Achermann, P., Jeanmonod, D., Gianotti, L.R., Pizzagalli, D. (2001). Brain sources of EEG gamma frequency during volitionally meditation-induced, altered states of consciousness, and experience of the self. *Psychiatry Research, 108:* 111-21.

Leotti, L.A., Wager, T.D. (2010). Motivational Influences on Response Inhibition Measures. *Journal of Experimental Psychology: Human Perception and Performance,* 36(2): 430-37.

Lepage, M., Habib, R., Tulving, E. (1998). Hippocampal PET activations of memory encoding and retrieval: The HIPER model. *Hippocampus*, 8: 313-22.

Lepage, M., Ghaffar, O., Nyberg, L., Tulving, E. (2000). Prefrontal cortex and episodic memory retrieval mode. *Proceedings of National Academy of Science, U.S.A.*, 97: 506-11.

Leveroni, C.L., Seidenberg, M., Mayer, A.R., Mead, L.A., Binder, J.R., Rao, S.M. (2000). Neural systems underlying the recognition of familiar and newly learned faces. *Journal of Neuroscience*, 20: 878-86.

Levin, H.S., Papanicolaou, A., Eisenberg, H.M. (1984). Observations on amnesia after nonmissile head injury. In: L.R. Squire, N. Butters (eds.), *Neuropsychology of Memory*. London: Guilford Press. 247-57.

Levin, H.S. (1990). Memory deficit after closed head injury. *Journal of Clinical & Experimental Neuropsychology*, 12(1): 129-53.

Lezak, M.D., Howieson, D.B., Loring, D.W. (2004). *Neuropsychological Assessment* (4th ed.). New York: Oxford University Press.

Lezak, M.D. (1982). Neuropsychological Assessment. 2nd ed. Oxford University Press.

Lezak, M.D. (1995). Neuropsychological Assessment. Third Edition. New York: Oxford University Press.

Lhermitte, F., Pillon, B., Serdaru, M. (1986). Human autonomy and the frontal lobes. Part I: Imitation and utilization behavior: A neuropsychological study of 75 patients. *Annals of Neurology*, 19(4): 326-34.

Lhermitte, F. (1983). 'Utilization behaviour' and its relation to lesions of the frontal lobes. *Brain*, 106: 237-55.

Libet, B. (1978). Neuronal vs. subjective timing, for a conscious sensory experience. P.A. Buser, A. Rougeul-Buser (Eds.), *Cerebral Correlates of Conscious Experience*, 69-82, Amsterdam/New York: North Holland.

Libet, B., Gleason, C.A., Wright, E.W. Jr., Pearl, D.K. (1983). Time of conscious intention to act in relation to onset of cerebral activity (readiness potential). *Brain*, 106: 623-42.

Libet, B. (1985). Unconscious cerebral initiative and the role of conscious will in voluntary action. *The Behavioural and Brain Sciences*, 8: 529-39; with open peer commentary: 539-58; and Libet's reply, *Theory and evidence relating cerebral processes to conscious will*. 558-66.

Libet, B. (1999). Do we have free will? *Journal of Consciousness Studies*, 6: 47-57.

Libet, B. (2001). Consciousness, free action and the brain. *Journal of Consciousness Studies*, 8: 59-65.

Liebenthal, E., Binder, J.R., Spitzer, S.M., Possing, E.T., Medler, D.A. (2005). Neural substrates of phonemic perception. *Cerebral Cortex*, 15: 1621-31.

Liégeois-Chauvel, C., de Graaf, J.B., Laguitton, V., Chauvel, P. (1999). Specialization of left auditory cortex for speech perception in man depends on temporal coding. *Cerebral Cortex*, 9(5): 484-96.

Linehan, M.M. (1993). Cognitive behavioural treatment of borderline personality disorder. Nueva York: Guilford Press.

Liston, C., Matalon, S., Hare, T.A., Davidson, M.C., Casey, B.J. (2006). Anterior Cingulate and Posterior Parietal Cortices Are Sensitive to Dissociable Forms of Conflict in a Task-Switching Paradigm. *Neuron*, 50(4): 643-53.

Liu, G., Chua, R., Enns, J.T. (2008). Attention for perception and action: task interference for action planning, but not for online control. *Experimental Brain Research*, 185(4): 709-17.

Lorber, M.F. (2004). Psychophysiology of aggression, psychopathy, and conduct problems: a meta-analysis. *Psychological Bulletin*, 130: 531-52.

Lorenz, Konrad (1973). *Behind the Mirror, A Search for a Natural History of Human Knowledge*. R. Piper & Co., Verlag. English translation (1977), Methuen & Co.

Lou, H.C., Kjaer, T.W., Friberg, L., Wildschiodtz, G., Holm, S., Nowak, M. (1999). A 15O-H2O PET study of meditation and the resting state of normal consciousness. *Human Brain Mapping, 7:* 98-105.

Lovblad, K., Dierks, T. (2004). Pathways that make voices: white matter changes in auditory hallucinations. *Archives of General Psychiatry,* 61(7): 658-68.

Lu, J., Greco, M.A., Shiromani, P., Saper, C.B. (2000). Effect of lesions of the ventrolateral preoptic nucleus on NREM and REM sleep. *Journal Neuroscience,* 20: 3830-42.

Lucas, R.E., Le, K., Dyrenforth, P.S. (2008). Explaining the extraversion/positive affect relation: Sociability cannot account for extraverts greater happiness. *Journal of Personality,* 76: 387-414.

Lutz, A., Greischar, L.L., Rawlings, N.B., Ricard, M., Davidson, R.J. (2004). Long-term meditators self-induced high-amplitude gamma synchrony during mental practice. *Proceedings of the National Academy of Sciences, U.S.A., 101*: 16369-73.

Lutz, A., Greischar, L., Ricard, M., Converse, A., Davidson, R.J. (2003). *Comparative study of synchrony patterns during three meditative states: Preliminary data.* Paper presented at the meeting of the Society for Neuroscience, New Orleans, LA.

Luu, P., Posner, M.I. (2003). Anterior cingulate cortex regulation of sympathetic activity. *Brain,* 126: 2119-20.

Luria, A.R. (1966a). Higher Cortical Functions in Man. Basic Books, New York.

Luria, A.R. (1966b). Human Brain and Psychological Processes. Harper & Row.

Luria, A.R. (1969). Frontal lobe syndromes. In P.J. Vinken and G.W. Bruyn (Eds.), *Handbook of Clinical Neurology, II.* New York: Elsevier.

Luria, A.R. (1970). The functional organization of the brain. *Scientific American*, 222(3): 66-78.

Luria, A.R. (1973). *The Working Brain.* Basic Books.

Luria, A.R. (1999). Outline for the neuropsychological examination of patients with local brain lesions. *Neuropsychology Review,* 9(1): 9-22.

Ma, S.H., Teasdale, J.D. (2004). Mindfulness-based cognitive therapy for depression: Replication and exploration of differential relapse prevention effects. *Journal of Consulting and Clinical Psychology,* 72(1): 31-40.

Mace, C.J., Trimble, M.R. (1991). Psychosis following temporal lobe surgery: a report of six cases. *J. Neurology, Neurosurgery & Psychiatry*, 54: 639-44.

MacLean, P.D. (1990). The Triune Brain in Evolution: Role in Paleocerebral Functions, Springer.

Macpherson, J.M., Marangoz, C., Miles, T.S., Wiesendanger, M. (1982). Microstimulation of the supplementary motor area (SMA) in the awake monkey. *Experimental Brain Research*, 45: 410-16.

Maguire, E.A., Frith, C.D. (2003). Lateral asymmetry in the hippocampal response to the remoteness of autobiographical memories. *Journal of Neuroscience*, 23: 5302-07.

Madhavi, R., Mukundan, C.R. (1999). *Slow DC Potentials and the Study of Volition.* Unpublished Ph.D. thesis submitted to National Institute of Mental Health & Neuro Sciences, Deemed University, Bangalore.

Makris, N., Kennedy, D.N., McInerney, S., Sorensen, A.G., Wang, R., Caviness, V.S. Jr, Pandya, D.N. (2005). Segmentation of subcomponents within the superior longitudinal fascicle in humans: a quantitative, in vivo, DT-MRI study. *Cerebral Cortex,* 15(6): 854-69.

Malia, K., Powell, G., Torode, S. (1995). Personality and psychosocial function after brain injury. *Brain Injury,* 9(7): 697-12.

Mandler, G. (1980). Recognizing: The judgment of prior occurrence. *Psychological Review*, 87: 252-71.

Mandler, G. (1984). *Mind and Body: Psychology of emotion and stress.* New York: Norton.

Manicavasgar, V., Parker, G., Perich, T. (2011). Mindfulness-based Cognitive Therapy Vs. Cognitive Behaviour Therapy as a Treatment for Non-Melancholic Depression. *Journal of Affective Disorders,* 130(1-2): 138-44.

Mansouri, F.A., Tanaka, K., Buckley, M.J. (2009). Conflict-induced behavioural adjustment: a clue to the executive functions of the prefrontal cortex. *Nature Reviews Neuroscience*, 10: 141-52.

Markowitsch, H.J., Vandekerckhove, M.M., Lanfermann, H., Russ, M.O. (2003): Engagement of lateral and medial prefrontal areas in the ecphory of sad and happy autobiographical memories. *Cortex,* 39(4-5): 643-65.

Marois, R., Chun, M.M. (2000). Neural Correlates of the Attentional Blink. *Neuron*, 28: 299-308.

Marsh, R.L., Hicks, J.L., Taylor, T.D. (2002). Source monitoring does not alleviate (and may exacerbate) the occurrence of memory conjunction errors. *Journal of Memory and Language*, 47(2): 315-26.

Marteniuk, R.G., MacKenzie, C.L., Baba, D.M. (1984). Bimanual movement control: information processing and interaction effects. *Quarterly Journal of Experimental Psychology,* 36A: 335-65.

Martí-Fàbregas, J., Cocho, D., Lleó, A., Martí-Vilalta, J.L. (2000). Transcranial Doppler recording in a patient with transient positional cerebral ischemia. *Neurology,* 12; 55(5): 731-32.

Martin, R.C., He, T. (2004). Semantic short-term memory and its role in sentence processing: a replication. *Brain Language*, 89: 76-82.

Masayuki, K. (2006). Functional Organization of the Human Gustatory Cortex. *Journal of Oral Biosciences,* 48(4): 244-60.

Mashour, G.A. (2004a). Consciousness unbound: toward a paradigm of general anesthesia. *Anesthesiology*, 100: 428-33.

Mashour, G.A. (2004b). The cognitive binding problem: from Kant to quantum neurodynamics. *NeuroQuantology*, 1: 29-38.

Mashour, G.A., Walker, E.E., Martuza, R.L. (2005). Psychosurgery: past, present, and future. *Brain Research Reviews*, 48: 409-19.

Maslow, A.H. (1987). Motivation and Personality. Third Ed. NY: Addison-Wesley.

Matsuhashi, M., Hallett, M. (2008). The timing of the conscious intention to move. *European Journal of Neuroscience*, 28(11): 2344-51.

Max, J.E., Robertson, B.A., Lansing, A.E. (2001). The phenomenology of personality change due to traumatic brain injury in children and adolescents. *Journal of Neuropsychiatry Clinical Neuroscience*, 13(2): 161-70.

Mellet, E., Tzourio-Mazoyer, N., Bricogne, S., Mazoyer, B., Kosslyn, S.M., Denis, M. (2000). Functional anatomy of high-resolution visual mental imagery. *Journal of Cognitive Neuroscience*, 12: 98-109.

Meltzoff, A.N., Brooks, R. (2001). 'Like me' as a building block for understanding other minds: bodily acts, attention and intention. In B.F. Malle, L.J. Moses, D.A. Baldwin (Eds.), *Intentions and Intentionality: Foundations for Social Cognition*, 171-92. MIT Press.

"Max Wertheimer memorial issue", *Psychological Research*, 51(2): 43-85 (1989).

McCarthy, G., Puce, A., Constable, R.T., Krystal, J.H., Gore, J.C., Goldman-Rakic, P. (1996). Activation of human prefrontal cortex during spatial and nonspatial working memory tasks measured by functional MRI. *Cerebral Cortex*, 6: 600-11.

McCarthy, R., Warrington, E.K. (1984). A two-route model of speech production. Evidence from aphasia. *Brain*, 107, 463-85.

McDaniel, M.A., Einstein, G.O. (2007). *Prospective memory: An overview and synthesis of an emerging field.* Sage Publications.

McDaniel, M.A., Einstein, G.O., Graham, T., Rall, E. (2004). Delaying execution of intentions: Overcoming the costs of interruptions. *Applied Cognitive Psychology*, 18: 533-47.

McDermott, K.B., Buckner, R.L., Petersen, S.E., Kelley, W.M., Sanders, A.L. (1999). Set- and code-specific activation in frontal cortex: an fMRI study of encoding and retrieval of faces and words. *Journal Cognitive Neuroscience,* 11: 631-40.

McGaugh, J.L. (2000). Memory—a Century of Consolidation. *Science,* 287(5451): 248-51.

McGuire, P.K., Silbersweig, D.A., Frith, C.D. (1996a). Functional neuroanatomy of verbal self-monitoring.*Brain*, 119(Pt 3): 907-17.

McGuire, P.K., Silbersweig, D.A., Wright, I., Murray, R.M., Frackowiak, R.S.J., Frith, C.D. (1996b). The neural correlates of inner speech and auditory verbal imagery in schizophrenia: Relationship to auditory verbal hallucinations. *British Journal of Psychiatry*, 169(2): 148-59.

McGinty, D., Szymusiak, R. (2000). The sleep-wake switch: A neuronal alarm clock. *Nature Medicine,* 6: 510-11.

McKinlay, W.W., Brooks, D.N., Bond, M.R., Martinage, D.P., Marshall, M.M. (1981). The short-term outcome of severe blunt head injury as reported by relatives of the injured persons. Journal of Neurology, *Neurosurgery & Psychiatry*, 44(6): 527-33.

McElree, B. (2001). Working memory and focal attention. *Journal of Experimental Psychology: Learning, Memory, & Cognition*, 27(3): 817-35.

McDermid Vaz, S.A., Heinrichs, R.W. (2002). Schizophrenia and memory impairment: evidence for a neurocognitive subtype. *Psychiatry Research,* 113(1-2): 93-105.

McNabb, A.W., Carroll, W.M., Mastaglia, F.L. (1988). "Alien hand" and loss of bimanual coordination after dominant anterior cerebral artery territory infarction. *Journal of Neurology, Neurosurgery, and Psychiatry,* 51(2): 218-22.

Mendez, M.F., Adams, N.L., Lewandowski, K.S. (1989). Neurobehavioral changes associated with caudate lesions. *Neurology,* 19: 349-54.

Meredith, M.A., Stein, B.E. (1986). Visual, auditory, and somatosensory convergence on cells in superior colliculus results in multisensory integration. *Journal of Neurophysiology*, 56: 640-62.

Meredith, M.A. (2004). Cortico-cortical connectivity and the architecture of cross-modal circuits. In C. Spence, G. Calvert, B. Stein. (Eds.), *Handbook of Multisensory Processes*. Cambridge, MA: MIT Press. 343-55.

Mesulam, M.M. (1998). From Sensation to Cognition. *Brain*, 121: 1013-52.

Mesulam, M.M. (1981). A cortical network for directed attention and unilateral neglect. *Archives of Neurology,* 10: 304-25.

Meyer, M., Zaehle, T., Gountouna, V.E., Barron, A., Jancke, L., Turk, A. (2005). Spectro-temporal processing during speech perception involves left posterior auditory cortex. *NeuroReport,* 16: 1985-89.

Miller, G.A. (1956). The Magical Number Seven, Plus or Minus Two: Some Limits on our Capacity for Processing Information. *Psychological Review*, 63: 81-97.

Millis, S.R., Rosenthal, M., Novack, T.A., Sherer, M., Nick, T.G., Kreutzer, J.S., High, W.M. Jr, Ricker, J.H. (2001). Long-term neuropsychological outcome after traumatic brain injury. *Journal of Head Trauma and Rehabilitation,* 16(4): 343-55.

Miller, E.K., Cohen, J.D. (2001). An integrative theory of prefrontal cortex function. *Annual Review of Neuroscience,* 24(1): 167-202.

Miller, G.A., Galanter, E., Pribram, K.H. (1960). Plans and the Structure of Behavior. Holt, Rinehart & Winston, New York. 65.

Miller, F.D., Hicks, S.P., D'Amato, C.J., Landis, J.R. (1984). A descriptive study of neuritic plaques and neurofibrillary tangles in an autopsy population. *American Journal of Epidemiology,* 120(3): 331-41.

Miller, M.B., Kingstone, A., Gazzaniga, M.S. (2002). Hemispheric encoding asymmetry is more apparent than real. *Journal of Cognitive Neuroscience,* 14: 702-08.

Milner, B. (2005). The medial temporal-lobe amnesic syndrome. *Psychiatric Clinics of North America,* 28(3): 599-611.

Milner, B., Petrides, M., Smith, M.L. (1985). Frontal lobes and the temporal organization of memory. *Human Neurobiology,* 4(3): 137-42.

Milner, A.D., Paulignan, Y., Dijkerman, H.C., Michel, F., Jeannerod, M. (1999). A paradoxical improvement of misreaching in optic ataxia: New evidence for two separate neural systems for visual localization. *Proceedings of the Royal Society*, London. B 266: 2225-29.

Milner, A.D., Perrett, D.I., Johnston, R.S., Benson, P.J., Jordan, T.R., Heeley, D.W., Bettucci, D., Mortara, F., Mutani, R., Terazzi, E., Davidson, D.L.W. (1991). Perception and action in "visual form agnosia". *Brain,* 114(Pt 1B): 405-28.

Mitchell, R.L., Elliott, R., Barry, M., Cruttenden, A., Woodruff, P.W. (2003). The neural response to emotional prosody, as revealed by functional magnetic resonance imaging. *Neuropsychologia*, 41: 1410-21.

Miyaki, A., Friedman, N.P., Emerson, M.J., Witzki, A.H., Howerter, A., Wagner, T.D. (2000). The unity and diversity of executive functions and their contributions to complex 'frontal lobe' tasks: A latent variable analysis. *Cognitive Psychology,* 41(1): 49-100.

Monsell, S. (2003). Task switching. *TRENDS in Cognitive Sciences,* 7(3): 134-40.

Moore, J., Haggard, P. (2008). Awareness of action: Inference and prediction. *Consciousness and Cognition, 17*: 136-44.

Moore, J.W., Lagnado, D., Deal, D.C. Haggard, P. (2009). Feelings of control: contingency determines experience of action. *Cognition,* 110(2): 279-83.

Morecraft, R.J., Geula, C., Mesulam, M.M. (1992). Cytoarchitecture and neural afferents of orbitofrontal cortex in the brain of the monkey. *Journal of Comparative Neurology*, 15; 323(3): 341-58.

Morin, A. (1993). Self-talk and self-awareness: On the nature of the relation. *The Journal of Mind and Behavior*, 14: 223-34.

Morin, A. (1995). Characteristics of an effective internal dialogue in the acquisition of self information. *Imagination, Cognition and Personality*, 15(1): 45-58.

Morris, J.S., Ohman, A., Dolan, R.J. (1998). Conscious and unconscious emotional learning in the human amygdala. *Nature*, 4; 393(6684): 467-70.

Moscovitch, M. (1992). Memory and working with memory: A component process model based on modules and central systems. *Journal of Cognitive Neuroscience,* 4: 257-67.

Moscovitch, M. (1994). Memory and working with memory: Evaluation of a component process model and comparisons with other models. In D.L. Schacter and E. Tulving (Eds.), *Memory Systems* 269-310. Cambridge: MIT Bradford Press.

Moscovitch, M., Nadel, L. (1998). Consolidation and the hippocampal complex revisited: In defense of the multiple-trace model. *Current Opinion in Neurobiology,* 8: 297-300.

Moscovitch, M., Winocur, G. (2002). The frontal cortex and working with memory. In D.T. Stuss, R.T. Knight (Eds.), *Principles of Frontal Lobe Function,* 188-209. New York: University Press.

Moscovitch, M., Rosenbaum, R.S., Gilboa, A., Addis, D.R., Westmacott, R., Grady, C., McAndrews, M.P., Levine, B., Black, S., Winocur, G., Nadel, L. (2005). Functional neuroanatomy of remote episodic, semantic and spatial memory: A unified account base on multiple trace theory. *Journal of Anatomy*, 207: 35-66.

Mostofsky, S.H., Simmonds, D.J. (2008). Response inhibition and response selection: two sides of the same coin. *Journal of Cognitive Neuroscience,* 20(5): 751-61.

Mukundan, C.R. (2013). Neurocognitive aspects of perception. In S. Painadath SJ, M.N. Sreekala (Eds.), *Perception: An Interdisciplinary Exploration*, ISPCK/Sameeksha, Cambridge Press, New Delhi. 189-205.

Mukundan, C.R., Kamarajan, C., Ajayan, P., Roopesh, B.N., Sharma, M. (2013). Frontal Cortex and Recognition: Neurocognitive Findings of Hypnosis. *Indian Journal of Health and Welfare,* 4(4): 703-10.

Mukundan, C.R. (2012). Restoration of cognitive functions using computer aided programs in patients afflicted with traumatic brain injury and other brain lesions. In Jamuna, R. (Ed.), *Neuropsychological Rehabilitation—Principles and Applications*. Elsevier Publication. 11-32.

Mukundan, C.R. (2011a). Scientific methods of extraction of information from suspects: An analysis of current trends. *Indian Journal of Clinical Psychology*, 38(2): 129-40.

Mukundan, C.R. (2011b). Experiencing: Method of establishing contact with reality and its self-verification. In: A.K. Chouhan, S.S. Nathawat (Eds.), *New Facets of Positivism.* Macmillan Publishers India, Delhi. 393-404.

Mukundan, C.R., Hemalata, M. (2011c). Neurocognitive deficits and their restoration leading to rehabilitation in brain damaged patients. in C.R. Mukundan, Tej Behadur Singh (Consultant Editors) and Vibha Sharma, Shahazadi Malhotra (Eds). *Clinical Neuropsychology: Assessment and Rehabilitation—A Practical Approach*. Rashtra Bhasha Offset Press, Agra. 57-109.

Mukundan, C.R., Ajayan, P. (2011c). Awareness and Self-Image. *Indian Journal of Clinical Psychology*, 38(1): 37-48.

Mukundan, C.R. (2010). Reading from memory: a paradigm shift for deception detection in investigative psychology. *Amity Journal of Applied Psychology*, 1(1): 24-34.

Mukundan, C.R. (2009). Neural Correlates of Experience. In A. Surila, Ira Das, K. Kavita, K. Surat (Eds.), *Health Psychology*. Allied Publishers, New Delhi. 46-58.

Mukundan, C.R. (2008). Brain Electrical Oscillations Signature Profiling for Crime Investigation. In V. Veeraraghavan (Ed.), *Handbook of Forensic Psychology*. Selective & Scientific Books, New Delhi. 123-46.

Mukundan C.R. (2007a). *Brain Experience: Neuroexperiential Perspectives of Brain-Mind*. Atlantic Publishers, New Delhi.

Mukundan, C.R. (2007b). Brain Signature Profiling for Crime Detection. In: Krian Rao, Indira Jai Prakas, K. Srinivasan (Eds.), *Mindscapes: Global Perspectives on Psychology in Mental Health*. NIMHANS Publication. 282-97.

Mukundan, C.R. (1999a). Power of Words: Neuro-cognitive Approach for Understanding Brain Mechanisms of Awareness. In: Sangeetha Menon, M.G. Narasimhan, *Scientific and Philosophical Studies on Consciousness*. National Institute of Advanced Studies, Bangalore, India. 127-36.

Mukundan, C.R., Mukundan, H. (1999b). Encoding, memory, and retrieval: Hypothetical issues and clinical findings. In: S.K. Misra (Ed.), *Biology and Behaviour*. New Delhi: Concept Publishers.

Mukundan, C.R., Ramachandra, S., Singh, S., Sharma, M., Kamaraj, C. (1999c). Brain mechanisms of hypnosis: P300 studies. *Indian Journal of Clinical Psychology*, 26(1): 13-23.

Mukundan, C.R. (1998). From perception to thinking–Verbal adaptation in human brain. In: J.R. Isaac, H. Purendu (Eds.), *Proceedings of International Conference on Cognitive Systems*. New Delhi: Allied Publishers. XXXIX-XIII.

Mukundan, C.R. (1997). On mind, memory and brain. *Indian Journal of Clinical Psychology*, 24: 103-12.

Mukundan, C.R. (1996). NIMHANS neuropsychological battery: test descriptions, instructions, clinical data and interpretation. In *Proceedings of the National Workshop in Clinical Neuropsychology: 24-29 October NIMHANS, Bangalore, India*. Bangalore: NIMHANS Publications.

Mukundan, C.R. (1996a). Some psychophysiological and neuropsychological aspects of alcohol dependence. In: R. Ray, R.W. Pickens (Eds.), *Proceedings of Indo-US symposium on alcohol and drug abuse*. NIMHANS Publication, Bangalore. 227-36.

Mukundan, C.R., Rao, S.L., Jain, V.K., Jayakumar, P.N., Shilaja, K. (1991). Neuropsychological assessment: a cross validation study with neuroradiological/operative findings in patients with cerebral hemisphere lesions. *Pharmacopsychoecologia*, 4: 33-39.

Mukundan, C.R., Narayana Reddy, G.N., Hegde, A.S., Jayathi, Shankar (1990). Effects of long-term recovery on the middle latency components of evoked potential responses in head injury patients. *Pharmacopsychoecologia*, 2: 49-56.

Mukundan, C.R., Narayana Reddy, G.N., Hegde, A.S., Jayanthi, Shankar, Kaliaperumal, V.G. (1987). Neuropsychological and clinical recovery in patients with head trauma. *NIMHANS Journal*, 5(1): 23-31.

Mukundan, C.R. (1986a) *Evoked Potentials: Basic Principles and Methods*. NIMHANS Publications, No. 11.

Mukundan, C.R. (1986b). Computed EEG in schizophrenics. *Biological Psychiatry*, 21: 1225-28.

Mukundan, C.R., Singh, J., Ray, R., Desai, N. (1986c). Bereitschaftspotential in alcoholics. *Biological Psychiatry*, 21: 1090-92.

Mukundan, C.R. (1986d). Middle latency components of evoked potential responses in schizophrenics. *Biological Psychiatry*, 21: 1097-1100.

Mukundan, C.R., Murthy, V.N. (1979a). Lateralizing and localizing cerebral lesions by a battery of neuropsychological tests. Paper presented in the Joint Conference of Neurology, Psychiatry, Clinical Psychology and Psychiatric Social Work Societies of India, at National Institute of Mental Health & Neuro Sciences, Bangalore, December 1979.

Mukundan, C.R., Murthy, V.N., Hemalata, M. (1979b). Battery of tests of learning and memory function for assessing temporal lobe involvement. Paper presented in the Joint conference of Indian Societies of Neurology, Psychiatry, Clinical Psychology, and Psychiatric Social Work Societies of India, at National Institute of Mental Health & Neuro Sciences, Bangalore, December 1979.

Muller, V.A., Brass, M., Waszak, F., Prinz, W. (2007). The role of the pre-SMA and the rostral cingulate zone in internally selected actions. *NeuroImage*, *37*: 1354-61.

Mushiake, H., Inase, M., Tanji, J. (1991). Neuronal activity in the primate premotor, supplementary, and precentral motor cortex during visually guided and internally determined sequential movements. *Journal of Neurophysiology*. 66(3): 705-18.

Murthy, V.N., Fetz, E.E. (1992). Coherent 25- to 35-Hz oscillations in the sensorimotor cortex of awake behaving monkeys. *Proceedings of National Academy of Sciences, U.S.A.* 89: 5670-74.

Murray, E.A., Coulter, J.D. (1981). Supplementary sensory are: The medial parieztal cortex in the monkey. In C.N. Woolsey (Ed), *Cortical Sensory Organization*, vol. 1: Multiple Somatic Areas, Humana Press.

Nachev, P., Kennard, C., Husain, M. (2008). Functional role of the supplementary and presupplementary motor areas. *Nature Reviews Neuroscience,* 9: 856-69.

Nagai, Y., Critchley, H.D., Featherstone, E., Fenwick, P.B., Trimble, M.R., Dolan, R.J. (2004). Brain activity relating to the contingent negative variation: an fMRI investigation. *NeuroImage.* 21(4): 1232-41.

Naghavi, H.R., Nyberg, L. (2005). Common fronto-parietal activity in attention, memory, and consciousness: shared demands on integration? *Consciousness & Cognition*, 14(2): 390-425.

Nakai, T., Matsuo, K., Kato, C., Matsuzawa, M., Okada, T., Glover, G.H., Moriya, T., Inui, T. (1999). A functional magnetic resonance imaging study of listening comprehension of languages in human at 3 tesla: comprehension level and activation of the language areas. *Neuroscience Letters*, 263: 33-36.

Narayanan, N.S., Prabhakaran, V., Bunge, S.A., Christoff, K., Fine, E.M., Gabrieli, J.D. (2005). The role of the prefrontal cortex in the maintenance of verbal working memory: an event-related FMRI analysis. *Neuropsychology*, 19(2): 223-32.

Narr, K.L., Woods, R.P., Thompson, P.M., Szeszko, P., Robinson, D., Dimtcheva, T., Gurbani, M., Toga, A.W., Bilder, R.M. (2007). Relationships between IQ and Regional Cortical Grey Matter Thickness in Healthy Adults. *Cerebral Cortex*, 17(9): 2163-71.

Nash, J. (1950a). Equilibrium points in n-person games. *Proceedings of the National Academy of Sciences*, USA, 36(1): 48-49.

Nash, J. (1950b). The Bargaining Problem. *Econometrica*, 18: 155-62.

Nash, J. (1951). Non-cooperative Games. *Annals of Mathematics*, 54: 286-95.

Newberg, A., Alavi, A., Baime, M., Pourdehnad, M., Santanna, J., d'Aquili, E. (2001). The measurement of regional cerebral blood flow during the complex cognitive task of meditation: A preliminary SPECT study. *Psychiatry Research, 106:* 113-22.

Newberg, A., Pourdehnad, M., Alavi, A., d'Aquili, E.G. (2003). Cerebral blood flow during meditative prayer: Preliminary findings and methodological issues. *Perceptual and Motor Skills*, 97: 625-30.

Niebur, E., Koch, C., Rosin, C. (1993). An oscillation-based model for the neuronal basis of attention. *Vision Research*, 33: 2789-2802.

Nieuwenhuys, R., Ten Donkelaar, H.J., Nicholson, C. (1998). The Central Nervous System of Vertebrates, Vol. 3, Berlin: Springer.

Nolte, John (2002). *The Human Brain: An Introduction to Its Functional Anatomy*, 5th Ed. St. Louis: Mosby, 410-47.

Noel, A., Quinette, P., Guillery-Girard, B., Dayan, J., Piolino, P., Marquis, S., De La Sayette, V., Viader, F., Desgranges, B., Eustache, F. (2008). Psychopathological factors, memory disorders and transient global amnesia. *The British Journal of Psychiatry*, 193(2): 145-51.

Norman, J. (2002). Two visual systems and two theories of perception: An attempt to reconcile the constructivist and ecological approaches. *Behavioral and Brain Sciences. Cambridge University Press*. 25: 73-144.

Norman, D.A. (1968). Toward a theory of memory and attention. *Psychological Review*, 75: 522-36.

Nyberg, L., Eriksson, J., Larsson, A., Marklund, P. (2006). Learning by doing versus learning by thinking: An fMRI study of motor and mental training. *Neuropsychologia*, 44(5): 711-17.

Nyberg, L., Cabeza, R., Tulving, E. (1996a). PET studies of encoding and retrieval: the HERA model. *Psychonomic Bulletin & Review*, 3: 135-48.

Nyberg, L., McIntosh, A.R., Cabeza, R., Habib, R., Houle, S., Tulving, E. (1996b). General and specific brain regions involved in encoding and retrieval of events: what, where, and when. *Proceedings of National Academy of Science, U.S.A.*, 93: 11280-85.

Obhi, S.S., Haggard, P. (2004). Internally generated and externally triggered actions are physically distinct and independently controlled. *Experimental Brain Research, 156*: 518-23.

Obleser, J., Zimmermann, J., Van Meter, J., Rauschecker, J.P. (2007). Multiple stages of auditory speech perception reflected in event-related FMRI. *Cerebral Cortex*, 17: 2251-57.

Ochsner, K.N., Bunge, S.A., Gross, J.J., Gabrieli, J.D.E. (2002). Rethinking feelings: An fMRI study of the cognitive regulation of emotion. *Journal of Cognitive Neuroscience*, 14: 1215-29.

Oddy, M., Coughlan, T., Tyerman, A., Jenkins, D. (1985). Social adjustment after closed head injury: a further follow-up seven years after injury. *Journal of Neurology, Neurosurgery & Psychiatry,* 48(6): 564-68.

Ohman, A., Soares, J.J. (1998). Emotional conditioning to masked stimuli: expectancies for aversive outcomes following nonrecognized fear-relevant stimuli. *Journal of Experimental Psychology: General,* 127(1): 69-82.

O'Hara, P.A. (2008). Principle of circular and cumulative causation: fusing Myrdalian and Kaldorian growth and development dynamics. *Journal of Economic Issues*, 42(2): 375-87.

Olney, R.K., Murphy, J., Forshew, D., Garwood, E., Miller, B.L., Langmore, S., Kohn, M.A., Lomen-Hoerth, C. (2005). The effects of executive and behavioral dysfunction on the course of ALS. *Neurology,* 65(11): 1774-77.

Osaka, N., Osaka, M., Kondo, H., Morishita, M., Fukuyama, H., Shibasaki, H. (2004). The neural basis of executive function in working memory: an fMRI study based on individual differences. *NeuroImage,* 21(2): 623-31.

Oudman, E., Van der Stigchel, S., Wester, A.J., Kessels, R.P., Postma, A. (2011). Intact memory for implicit contextual information in Korsakoff's amnesia. *Neuropsychologia*, 49(10): 2848-55.

Owen, A.M., McMillan, K.M., Laird, A.R., Bullmore, E. (2005). N-back working memory paradigm: a meta-analysis of normative functional neuroimaging studies. *Human Brain Mapping,* 25(1): 46-59.

Owen, A.M., Morris, R.G., Sahakian, B.J., Polkey, C.E., Robbins, T.W. (1996). Double dissociations of memory and executive functions in working memory tasks following frontal lobe excisions, temporal lobe excisions or amygdalo-hippocampectomy in man. *Brain*, 119: 1597-615.

Owen, A.M., Stern, C.E., Look, R.B., Tracey, I., Rosen, B.R., Petrides, M. (1998). Functional organization of spatial and nonspatial working memory processing within the human lateral frontal cortex. *Proceedings of National Academy of Sciences, U.S.A.*, 95: 7721-26.

Oyebode, F. (2008). The neurology of psychosis. *Medical Principles and Practice*, 17(4): 263-69.

Pakkenberg, B. and Gundersen, H.J.G. (1997). Neocortical neuron number in humans: effect of sex and age. *Journal of Comparative Neurology*, 384: 312-20.

Pakkenberg, B., Pelvig, D., Marner, L., Bundgaard, M.J., Gundersen, H.J.G., Nyengaard, J.R. and Regeur, L. (2003). Aging and the human neocortex. *Experimental Gerontology*, 38: 95-99.

Paller, K.A., Hutson, C.A., Miller, B.B., Boehm, S.G. (2003). Neural manifestations of memory with and without awareness. *Neuron*, 38, 507-16.

Paller, K.A., Acharya, A. (1997). Functional neuroimaging of cortical dysfunction in alcoholic Korsakoff's syndrome. *Journal of Cognitive Neuroscience*, 9(2): 277-93.

Pandya, D.N., Kuypers, H.G.J.M. (1969). Corticocortical connections in the rhesus monkey. *Brain Research*, 13: 13-36.

Parvizi, J., Damasio, A. (2001). Consciousness and the brainstem.*Cognition*, 79(1-2): 135-60.

Pastötter, B., Hanslmayr, S., Bäuml, K-H.T. (2010). Conflict processing in the anterior cingulate cortex constrains response priming. *NeuroImage*, 50, 1599-1605.

Patrick, C.J. (2006). Getting to the heart of psychopathy. In H. Herve, J.C. Yuille (Eds.), *Psychopathy: Theory, Research, and Social Implications*. Hillsdale, NJ, Erlbaum. 207-52.

Paulesu, E., Frith, C.D., Frackowiak, R.S.J. (1993). The neural correlates of the verbal component of working memory. *Nature*, 362: 342-45.

Paulus, M.P., Hozack, N.E., Zauscher, B.E., Frank, L., Brown, G.G., Braff, D.L., Schuckit, M.A. (2002). Behavioral and Functional Neuroimaging Evidence for Prefrontal Dysfunction in Methamphetamine-Dependent Subjects. *Neuropsychopharmacology*, 1: 53-63.

Paulsen, O., Sejnowski, T.J. (2000). Natural patterns of activity and long-term synaptic plasticity. *Current Opinion in Neurobiology,* 10(2): 172-79.

Pavlov, I.P. (1927/1960). *Conditional Reflexes.* New York: Dover Publications.

Pelczar, M., Politynska, B. (1997). Pathogenesis and psychosocial consequences of post-concussion syndrome. *Neurologia i neurochirurgia polska,* 31(5): 989-98.

Penfield, W. (1975). *The mystery of the mind: A critical study of consciousness and the human brain.* Princeton, N.J.: Princeton University Press.

Pernille, J.O., Westerberg, H., Klingberg, T. (2004). Increased prefrontal and parietal activity after training in working memory. *Nature Neuroscience*, 7(1): 75-79.

Pessoa, L. (2005). To what extent are emotional visual stimuli processed without attention and awareness? *Current Opinion in Neurobiology*, 15: 188-96.

Pessoa, L., McKenna, M., Gutierrez, E., Ungerleider, L.G. (2002). Neural processing of emotional faces requires attention. *Proceedings of National Academy of Sciences*, 99: 11458-63.

Petchprapai, N., Winkelman, C. (2007). Mild traumatic brain injury: determinants and subsequent quality of life. A review of the literature. *Journal of Neuroscience Nursing,* 39(5): 260-72.

Petersen, S.E., Fox, P.T., Posner, M.I., Mintun, M., Raichle, M.E. (1988). Positron emission tomographic studies of the cortical anatomy of single-word processing. *Nature*, 331: 585-89.

Petrides, M., Alivisatos, B., Meyer, E., Evans, A.C. (1993). Dissociation of the human mid-dorsolateral from posterior dorsolateral frontal cortex in memory processing. *Proceedings of the National Academy of Sciences*, *U.S.A.*, 90: 873-77.

Petrides, M., Milner, B. (1982). Deficits on subject ordered tasks after frontal and temporal lobe lesions in man. *Neuropsychologia,* 20: 249-62.

Petrides, M., Pandya, D.N. (2007). Efferent association pathways from the rostral prefrontal cortex in the macaque monkey. *Journal of Neuroscience,* 27(43): 11573-86.

Petrides, M., Pandya, D.N. (1983). Projections to the frontal cortex from the posterior parietal regions in the rhesus monkey. *Society for Neurosciences, Abstracts.* 9-40.

Petrovitch, H., White, L.R., Izmirilian, G., Ross, G.W., Havlik, R.J., Markesbery, W., Nelson, J., Davis, D.G., Hardman, J., Foley, D.J., Launer, L.J. (2000). Midlife blood pressure and neuritic plaques, neurofibrillary tangles, and brain weight at death: the HAAS. *Neurobiology of Aging*, 21(1): 57-62.

Phan, K.L., Fitzgerald, D.A., Nathan, P.J., Moore, G.J., Uhde, T.W., Tancer, M.E. (2005). Neural substrates for voluntary suppression of negative affect: A functional magnetic resonance imaging study. *Biological Psychiatry, 57:* 210-19.

Phelps, E.A. (2004). Human emotion and memory: interactions of the amygdala and hippocampal complex. *Current Opinion Neurobiology,* 14: 198-202.

Phelps, E.A., Delgado, M.R., Nearing, K.I., LeDoux, J.E. (2004). Extinction learning in humans: role of the amygdala and vmPFC. *Neuron*, 16; 43(6): 897-905.

Phillips, L.H., Wynn, V.E., McPherson, S., Gilhooly, K.J. (2001). Mental planning and the Tower of London task. *Quarterly Journal of Experimental Psychology—Section A—Human Experimental Psychology,* 54(2): 579-97.

Phillips, L.H., Wynn, V., Gilhooly, K.J., Della Sala, S., Logie, R.H. (1999). The role of memory in the "Tower of London task". *Memory*, 7(2): 209-31.

Phillips, M.L., Williams, L.M., Heining, M., Herba, C.M., Russell, T., Andrew, C., Bullmore, E.T., Brammer, M.J., Williams, S.C., Morgan, M., Young, A.W., Gray, J.A. (2004). Differential neural responses to overt and covert presentations of facial expressions of fear and disgust. *NeuroImage*, 21: 1484-96.

Picard, N., Strick, P.L. (2003). Activation of the supplementary motor area (SMA) during performance of visually guided movements. *Cerebral Cortex*, 13: 977-86.

Piet, J., Hougaard, E. (2011). The Effect of Mindfulness-Based Cognitive Therapy for Prevention of Relapse in Recurrent Major Depressive Disorder: a Systematic Review and Meta-Analysis. *Clinical Psychology Review*, 31(6): 1032-40.

Pine, D.S., Shaffer, D., Schonfeld, I.S., Davies, M. (1997). Minor physical anomalies: modifiers of environmental risks for psychiatric impairment? *J. Am. Academy Child Adolescent Psychiatry*, 36: 395-403.

Poeppel, D. (2003). The analysis of speech in different temporal integration windows: cerebral lateralization as "asymmetric sampling in time." *Speech Communication,* 41: 245-55.

Poeppel, D., Guillemin, A., Thompson, J., Fritz, J., Bavelier, D., Braun, A.R. (2004). Auditory lexical decision, categorical perception, and FM direction discrimination differentially engage left and right auditory cortex. *Neuropsychologia*, 42(2): 183-200.

Ponsford, J., Sloan, S., Snow, P. (1995). Traumatic Brain Injury: Rehabilitation for everyday adaptive living. Hillsdale (USA): Lawrence Erlbaum Associates.

Poundstone, W. (1992). *Prisoner's Dilemma.* New York: Doubleday. Nash, J. (1950a). 'Equilibrium Points in *n*-Person Games.' *Proceedings of National Academy of Science, U.S.A.,* 36: 48-49.

Porges, S.W. (2001). The polyvagal theory: phylogenetic substrates of a social nervous system. *International Journal of Psychophysiology,* 42: 123-46.

Porges, S.W. (1998). Love: an emergent property of the mammalian autonomic nervous system. *Psychoneuroendocrinology,* 23: 837-61.

Posner, M.I., Nissen, M.J., Klein, R.M. (1976) Visual Dominance: An Information-Processing Account of Its Origins and Significance. *Psychological Review,* 83(2): 157-71.

Posner, M.I., Snyder, C.R.R. (1975). Attention and cognitive control. In R.L. Solso (Ed.), *Information processing and cognition: the Loyola symposium*. Hillsdale, N.J: L. Erlbaum Associates.

Posner, M.I., Petersen, S.E. (1990). The attention system of the human brain. *A Review of Neuroscience*, 13: 25-42.

Posner, M.I., Rothbart, M.K. (1998). Attention, self-regulation and consciousness. *Phil. Transaction of Royal Society of London: B*, 353: 1915-27.

Pribram, K.H., Luria, A.R. (Eds.), *Psychophysiology of the Frontal Lobes* (293-314). Academic Press, New York.

Pribram, K.H. (1973). The primate frontal cortex-executive of the brain. In K.H. Price BH, M. Mesulam (1995). Psychiatric manifestations of right hemisphere infarctions. *Journal of Nervous and Mental Disorders,* 173: 610-14.

Prigatano, G.P., Borgaro, S., Baker, J., Wethe, J. (2005). Awareness and distress after traumatic brain injury. *Journal of Head Trauma Rehabilitation*, 20(4): 359-67.

Pritchard, T.C., Macaluso, D.A., Eslinger, P.J. (1999). Taste perception in patients with insular cortex lesions. *Behavioral neuroscience,* 113 (4): 663-71.

Pull, C.B. (2007). Combined pharmacotherapy and cognitive-behavioural therapy for anxiety disorders. *Current Opinion in Psychiatry*, 20: 30-35.

Pulvermüller, F. (1999). Words in the brain's language. *Behavioral and Brain Sciences,* 22: 253-336.

Quinette, P., Guillery-Girard, B., Dayan, J., de la Sayette, V., Marquis, S., Viader, Desgranges, B., Eustache, F. (2006). What does transient global amnesia really mean? Review of the literature and thorough study of 142 cases. *Brain,* 129(7): 1640-58.

Raichle, M.E., MacLeod, A.M., Snyder, A.Z., Powers, W.J., Gusnard, D.A., Shulman, G.L. (2001). A default mode of brain function. *Proceedings of National Academy of Science, U.S.A.*, 16; 98(2): 676-82.

Raine, A. (2008). From genes to brain to antisocial behavior. *Current Directions in Psychological Sciences,* 17: 323-28.

Raine, A., Yang, Y. (2006). Neural foundations to moral reasoning and antisocial behavior. *Social Cognitive Affective Neuroscience,* 1: 203-13.

Raine, A. (1993). *The Psychopathology of Crime: Criminal Behavior as a Clinical Disorder*. San Diego, Academic Press.

Rajah, M.N., D'Esposito, M. (2005). Region-specific changes in prefrontal function with age: a review of PET and fMRI studies on working and episodic memory. *Brain*, 128(9): 1964-83.

Rapp, M.A., Schnaider-Beeri, M., Purohit, D.P., Reichenberg, A., McGurk, S.R., Haroutunian, V., Harvey, P.D. (2010). Cortical neuritic plaques and hippocampal neurofibrillary tangles are related to dementia severity in elderly schizophrenia patients. *Schizophrenia Research*, 116(1): 90-96.

Ramnani, N., Owen, A.M. (2004). Anterior prefrontal cortex: insights into function from anatomy and neuroimaging. *Nature Reviews Neuroscience,* 5(3): 184-94.

Rapaport, W.J. (2005). Implementation is semantic interpretation: further thoughts. *Journal of Experimental & Theoretical Artificial Intelligence*, 17(4): 385-417.

Rapaport, W.J. (1999). Implementation is semantic interpretation, *The Monist,* 82: 109-30.

Rapaport, W.J. (1998). How minds can be computational systems, *Journal of Experimental and Theoretical Artificial Intelligence*, 10: 403-19.

Rapgay, L., Bystrisky, A. (2009). Classical mindfulness: an introduction to its theory and practice for clinical application. Proceedings of the Conference on longevity, regeneration and optimal health: integrating eastern and western perspectives Phoenicia, NY.

Rangaswami, M., Mukundan, C.R. (1999). *Slow DC Potentials and the Study of Volition.* Ph.D. thesis submitted to

National Institute of Mental Health & Neuro Sciences, Deemed University, Bangalore.

Raymond, J.E., Shapiro, K.L., Arnell, K.M. (1992). Temporal suppression of visual processing in n RSV.P task: An attentional blink? *Journal of Experimental Psychology, Human Perception & Performance,* 18: 849-60.

Rees, G., Frackowiak, R.S.J., Frith, C.D. (1997). Two modulatory effects of attention that mediate object categorization in human cortex. *Science*, 275: 835-38.

Reinkemeier, M., Markowitsch, H.J., Rauch, M., Kessler, J. (1997). Differential impairments in recalling people's names: a case study in search of neuroanatomical correlates. *Neuropsychologia,* 35: 677-84.

Repp, H., Knoblich, G. (2007). Toward a psychophysics of agency: Detecting gain and loss of control over auditory action effects. *Journal of Experimental Psychology: Human Perception & Performance, 33*: 469-82.

Richard, B., Grinder, J. (1975a). *The Structure of Magic I: A Book About Language and Therapy*. Palo Alto, CA: Science & Behavior Books.

Richard, B., Grinder, J. (1975b). *The Structure of Magic II: A Book About Communication and Change*. Palo Alto, CA: Science & Behavior Books.

Richardson, J.T.E., Barry, C. (1985). The effects of minor closed head injury upon human memory: further evidence on the role of mental imagery. *Cognitive Neuropsychology,* 2(2): 149-68.

Richer, F., Décary, A., Lapierre, M.F., Rouleau, I., Bouvier, G., Saint-Hilaire, J.M. (1993). Target detection deficits in frontal lobectomy. *Brain Cognition,* 21(2): 203-11.

Ritskes, R., Ritskes-Hoitinga, M., Stodkilde-Jorgensen, H., Baerentsen, K., Hartman, T. (2003). MRI scanning during Zen meditation: The picture of enlightenment? *Constructivism in the Human Sciences, 8*: 85-90.

Robertson, I.H. (1993). Cognitive rehabilitation in neurologic disease. *Current Opinion in Neurology,* 6(5): 756-60.

Robinson, D.L. (1999). The technical, neurological and psychological significance of 'alpha', 'delta' and 'theta' waves confounded in EEG evoked potentials: a study of peak latencies. *Clinical Neurophysiology,* 110: 1427-34.

Rodd, J.M., Davis, M.H., Johnsrude, I.S. (2005). The neural mechanisms of speech comprehension: fMRI studies of semantic ambiguity. *Cerebral Cortex*, 15: 1261-69.

Roder, B., Stock, O., Neville, H., Bien, S., Rosler, F. (2002). Brain activation modulated by the comprehension of normal and pseudo-word sentences of different processing demands: a functional magnetic resonance imaging study. *NeuroImage*, 15: 1003-14.

Rodriguez, E., George, N., Lachaux, J.P., Martinerie, J., Renault, B., Varela, F.J. (1999). Perception's shadow: Long-distance gamma band synchronization of human brain activity. *Nature,* 397: 430-33.

Rolls, E.T., Perrett, D., Thorpe, S.J., Puerto, A., Roper-Hall, A., Maddison, S. (1979). Responses of neurons in area 7 of the parietal cortex to objects of different significance. *Brain Research,* 15; 169(1): 194-98.

Ropper, A.H., Gorson, K.C. (2007). Clinical practice. Concussion. *New England Journal of Medicine,* 356(2): 166-72.

Ross, J.S., Tkach, J., Ruggieri, P.M., Lieber, M., Lapresto, E. (2003). The mind's eye: functional MR imaging evaluation of golf motor imagery. *AJNR American Journal of Neuroradiology,* 24: 1036-44.

Rosen, G., Hugdahl, K., Ersland, L., Lundervold, A., Smievoll, A.I., Barndon, R., Sundberg, H., Thomsen, T., Roscher, B.E., Tjolsen, A., Engelsen, B. (2001). Different brain areas activated during imagery of painful and non-painful 'finger movements' in a subject with an amputated arm. *Neurocase*, 7: 255-60.

Rothschild, B. (2000). *The Body Remembers: The Psychophysiology of Trauma and Trauma Treatment.* New York: W.W. Norton & Company.

Rubens, A.B. (1975). Aphasia with infarction in the territory of anterior cerebral artery, *Cortex,* 11: 239-50.

Rubia, K., Taylor, E., Smith, A.B., Oksanen, H., Overmeyer, S., Newman, S. (2001). Neuropsychological analyses of impulsiveness in childhood hyperactivity. *British Journal of Psychiatry*, 179: 138-43.

Rueckert, L., Grafman, J. (1996). Sustained attention deficits in patients with right frontal lesions. *Neuropsychologia*, 34(10): 953-63.

Ruchkin, D.S., Canoune, H., Johnson, R., Ritter, W. (1995). Working memory and preparation elicit different patterns of slow wave event related potentials. *Psychophysiology*, 32: 399-410.

Ruchkin, D.S., Johnson, R., Grafman, J., Caoune, H., Ritter, W. (1992). Distinctions and similarities among working memory process: An event related potential study. *Cognitive Brain Research,* 1: 53-66.

Ruchsow, M., Trippel, N., Groen, G., Spitzer, M., Kiefer, M. (2003). Semantic and syntactic processes during sentence comprehension in patients with schizophrenia: evidence from event-related potentials. *Schizophrenia Research*, 64: 147-56.

Ryan, L.M., Warden, D.L. (2003). Post concussion syndrome. *International Review of Psychiatry,* 15(4): 310-16.

Rypma, B., D'Esposito, M. (1999a). The roles of prefrontal brain regions in components of working memory: effects of memory load and individual differences. *Proceedings of National Academy of Science, U.S.A.,* 96: 6558-63.

Rypma, B., Prabhakaran, V., Desmond, J.E., Glover, G.H., Gabrieli, J.D.E. (1999b). Load-dependent roles of frontal brain regions in the maintenance of working memory. *NeuroImage,* 9: 216-26.

Sadock, B.J. Sadock, V.A. (2008). Kaplan and Sadock's Concise Textbook of Child and Adolescent Psychiatry. 1st (first) edition. Lippincott Williams & Wilkins.

Sala, S.D., Spinnler, H., Venneri, A. (1997). Persistent global amnesia following right thalamic stroke: an 11-year longitudinal study. *Neuropsychology*, 11(1): 90-103.

Saleem, K.S., Suzuki, W., Tanaka, K., Hashikawa, T. (2000). Connections between anterior inferotemporal cortex and superior temporal sulcus regions in the macaque monkey. *Journal of Neuroscience,* 20: 5083-5101.

Salmaso, D., Denes, G. (1982). Role of the frontal lobes on an attention task: A signal detection analysis. *Perceptual and Motor Skills,* 54: 1147-50.

Salmon, E., Van der Linden, M., Collette, F., Delfiore, G., Maquet, P., Degueldre, C., Luxen, A., Franck, G. (1996). Regional brain activity during working memory tasks. *Brain*, 119(Pt 5): 1617-25.

Sakai, K., Hikosaka, O., Takino, R., Miyauchi, S., Nielsen, M., Tamada, T. (2000). What and when: Parallel and convergent processing in motor control. *The Journal of Neuroscience*, 20: 2691-2700.

Sandel, S.L., Judge, J.O., Landry, N., Faria, L., Ouellette, R., Majczak, M. (2005). Dance and movement program improves quality-of-life measures in breast cancer survivors. *Cancer Nursing,* 28: 301-09.

Saper, C.B., Chou, T.C., Gooley, J. (2005a). The hypothalamic integrator for circadian rhythms. *Trends in Neuroscience,* 28: 152-57.

Saper, C.B., Chou, T.C., Scammell, T.E. (2001). The sleep switch: hypothalamic control of sleep and wakefulness. *Trends in Neuroscience,* 24: 726-31.

Saper, C.B., Scammell, T.E., Lu, J. (2005b). Hypothalamic regulation of sleep and circadian rhythms. *Nature,* 437: 1257-63.

Sarter, M., Bruno, J.P. (1998). Cortical afferents originating in the basal forebrain: Mediation of specific aspects of attentional processing versus general assumptions about cortical activation and behavioral state. *INABIS98 SYMPOSIUM.*

Sauseng, P., Klimesch, W., Schabus, M., Doppelmayr, M. (2005). Fronto-parietal EEG coherence in theta and upper alpha reflect central executive functions of working memory. *International Journal of Psychophysiology,* 57(2): 97-103.

Savard, G., Andermann, F., Olivier, A., Rémillard, G.M. (1991). Postictal psychosis after partial complex seizures: a multiple case study. *Epilepsia,* 32: 225-31.

Scepkowski, L.A., Cronin-Golomb, A. (2003). The alien hand: cases, categorizations, and anatomical correlates. *Behavioral Cognitive Neuroscience Review,* 2(4): 261-77.

Schiff, N.D. (2004). The neurology of impaired consciousness: Challenges for cognitive neuroscience. In M.S. Gazzaniga (Ed), *The Cognitive Neurosciences III.* MIT Press. 1121-32.

Segal, Z.V., Williams, J.M.G., Teasdale, J.D. (2002). Mindfulness-based cognitive therapy for depression: A new approach to preventing relapse. New York: The Guilford Press.

Suskauer, S.J., Simmonds, D.J., Fotedar, S., Blankner, J.G., Pekar, J.J., Denckla, M.B., Mostofsky, S.H. (2008). Functional Magnetic Resonance Imaging Evidence for Abnormalities in Response Selection in Attention Deficit Hyperactivity Disorder: Differences in Activation Associated with Response Inhibition but Not Habitual Motor Response. *Journal of Cognitive Neuroscience,* 20(3): 478-93.

Saykin, A.J., Johnson, S.C., Flashman, L.A., McAllister, T.W., Sparling, M., Darcey, T.M., Moritz, C.H., Guerin, S.J., Weaver, J., Mamourian, A. (1999). Functional differentiation of medial temporal and frontal regions involved in processing novel and familiar words: an fMRI study. *Brain,* 122: 1963-71.

Schabus, M., Gruber, G., Parapatics, S., Sauter, C., Klösch, G., Anderer, P., Klimesch, W., Saletu, B., Zeitlhofer, J. (2004). Sleep spindles and their significance for declarative memory consolidation. *SLEEP*, 27(8): 1479-85.

Schacter, D.L., Harbluk, J.L., McLachlen, D.R. (1984). Retrieval without recollection: an experimental analysis of source amnesia. *Journal of Verbal Learning and Verbal Behaviour*, 23(5): 593-611.

Schacter, D.L., Kaszniak, A.W., Kihlstrom, J.F., Valdiserri, M. (1991). The relation between source memory and aging. *Psychology of Aging*, 6(4): 559-68.

Schmidt, R.A. (1975). A schema theory of discrete motor skill learning. *Psychological Review*, 82: 225-60.

Schmidt, R.A., Lee, T.D. (2005). *Motor control and learning: A behavioural emphasis*. Champaign, IL: Human Kinetics.

Schöner, G. and Kelso, J.A.S. (1988). Dynamic pattern generation in behavioral and neural systems. *Science*, 239: 1513-20.

Schonwiesner, M., Rubsamen, R., vonCramon, D.Y. (2005). Hemispheric asymmetry for spectral and temporal processing in the human antero-lateral auditory belt cortex. *European Journal of Neuroscience*, 22: 1521-28.

Schott, J.M., Rossor, M.N. (2003). Physical Signs—The grasp and other primitive reflexes. *Journal of Neurology, Neurosurgery and Psychiatry*, 74: 558-60.

Schnyer, D.M., Verfaellie, M., Alexander, M.P., LaFleche, G., Nicholls, L., Kaszniak, A.W. (2004). A role for right medial prefontal cortex in accurate feeling-of-knowing judgements: Evidence from patients with lesions to frontal cortex. *Neuropsychologia*, 42: 957-66.

Scott, S.K., Blank, C.C., Rosen, S., Wise, R.J. (2000). Identification of a pathway for intelligible speech in the left temporal lobe. *Brain*, 123: 2400-06.

Scott, R., Lau, B.M., Shapiro, S., Carlson, L., Anderson, N.D., Carmody, J., Segal, Z.V., Abbey, S., Speca, M., Velting, D., Devins, G. (2004). Mindfulness: A proposed operational definition. *Clinical Psychology: Science & Practice*, 11(3): 230-41.

Sebanz, N., Lackner, U. (2007). Who's calling the shots? Intentional content and feelings of control. *Consciousness and Cognition*, *16*: 859-76.

Seltzer, B., Pandya, D.N. (1980). Converging visual and somatic sensory input to the intraparietal sulcus of the rhesus monkey. *Brain Research,* 192: 339-51.

Senge, P.M. (1990). *The Fifth Discipline: The Art and Practice of the Learning Organization.* Currency Doubleday, New York.

Shailaja, K., Mukundan, C.R. (1989). Frontal Lobe deficits. Unpublished Ph.D. thesis submitted to National Institute of Mental Health & Neuro Sciences, Bangalore University, Bangalore.

Shallice, T., Fletcher, P., Frith, C.D., Grasby, P., Frackowiak, R.S., Dolan, R.J. (1994). Brain regions associated with acquisition and retrieval of verbal episodic memory. *Nature,* 368: 633-35.

Shallice, T., Burgess, P.W., Schon, F., Baxter, D.M. (1989). The origins of utilization behaviour. *Brain,* 112(Pt 6): 1587-98.

Shallice, T. (1988). *From neuropsychology to mental structure.* Cambridge, UK: Cambridge University Press.

Shallice, T. (1982). Specific impairments of planning. Philosophical Transactions of the Royal Society of London. Series B, *Biological Sciences*, 298(1089): 199-209.

Shamay-Tsoory, S.G., Harari, H., Aharon-Peretz, J., Levkovitz, Y. (2010). The role of the orbitofrontal cortex in affective theory of mind deficits in criminal offenders with psychopathic tendencies. *Cortex*, 46(5): 668-77.

Shamay-Tsoory, S.G., Tomer, R., Berger, B.D., Goldsher, D., Aharon-Peretz, J. (2005). Impaired "affective theory of mind" is associated with right ventromedial prefrontal damage. *Cognitive Behavioral Neurology,* 18(1): 55-67.

Sharot, T., Phelps, E.A. (2004). How arousal modulates memory: disentangling the effects of attention and retention. *Cognitive Affectective Behavioral Neuroscience,* 4: 294-306.

Shastri, L., Ajjanagadde, V. (1993). From simple associations to systematic reasoning: a connectionist representation of rule, variables and dynamic bindings using temporal synchrony. *Behavioral and Brain Sciences,* 16: 417-94.

Shaw, N.A. (2002). The Neurophysiology of Concussion. *Progress in Neurobiology*, 67(4): 281-344.

Shekhar, R. (2008). Transient global amnesia—a review. *International Journal of Clinical Practice,* 62(6): 939-42.

Shergill, S.S., Bramer, M.J., Williams, S.C.R., Murray, R.M., McGuire, P.K. (2000). Mapping auditory hallucinations in schizophrenia using functional magnetic resonance imaging. *Archives of General Psychiatry,* 57: 1033-38.

Sherin, J.E., Shironmani, P.J., McCarley, R.W., Saper, C.B. (1996). Activation of ventrolateral preoptic neurons during sleep. *Science*, 71: 216-19.

Sherwood, D.E. (1994). Hand preference, practice order, and spatial assimilations in rapid bimanual movement. *Journal of Motor Behavior,* 26(2): 123-43.

Shiffrin, R.M., Schneider, W. (1977). Controlled and automatic human information processing II: Perceptual learning, automatic attending, and a general theory. *Psychological Review*, 84(2): 127-90.

Shibasaki, H., Barrett, G., Halliday, E., Halliday, A.M. (1980a). Components of the movement related cortical potentials and their scalp topography. *Electroencephalography Clinical Neurophysiology*, 49: 213-26.

Shibasaki, H., Barrett, G., Halliday, E., Halliday, A.M. (1980b). Cortical potentials following voluntary and passive finger movements. *Electroencephalography Clinical Neurophysiology*, 50: 201-13.

Shibasaki, H., Barrett, G., Halliday, E., Halliday, A.M. (1981). Cortical potentials associated with voluntary foot movements in man. *Electroencephalography Clinical Neurophysiology*, 52: 507-16.

Shibasaki, H., Sadato, N., Lyshkow, H., Yonekura, Y., Honda, M., Nagamine, T., Suwazono, S., Magata, Y., Ikeda, A., Miyazaki, M. (1993). Both primary motor cortex and supplementary motor area play an important role in complex finger movement. *Brain*, 116: 1387-98.

Shimamura, A.P., Janowsky, J.S., Squire, L.R. (1990). Memory for the temporal order of events in patients with frontal lobe lesions and amnesic patients. *Neuropsychologia*, 28(8): 803-13.

Siegrist, M. (1995). Inner speech as a cognitive process mediating self-consciousness and inhibiting self-deception. *Psychological Reports*, 76: 259-65.

Simone, P., Baylis, G. (1997). Selective attention in a reaching task: effect of normal ageing and Alzheimer's disease. *Journal of Experimental Psychology*, 23: 595-608.

Singer, W. (1994). Putative functions of temporal correlations in neocortical processing. In: C. Koch C., J. Davis (eds.), *Large Scale Neuronal Theories of the Brain* (201-38). Cambridge, Massachusetts Institute of Technology Press.

Singer, W. (1996). Neuronal synchronization: A solution to the binding problem? In: R. Llinas, P.S. Churchland (eds.), *The Mind-Brain Continuum* (101-30). Cambridge, Massachusetts Institute of Technology Press.

Singh, J., Mukundan, C.R., Das, B.S., Arya, B.Y.T. (1986). Contingent negative variations in patients with cortical lesions. *NIMHANS Journal*, 4: 23-32.

Singh, J., Knight, R.T. (1990). Frontal lobe contribution to voluntary movements in humans. *Brain Research*, 29; 531(1-2): 45-54.

Skeem, J.L., Polaschek, D.L.L., Patrick, C.J., Lilienfeld, S.O. (2011). Psychopathic personality: Bridging the gap between scientific evidence and public policy. *Psychological Science in the Public Interest,* 12(3): 95-162.

Skipper, J.I., Goldin-Meadow, S., Nusbaum, H.C., Small, S.L. (2007). Speech-associated gestures, Broca's area, and the human mirror system. *Brain and Language,* 101(3): 260-77.

Smith, E.E., Jonides, J. (1999a). Neuroimaging analyses of human working memory. *Proceedings of National Academy of Sciences, U.S.A.,* 95, 12061-68.

Smith, E.E., Jonides, J. (1999b). Storage and executive processes in the frontal lobes. *Science*, 283: 1657-61.

Smith, E.E., Jonides, J., Koeppe, R.A. (1996). Dissociating verbal and spatial working memory using PET. *Cerebral Cortex*, 6: 11-20.

Smith, E.E., Jonides, J., Marshuetz, C., Koeppe, R.A. (1998). Components of verbal working memory: Evidence from neuroimaging. *Proceedings of National Academy of Sciences, U.S.A.*, 95: 876-82.

Snowden, J.S., Bathgate, D., Varma, A., Blackshaw, A., Gibbons, Z.C., Neary, D. (2001). Distinct behavioural profiles in frontotemporal dementia and semantic dementia. *Journal of Neurology, Neurosurgery and Psychiatry*, 70: 323-32.

Sokolov, E.N. (1960). Neuronal models and the orienting reflex. In Mary A.B. Brazier (Ed.), *The Central Nervous System and Behavior*. NY: JosiahMacy, Jr. Foundation, 187-276.

Sokolov, E.N. (1963). *Perception and the Conditioned Reflex*. Oxford, Pergamon.

Solodkin, A., Hlustik, P., Chen, E.E., Small, S.L. (2004), Fine modulation in network activation during motor execution and motor imagery. *Cerebral Cortex*, 14: 1246-55.

Soon, C.S., Brass, M., Heinze, H.J., Haynes, J.D. (2008). Unconscious determinants of free decisions in the human brain. *Nature Neuroscience*, 11(5): 543-45.

Speedie, L.J., Heilman, K.M. (1982a). Anterograde deficits for visuospatial material after infarction of the right thalamus. *Achieves of Neurology*, 40: 183-86.

Speedie, L.J., Heilman, K.M. (1982b). Amnestic disturbance following infarction of the left dorsomedial nucleus of the thalamus. *Neuropsychologia*, 20(5): 597-604.

Spence, C. (2009). Explaining the Colavita visual dominance effect. *Progress in Brain Research*, 176: 245-58.

Sperry, R.W. (1950). Neural basis of the spontaneous optokinetic response produced by visual inversion. *Journal of Comparative and Physiological Psychology*, 43: 482-89.

Sperry, R.W. (1952). Neurology and the mind-brain problem. *American Scientist,* 40: 291-312.

Spijkers, W., Spellerberg, S. (1995). On-line visual control of aiming movements? *Acta Psychologica* (Amst), 90(1-3): 333-48.

Spiegel, K., Leproult, R., L'Hermite-Baleriaux, M., Copinschi, G., Penev, P.D., Van Cauter, E. (2004). Leptin levels are dependent on sleep duration: relationships with sympathovagal balance, carbohydrate regulation, cortisol, and thyrotropin. *Journal of Clinical Endocrinology Metabolism*, 89: 5762-71.

Squire, L.R. (1992). Memory and the hippocampus: a synthesis from findings with rats, monkeys, and humans. *Psychological Review*, 99: 195-231.

Squire, L.R., Ojemann, J.G., Miezin, F.M., Petersen, S.E., Videen, T.O., Raichle, M.E. (1998). Activation of the hippocampus in normal humans: a functional anatomical study of memory. *Proceedings of National Academy of Science, U.S.A.*, 89: 1837-41.

Starkstein, S.E., Robinson, R.G. (1997). Mechanism of disinhibition after brain lesions. *Psychological Bulletin*, 80: 539-56.

Steinvorth, S., Corkin, S., Halgren, E. (2006). Ecphory of autobiographical memories: an fMRI study of recent and remote memory retrieval. *NeuroImage*, 30(1): 285-98.

Steriade, M. (2006). Grouping of brain rhythms in corticothalamic systems. *Neuroscience,* 137(4): 1087-106.

Steriade, M., McCarley, R.W. (1990). Brainstem control of wakefulness and sleep. NY: Plenum Press.

Stevens, J. (1990). Psychiatric consequences of temporal lobectomy for intractable seizures: a 20-30-year follow-up of 14 cases. *Psychological Medicine,* 20: 529-45.

Stevens, A.A. (2004). Dissociating the cortical basis of memory for voices, words and tones. *Brain Research Cognitive Brain Research*, 18: 162-71.

Stigsdotter, A., Bäckman, L. (1995). Effects of multifactorial memory training in old age: generalizability across tasks and individuals. The *Journals of Gerontology. Series B, Psychological Sciences and Social Sciences*, 50b3: 134-40.

Storandt, M., Mintun, M.A., Head, D., Morris, J.C. (2009). Cognitive decline and brain volume loss as signatures of cerebral amyloid-beta peptide deposition identified with Pittsburgh compound B: cognitive decline associated with Abeta deposition. *Archives of Neurology,* 66(12): 1476-81.

Stinus, L., Kelley, A.E., Iversen, S.D. (1978). Increased spontaneous activity following substance P infusion into A10 dopaminergic area. *Nature,* 7; 276(5688): 616-18.

Storandt, M. (2008). Cognitive Deficits in the Early Stages of Alzheimer's Disease, Current Directions In Psychological Science, *Association for Psychological Science,* 17(3): 198-202.

Storandt, M., Grant, E.A., Miller, J.P., Morris, J.C. (2006). Longitudinal course and neuropathological outcomes in original vs. revised MCI and in preMCI. *Neurology,* 67: 467-73.

Stuss, D.T., Benson, D.F. (2008). *The Frontal Lobes.* Raven Press, New York.

Swinnen, S.P., Li, Y., Dounskaia, N., Byblow, W., Stinear, C., Wagemans, J. (2004). Perception-action coupling during bimanual coordination: the role of visual perception in the coalition of constraints that govern bimanual action. *Journal of Motor Behavior,* 36(4): 394-98, 402-07; discussion 408-17.

Tanaka, K. (1993). Neuronal mechanisms of object recognition. *Science*, *262*: 685-88.

Tanoue, R.T., Jones, K.T., Peterson, D.J., Berryhill, M.E. (2013). Differential frontal involvement in shifts of internal and perceptual attention. *Brain Stimulus,* 6(4): 675-82.

Taylor, K.I., Regard, M. (2003). Language in the right cerebral hemisphere: Contributions from reading studies. *Physiology,* 18(6): 257-61.

Taylor, S., Woody, S., Koch, W.J., McLean, P., Paterson, R.J., Anderson, K.W. (1997). Cognitive restructuring in the treatment of social phobia. *Behavior Modification*, 21: 487-511.

Teasdale, G., Jennett, B. (1974). Assessment of coma and impaired consciousness. A practical scale. *The Lancet,* 13(2): (7872): 81-84.

Tekin, S., Cummings, J.L. (2002). Frontal-subcortical neuronal circuits and clinical neuropsychiatry, an update. *Journal of Psychosomatic Research,* 53: 647-54.

Teuber, H.L. (1963). Maze perception and its disturbance after brain injury in Man. *Neuropsychologia,* 1: 47-57.

Teuber, H.L. (1964). The riddle of the frontal lobe in man. In J.P. Warren and K. Akerts (Eds), *The Frontal Granular Cortex and Behavior*. New York: McGraw-Hill.

Theeuwes, J. (1991). Exogenous and endogenous control of attention—the effect of visual onsets and offsets. *Perception & Psychophysics,* 49(1): 83-90.

Thompson, C., Henry, J.D., Rendell, P.G., Withall, A., Brodaty, H. (2010). Prospective memory function in mild cognitive impairment and early dementia. *Journal of the International Neuropsychological Society*, 16: 318-25.

Thorndike, E.L. (1901). Animal intelligence: An experimental study of the associative processes in animals. *Psychological Review Monograph Supplement*, 2: 1-109.

TIFAC-DFS Project Report (2008). Technology Information Forecasting & Assessment Council—Directorate of Forensic Sciences, Gandhinagar (TIFAC-DFS): Project Report on *Normative Data for Brain Electrical Activation Profiling.*

Till, C., Colella, B., Verwegen, J., Green, R.E. (2008). Postrecovery Cognitive Decline in Adults With Traumatic Brain Injury. *Archives of Physical Medicine and Rehabilitation,* 89, Suppl 2: 25-34.

Tipper, S.P., Howard, L.A., Houghton, G. (2000). Behavioral consequences of selection from neural population codes. In S. Monsell, J. Driver (Eds.), *Control of Cognitive*

Processes: Attention and Performance. Cambridge MA, MIT Press.

Tiraboschi, P., Hansen, L.A., Thal, L.J., Corey-Bloom, J. (2004). The importance of neuritic plaques and tangles to the development and evolution of AD. *Neurology*, 62(11): 1984-89.

Toplak, M.E., Jain, U., Tannock, R. (2005). Executive and motivational processes in adolescents with Attention-Deficit-Hyperactivity Disorder (ADHD). *Behavioral and Brain Functions,* 1: 8-20.

Troyer, A.K., Craik, F.I. (2000). The effect of divided attention on memory for items and their context. *Canadian Journal of Experimental Psychology*, 54(3): 161-71.

Tucker, A., Fishbein, W. (2009). The Impact of sleep duration and subject intelligence on declarative and motor memory performance: how much is enough? *Journal of Sleep Research,* 304-12.

Trevarthen, C. (1979). Communication and cooperation in early infancy. In M. Bullowa (Ed), *Before Speech: The Beginning of Human Communication*) (321-47). Cambridge University Press.

Tulving, E. (2002). Episodic memory: from mind to brain. *Annual Review of Psychology*, 53: 1-25.

Tulving, E. (Eds). (1994). *Memory Systems*. MIT Bradford Press, Cambridge. 269-310.

Tulving, E. (1972). Episodic and semantic memory. In E. Tulving and W. Donaldson (Eds.), *Organization of Memory* (381-403). New York: Academic Press.

Tulving, E. (1987). Multiple memory systems and consciousness. *Human Neurobiology,* 6: 67-80.

Tulving, E., Markowitsch, H.J., Kapur, S., Habib, R., Houle, S. (1994a). Novelty encoding networks in the human brain: positron emission tomography data. *Neuroreport,* 20; 5(18): 2525-28.

Tulving, E., Kapur, S., Craik, F., Moscovitch, M., Houle, S. (1994b). Hemispheric encoding/retrieval asymmetry in episodic memory: Positron Emission Tomography Findings. *Proceedings of National Academy of Sciences, U.S.A.*, 91: 2016-20.

Tulving, E., Kapur, S., Markowitsch, H.J., Craik, F.I.M., Habib, R., Houle, S. (1994c). Neuroanatomical correlates of retrieval in episodic memory: auditory sentence recognition. *Proceedings of the National Academy of Sciences, U.S.A.*, 91: 2012-15.

Turken, A.U., Swick, D. (1999). Response selection in the human anterior cingulate cortex. *Nature Neuroscience,* 2: 920-24.

Turner, M.E., Pratkanis, A.R. (1998). Twenty-five years of groupthink theory and research: lessons from the evaluation of a theory, *Organizational Behavior and Human Decision Processes,* 73: 105-15.

Turriziani, P., Carlesimo, G.A., Perri, R., Tomaiuolo, F., Caltagirone, C. (2003). Loss of spatial learning in a patient with topographical disorientation in new environments. *Journal of Neurology, Neurosurgery & Psychiatry,* 74(1): 61-69.

Ullman, M.T. (2004). Contributions of memory circuits to language: the declarative/procedural model. *Cognition*, 92: 231-70.

Umeda, S., Akine, Y., Kato, M., Muramatsu, T., Mimura, M., Kandatsu, S., Tanada, S., Obata, T., Ikehira, H., Suhara, T. (2005). Functional network in the prefrontal cortex during episodic memory retrieval. *Neuroimage,* 26(3): 932-40.

Vandana, V., Mukundan, C.R., Nagaraja, D. (1996). Contingent Negative Variation in Dementia. *NIMHANS Journal,* 14(2): 133-38.

Vandekerckhove, M.M., Markowitsch, H.J., Mertens, M. Woermann, F.G. (2005). Bi-hemispheri engagement in the retrieval of autobiographical episodes. *Behavioral Neurology,* 16(4): 203-10.

van der Naalt, J. (2001). Prediction of outcome in mild to moderate head injury: A review. *Journal of Clinical and Experimental Neuropsychology*, 23(6): 837-51.

van den Bosch, G.E., Marroun, H.E., Schmidt, M.N., Tibboel, D., Manoach, D.S., Calhoun, V.D., White, T.J. (2012). Brain connectivity during verbal working memory in children and adolescents. *Human Brain Mapping*, doi: 10.1002/hbm.22193. [Epub ahead of print]

Verhaeghen, P., Marcoen, A., Goossens, L. (1992). Improving memory performance in the aged through mnemonic training: a meta-analytic study. *Psychology and Aging*, 72: 242-51.

Verschueren, S.M., Swinnen, S.P., Cordo, P.J., Dounskaia, N.V. (1999). Proprioceptive control of multijoint movement: unimanual circle drawing. *Experimental Brain Research*, 127(2): 171-81.

von der Malsburg, C. (1996). The binding problem of neural networks. In: R. Llinas P.S. Churchland (Eds.), *The Mind-Brain Continuum: Sensory Processes* (131-46). Cambridge, MA: MIT Press.

Vreeling, F.W., Jolles, J., Verhey, F.R., Houx, P.J. (1993). Primitive reflexes in healthy, adult volunteers and neurological patients: methodological issues. *Journal of Neurology*, 240(8): 495-504.

Vuilleumier, P., Armony, J.L., Clarke, K., Husain, M., Driver, J., Dolan, R.J. (2002). Neural response to emotional faces with and without awareness: Event-related fMRI in a parietal patient with visual extinction and spatial neglect. *Neuropsychologia*, 40: 2156-66.

Vuilleumier, P., Armony, J.L., Driver, J., Dolan, R.J. (2003). Distinct spatial frequency sensitivities for processing faces and emotional expressions. *Nature Neuroscience*, 6: 624-31.

Wadhavan, J.M., Mukundan, C.R. (1985). Isolation: An experimental study of psychological and psychophysiological factors. Unpublished Ph.D. thesis submitted to National Institute of Mental Health & Neuro Sciences, Bangalore University, Bangalore.

Wagner, A.D., Poldrack, R.A., Eldridge, L.L., Desmond, J.E., Glover, G.H., Gabrieli, J.D. (1998). Material-specific lateralization of prefrontal activation during episodic encoding and retrieval. *NeuroReport,* 9: 3711-17.

Wagner, A.D., Pare-Blagoev, E.J., Clark, J., Poldrack, R.A. (2001). Recovering meaning: left prefrontal cortex guides controlled semantic retrieval. *Neuron*, 31: 329-38.

Walcott, C.M., Landau, S. (2004). The relation between disinhibition and emotion regulation in boys with attention deficit hyperactivity disorder. *Journal of Clinical Child and Adolescent Psychology,* 33: 772-82.

Ward, J. (2006). *The Student's Guide to Cognitive Neuroscience.* Psychology Press, U.K.

Wallace, B. Alan (2006). *The attention revolution: Unlocking the power of the focused mind.* Boston, Wisdom Publications.

Weber, S., Habel, U., Amunts, K., Schneider, F. (2008). Structural brain abnormalities in psychopaths—a review. *Behavioral Sciences & the Law,* 26(1): 7-9.

Wechsler, D. (1987). *Wechsler Memory Scale*—Revised. San Antonio, TX: Psychological Corporation.

Wechsler, D. (1981). *Manual for the Wechsler Adult Intelligence Scale*—Revised. New York: Psychological Corporation.

Weintraub, S., Mesulam, M.M. (1987). Right cerebral dominance in spatial attention: Further evidence based on ipsilateral neglect. *Archives of Neurology,* 44: 621-25.

Wenke, D., Waszak, F., Haggard, P. (2009). Action selection and action awareness. *Psychological Research,* 73: 602-12.

Wertheimer, M. (2000). *A Brief History of Psychology.* 4th edition. Fort Worth TX: Harcourt Brace.

Weyhenmeyer, J.A., Gallman, E.A. (2007). *Rapid Review of Neuroscience* (102). Mosby Elsevier.

Wexler, M.N., Fraser, S. (1995). Expanding the groupthink explanation to the study of contemporary cults. *Cultic Studies Journal,* 12(1): 49-71.

Whalen, P.J., Rauch, S.L., Etcoff, N.L., McInerney, S.C., Lee, M.B., Jenike, M.A. (1998). Masked presentations of emotional facial expressions modulate amygdala activity without explicit knowledge. *Journal of Neuroscience*, 18(1): 411-18.

Wickelgren I. (1997). Getting a grasp on working memory. *Science*, 275: 1580-82.

Wilkins, A.J., Shallice, T., McCarthy, R. (1987). Frontal lesions and sustained attention. *Neuropsychologia,* 25(2): 359-65.

Windmann, S., Kruger, T. (1998). Subconscious detection of threat as reflected by an enhancedresponse bias. *Conscious Cognition*, 7: 603-33.

Wiesendanger, M., Serrien, D.J. (2001). Toward a physiological understanding of human dexterity. *News in Physiological Sciences,* 16: 228-33.

Wildgruber, D., Kischka, U., Ackermann, H., Klose, U., Grodd, W. (1999). Dynamic pattern of brain activation during sequencing of word strings evaluated by fMRI. *Brain Research Cognitive Brain Research,* 7: 285-94.

Willcutt, E.G., Doyle, A.E., Nigg, J.T., Faraone, S.V., Pennington, B.F. (2005). Validity of the executive function theory of attention-deficit hyperactivity disorder: a meta-analytic review. *Biological Psychiatry,* 57(11): 1336-46.

Wilkins, A.J., Shallice, T., McCarthy, R. (1987). Frontal lesions and sustained attention. *Neuropsychologia,* 25: 359-65.

Williams, R.W., Herrup, K. (1988). The control of neuron number. *Annual Review of Neuroscience,* 11: 423-53.

Wise, R., Hadar, U., Howard, D., Patterson, K. (1991). Language activation studies with positron emission tomography. Ciba Found Symp, 163: 218-28; discussion 228-34.

Wilson, B.A. (1996). Rehabilitation and management of memory problems. *Acta Neurologica Belgica*, 96(1): 51-54.

Wolfram, S. (1998). Predictive Reward Signal of Dopamine Neurons. *The Journal of Neurophysiology*, 80(1): 1-27.

Wright, R.D., Ward, L.M. (2008). *Orienting of Attention.* Oxford University Press.

Yerkes, R.M., Dodson, J.D. (1908). The relation of strength of stimulus to rapidity of habit-formation. *Journal of Comparative Neurology and Psychology,* 18: 459-82.

Yook, K., Lee, S.H., Ryu, M., Kim, K.H., Choi, T.K., Suh, S.Y., Kim, Y.W., Kim, B., Kim, M.Y., Kim, M.J. (2008). Usefulness of mindfulness-based cognitive therapy for treating insomnia in patients with anxiety disorders: A pilot study. *The Journal of Nervous and Mental Disease, 196*: 501-03.

Yu, Gao, Raine, A., Venables, P.H., Dawson, M.E., Mednick, S.A. (2010). Association of Poor Childhood Fear Conditioning and Adult Crime. *American Journal of Psychiatry,* 167: 56-60.

Zaehle, T., Wustenberg, T., Meyer, M., Jancke, L. (2004). Evidence for rapid auditory perception as the foundation of speech processing: a sparse temporal sampling fMRI study. *European Journal of Neuroscience,* 20: 2447-56.

Zafeiriou, D.I. (2004). Primitive reflexes and postural reactions in the neurodevelopmental examination. *Pediatric Neurology*, 31(1): 1-8.

Zald, D.H. (2003). The human amygdala and the emotional evaluation of sensory stimuli. *Brain Research Brain Research Review,* 41: 88-123.

Zatorre, R.J., Belin, P. (2001). Spectral and temporal processing in human auditory cortex. *Cerebral Cortex*, 11: 946-53.

Zatorre, R.J., Belin, P., Penhune, V.B. (2002). Structure and function of auditory cortex: music and speech. *Trends in Cognitive Science,* 6: 37-46.

Zwil, A.S., Sandel, M.E., Kim, E. (1993). Organic and psychological sequelae of traumatic brain injury: the postconcussional syndrome in clinical practice. *New Directions for Mental Health Services*, (57): 109-15.

Subject Index